Neuroanatomy

AN ILLUSTRATED COLOUR TEXT

Neuroanatomy

AN ILLUSTRATED COLOUR TEXT

Sixth Edition

Alan R Crossman PhD DSc
Emeritus Professor of Anatomy
The University of Manchester
Manchester, UK

David Neary MD FRCP
Honorary Professor of Neuroscience
Manchester, UK

Illustrated by Ben Crossman MA

For additional online content visit StudentConsult.com

ELSEVIER

ELSEVIER

ISBN: 9780702074622

Notices

Practitioners and researchers must always rely on their own experience and knowledge in evaluating and using any information, methods, compounds or experiments described herein. Because of rapid advances in the medical sciences, in particular, independent verification of diagnoses and drug dosages should be made. To the fullest extent of the law, no responsibility is assumed by Elsevier, authors, editors or contributors for any injury and/or damage to persons or property as a matter of products liability, negligence or otherwise, or from any use or operation of any methods, products, instructions, or ideas contained in the material herein.

your source for books, journals and multimedia in the health sciences
www.elsevierhealth.com

Working together to grow libraries in developing countries

www.elsevier.com • www.bookaid.org

The publisher's policy is to use paper manufactured from sustainable forests

Printed in China
Last digit is the print number: 9   8   7   6   5   4   3   2   1

Senior Content Strategist: Jeremy Bowes
Senior Content Development Specialist: Kim Benson
Project Manager: Julie Taylor
Design: Brian Salisbury
Illustrator: Ben Crossman
Marketing Manager: Deborah Watkins

Preface to the sixth edition

A basic knowledge of human neuroanatomy is an essential prerequisite for medical students about to embark upon clinical studies. Without such knowledge it is impossible to understand the myriad of clinical signs and symptoms that arise from disorders of the nervous system. This book has been designed primarily for medical students, but neuroanatomy is an important subject also for students of basic neuroscience and of many subjects allied to medicine.

In revising and updating *Neuroanatomy* for a sixth edition, we have retained our original intention to produce a relevant, clear, succinct and well-illustrated account of the anatomy of the human nervous system.

Relevance is, perhaps, the most important feature. Neuroanatomy is an extensive subject, and the pace of research in both the basic and clinical sciences means that it is ever-expanding. At the same time, students are under pressure and neuroanatomy will almost certainly not be the only subject that they are studying.

Although the question "What do I need to know?" is anathema to some educators, it is perfectly understandable. What to include and what to leave out is, of course, a matter of judgement. Our approach has been to include what we consider to be essential material, correlating, wherever possible, anatomical structure with function and, where applicable, relating it to clinical significance. We believe that the breadth and depth of coverage of the subject in *Neuroanatomy* are sufficient to enable students to commence their training in clinical neuroscience with confidence.

Clarity is also of great importance. Neuroanatomy is a complex subject and one with which students often find difficulty. We have made every effort, therefore, to avoid vagueness, opacity and ambiguity and to make descriptions and concepts as straightforward as possible. Not only does *Neuroanatomy* focus on the essential material but the text is also deliberately succinct and to the point.

The internal anatomy of the central nervous system – its nuclei, nerve fibre tracts and, particularly, their connections – cannot always be readily visualised in dissections, brain sections or scans. As a consequence, clear, uncomplicated and explicit illustrations are an absolute necessity. The illustrations have always been a strong point of the book – and one of the features that has attracted most compliments from readers. Since the third edition, Ben Crossman has been responsible for illustration of the entire book. For this edition, some new figures have been introduced and virtually all of the figures have been revised to further improve clarity and aesthetic appearance. We are grateful to Ben for his artistic interpretation of our primitive sketches and his skillful enhancement and annotation of the photographs of anatomical specimens.

A R Crossman
D Neary
Manchester 2018

Preface to the first edition

This book has been written primarily for undergraduate medical students. At the same time, we have borne in mind students following other health science courses where a basic understanding of the nervous system and its major disorders is required, and also students of basic neuroscience, who are invariably intrigued and edified by discussion of the disorders which afflict the human nervous system.

The book has been prepared during a period of widespread debate on, and evolution in, the substance and style of medical education. There are several driving forces for change, one being the recognition that unreasonable and unnecessary demands are often being made of students in the sheer volume of information which they are required to assimilate. This has prompted students, educators and health professionals alike to question, across the whole curriculum, the depth of knowledge which is required by the newly-qualified doctor and the means by which it should be achieved. The General Medical Council has

recommended the development of a system-based core curriculum and has emphasised the crucial importance of integration between basic science and clinical medicine. These proposals have been welcomed and amplified, with respect to the teaching of neurology, by the Association of British Neurologists.

No area of medical science lends itself better than neuroscience to such a system-based, integrated approach and this has been the principal philosophy guiding the preparation of this book. Neuroscience, with all its sub-specialities both basic and clinical, is an enormous field where the growth of knowledge through research is exponential. This creates a great challenge to the medical educator in selecting what should comprise the core curriculum. It also signifies the potential for future advances in the diagnosis, prevention and treatment of neurological disease, recognised by the designation of the 1990s as the 'Decade of the Brain'.

Neuroanatomy is the cornerstone upon which is built an understanding of the

nervous system and its disorders. The aim of this book, therefore, is to provide a clear and concise account of the anatomy of the human nervous system in sufficient detail to understand its main functions and the common disorders by which it is affected. An important feature of the book is the integration of neuroanatomy with illustrative clinical material. This has been done in order to show how a knowledge of neuroanatomy can help in the understanding of clinical symptoms and also to emphasise those areas of neuroanatomy which are particularly relevant to human neurological disease. We have introduced clinical concepts in the most elementary way to give a broad outline of the aetiology of nervous disease and the link with clinical diagnostic methods. Clinical material has been integrated as closely as possible with the relevant neuroanatomy. Furthermore, the clinical text has been boxed so that it is readily identifiable and can be easily selected to review or pass over. Each chapter also contains boxed summaries.

The purpose of these is to assist the reader in identifying key points and as an aid to revision.

Both neuroanatomy and clinical medicine are new to the student first entering medical school. By studying the introductory chapter and the summaries of later, more detailed, chapters the student will gain an overview of the scope and extent of the subject of neuroanatomy and will be introduced to the basic concepts underlying the clinical diagnosis of neurological disease. For those unfamiliar with clinical terminology a glossary has been provided to explain the meaning of commonly used expressions. As more detailed knowledge of neuroanatomy is gained, this will be enhanced and illuminated by reference to the selected clinical material which exemplifies the relevance of neuroanatomy to clinical neurology. Later, when students enter neurological training, they need to refresh in their minds the basic principles of neuroanatomy and link these to clinical diagnostic methods. At this time, the systematic study of patients with individual neurological diseases can be greatly enhanced by returning to the detailed anatomy of diseased structures.

A R Crossman
D Neary
Manchester 1995

Acknowledgements

As in the past, we are indebted to colleagues Professor David J Brooks, Professor Marco Catani, Professor Paul D Griffiths, Professor Alan Jackson, Professor David Mann, Dr R Anne McKinney and Professor Gary C Schoenwolf for providing scans and other images which enhance the illustration of this book. We are also most grateful to Dr Adrianne Noe and Archibald J Fobbs for providing photographs of brain sections from the Yakovlev-Haleem Collection held in the National Museum of Health and Medicine, Armed Forces Institute of Pathology, Washington DC, USA. We would also like to thank the numerous academic colleagues and medical students around the world who have sent constructive comments on previous editions and suggestions for improvement.

The authors greatly appreciate the continued enthusiasm of Elsevier for *Neuroanatomy* over a period of more than two decades. In the preparation of this sixth edition we wish to thank colleagues at Elsevier, in particular Senior Content Strategist Jeremy Bowes and Senior Content Development Specialist Dr Kim H Benson, for their encouragement and support.

A R Crossman
D Neary
Manchester 2018

Contents

Introduction and overview

The nervous system of all animals functions to detect changes in the internal and external environments and to bring about responses in muscles, organs and glands that are appropriate for the preservation of the individual and the propagation of the species. In relatively primitive species such functions are focused primarily on:

- Maintenance of the internal environment (homoeostasis)
- Perception of, and response to, external stimuli/threats
- Finding food
- Mating

With ascent of the evolutionary scale there is, in addition, an increasing capacity for 'higher functions' of the nervous system, such as learning, memory, cognition and, ultimately, self-awareness, intellect and personality. At the pinnacle of this

process, the human nervous system is the most complex and versatile product of evolution.

Although a great deal is known about how the nervous system works, much still awaits elucidation. Indeed, the anatomical, physiological, biochemical and molecular basis of neural function remain areas of intense research activity in both the basic and clinical sciences.

The nervous system can be damaged by inherited and developmental abnormalities, by disease and traumatic injury and by neurodegenerative processes associated with ageing. The prevention, diagnosis and treatment of neurological disorders are, therefore, of immense socio-economic importance. A knowledge of neuroanatomy and its correlation with function and dysfunction is fundamental to the practice of clinical

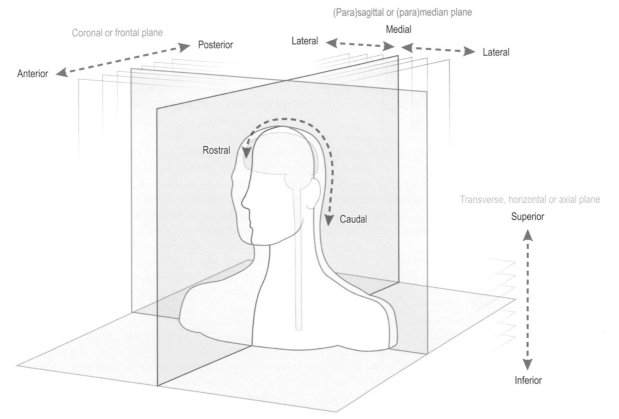

Fig. 1.1 Neuroanatomical terminology for planes, directions and relationships.

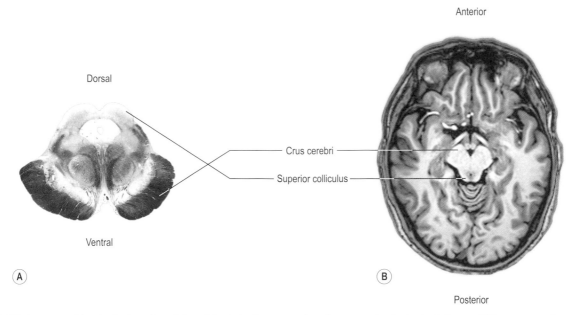

Fig. 1.2 (A) Transverse histological section of the midbrain in the conventional neuroanatomical orientation and (B) corresponding axial MRI scan in conventional neuroradiological orientation.

neurosciences and to the prospect of future advances in the prevention and treatment of neurological disorders.

Neuroanatomical terminology and conventions

The formal names given to parts of the body are agreed internationally by the Federative Committee on Anatomical Terminology and have been published as the Terminologia Anatomica (1998; Thieme). The names of many structures in the nervous system have a Greek or Latin origin and are unique to neuroanatomy. Often the name is descriptive of some perceived physical characteristic, such as shape (e.g. 'hippocampus', meaning sea-horse) or colour (e.g. 'substantia nigra', meaning black substance). Some structures are known by eponyms, usually in recognition of the person who first described them or whose work on them was particularly prominent (e.g. circle of Willis; foramen of Monro). Many of the latter names are considered to be anachronistic, but some remain in common usage.

In anatomy generally, the location and relationships of structures are described with reference to three orthogonal planes: sagittal or median, horizontal or transverse (called axial in radiology) and coronal or frontal (Fig. 1.1). Directions and relationships are designated as medial or lateral, superior or inferior and anterior or posterior, with reference to the orientation of these planes. There is, however, an additional terminological complication when describing the brain and spinal cord, as explained below.

In neuroanatomy, the positional/directional terms – rostral, caudal, dorsal and ventral – are also commonly used. These terms have their origin in embryology and mean, respectively, towards the head end (rostral), tail end (caudal), back (dorsal) and belly (ventral). If the long axis of the brain and spinal cord were to remain in a straight line during embryological development then, in the adult, rostral would simply equate to superior, caudal to inferior, dorsal to posterior and ventral to anterior. For all intents and purposes, this is what happens with the spinal cord but the long axis of the brain, on the other hand, undergoes considerable distortion and, in particular, the brainstem becomes flexed at several points (see Fig. 1.12). In neuroanatomy, therefore, it is customary to use the terms that are common to all anatomy when describing a position in space and to reserve the terms 'rostral, caudal, dorsal and ventral' for the description of location and direction relative to the long axis of the nervous system.

In neuroanatomy, horizontal or transverse sections through the spinal cord and lower part of the brain (brainstem) are usually depicted/orientated with dorsal at the top and ventral at the bottom (Fig. 1.2A). The convention in clinical neuroradiology, on the other hand, is that axial images are orientated as if looking from the subject's feet towards the head, with anterior at the top of the image. In sections that contain the brainstem, therefore, the dorsal aspect of the brainstem is towards the bottom of the image and the ventral aspect is towards the top (Fig. 1.2B). This convention means that left and right are also reversed.

Components and organisation of the nervous system

Neurones and neuroglia

The basic structural and functional unit of the nervous system is the **nerve cell** or **neurone** (Figs 1.3, 1.4), of which the human nervous system is estimated to contain about 10^{10}. The functions of the neurone are to receive and integrate incoming information from **sensory receptors** and other neurones and to transmit information to other neurones or non-neural structures that are under neural control (muscles, organs and glands – sometimes referred to as '**effector organs**'). Neuronal structure is highly specialised to fulfil these functions. Each neurone is a separate physical entity with a limiting cell membrane. Information is passed between neurones at specialised regions called **synapses** where the membranes of adjacent cells are in close apposition (Fig. 1.3).

There is wide diversity in the size and shape of neurones in different parts of the nervous system, but all share certain common characteristics. There is a single cell body from which a variable number of branching processes emerge. Most of these processes are receptive in function and are known as **dendrites**. The dendrites possess synapses, sometimes many thousands of them, through which they receive incoming information from other nerve cells. In sensory neurones, the dendrites may be

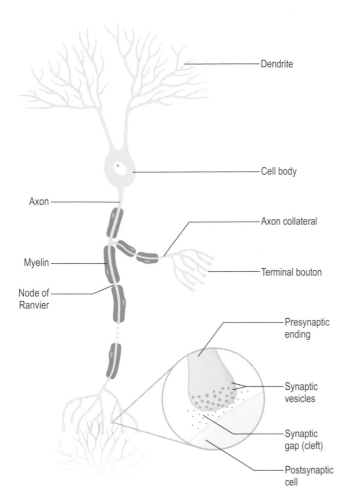

Fig. 1.3 **Schematic representation of the basic structure of the neurone and the synapse.**

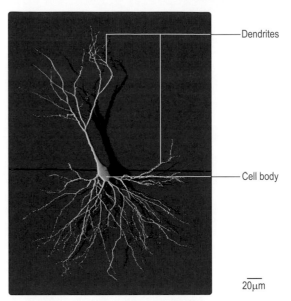

Fig. 1.4 **Pseudocoloured three-dimensional reconstruction of a neurone from the hippocampus, imaged by confocal laser scanning microscopy.** One of the processes at the base of the neurone is the axon. *(Courtesy of Dr R A McKinney, Brain Research Institute, University of Zurich, Switzerland.)*

further specialised to detect changes in the external or internal environment. One of the processes attached to the cell body is called the **axon** (nerve fibre) and this carries information away from the cell body. Axons are highly variable in length and may divide into several branches, or collaterals, through which information can be distributed to a number of different destinations simultaneously. At the end of the axon, synaptic specialisations called nerve terminals (presynaptic endings; **terminal boutons**) occur, from which information is transferred, usually to the dendrites of other neurones. In efferent or motor neurones, which control non-neural structures such as muscle cells, the axonal endings may be further specialised (e.g. the neuromuscular junction).

Information is coded and distributed within neurones by changes in electrical charge. The cell membrane of neurones is polarised, which means that an electrical potential difference (the membrane potential) exists across it. In the resting state, this potential difference (the **resting potential**) is of the order of 60–70 millivolts (mV), the inside of the cell being negative with respect to the outside. When a neurone is stimulated or excited above a certain threshold level, there is a brief reversal of the polarity of its membrane potential, termed the **action potential**. Action potentials are propagated down the axon and invade the nerve terminals. At most synapses, transmission of information between neurones occurs by chemical rather than electrical means. Invasion of nerve terminals by an action potential causes the release of specific chemicals (**neurotransmitters**) that are stored in **synaptic vesicles** in the presynaptic ending. The neurotransmitter

diffuses across the narrow gap between pre- and postsynaptic membranes and binds to specific receptors on the postsynaptic cell, inducing changes in the membrane potential. The change may be either to depolarise the membrane, thus moving towards the threshold for production of action potentials, or to hyperpolarise and, thus, stabilise the cell.

The other major cellular components of the nervous system are **neuroglial cells**, or **glia**, which outnumber neurones by about an order of magnitude. Unlike neurones, neuroglia do not have a direct role in information processing but they fulfil a number of other roles that are essential for the normal functioning of the nervous system. One type of glial cell (the oligodendrocyte) is responsible for the production of myelin, a structure high in lipoprotein that ensheathes many axons and greatly increases the speed of conduction of action potentials.

Central and peripheral nervous systems

At a simple anatomical level, the nervous system (Fig. 1.5) is divided into the **central nervous system** (**CNS**) and the **peripheral nervous system** (**PNS**). The central nervous system consists of the brain and spinal cord, lying within the protection of the cranium and vertebral column, respectively. It is the most complex part of the nervous system, containing the majority of nerve cell bodies and synaptic connections. The peripheral nervous system constitutes the link between the CNS and structures in the periphery of the body, from which it receives sensory information and to which it sends controlling impulses. The peripheral nervous system consists of nerves joined to the brain and spinal cord (**cranial** and **spinal nerves**) and their ramifications within the body. Spinal nerves serving the upper or lower limbs coalesce to form the **brachial** or **lumbar plexus**, respectively, within which fibres are redistributed into named **peripheral nerves**. The PNS also includes many peripherally located nerve cell bodies, some of which are aggregated within structures called **ganglia**.

Somatic and autonomic nervous systems

At a functional level, neurones that are concerned with detecting changes in the external environment, or with the control of

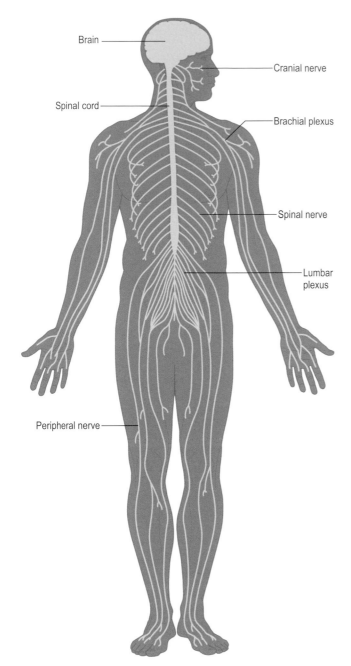

Fig. 1.5 Central and peripheral nervous systems.

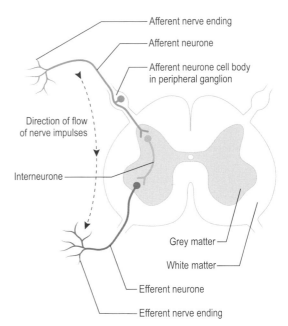

Fig. 1.6 The general arrangement of afferent, efferent and interneurones.

movement, are collectively referred to as the **somatic nervous system**. Neurones that detect changes in, and control the activity of, the viscera are collectively referred to as the **autonomic nervous system**. Somatic and autonomic components are present in both the central and peripheral nervous systems. The autonomic nervous system is divided into two anatomically and functionally distinct parts, namely the **sympathetic** and **parasympathetic divisions**, which generally have opposing (antagonistic) effects on the structures that they innervate. The autonomic nervous system innervates smooth muscle, cardiac muscle and secretory glands. It is an important part of the homeostatic mechanisms that control the internal environment of the body.

Afferent neurones, efferent neurones and interneurones

Nerve cells that carry information from peripheral receptors to the CNS are referred to as **afferent neurones** (Fig. 1.6). If the

information they carry reaches consciousness, they are also called **sensory neurones**. **Efferent neurones** carry impulses away from the CNS and if they innervate skeletal muscle to cause movement, they are also called **motor neurones**. The vast majority of neurones, however, are located entirely within the CNS and are referred to as **interneurones**. The terms 'afferent' and 'efferent' are also commonly used to denote the polarity of projections to and from structures within the CNS, even though the projections are entirely contained within the brain and spinal cord. The projections to and from the cerebral cortex, for example, are referred to as cortical afferents and efferents, respectively.

Grey and white matter, nuclei and tracts

The CNS is a highly heterogeneous structure in terms of the distribution of nerve cell bodies and their processes (Fig. 1.7). Some regions are relatively enriched in nerve cell bodies (e.g. the central portion of the spinal cord and the surface of the cerebral hemisphere) and are referred to as **grey matter**. Conversely, other regions contain mostly nerve processes (usually axons). These are often myelinated (ensheathed in myelin), which confers a paler coloration – hence the term **white matter**.

Nerve cell bodies with similar anatomical connections and functions (e.g. the motor neurones innervating a group of related muscles) tend to be located together in groups called nuclei. Similarly, nerve processes sharing common connections and functions tend to follow the same course, running in pathways or tracts (Fig. 1.7 and see Fig. 1.23).

Decussation of sensory and motor pathways

It is a general principle of the organisation of the CNS that pathways conveying sensory information to a conscious level (the cerebral hemisphere) cross over, or **decussate**, from one side of the CNS to the other. The same is true of descending pathways from the cerebral hemisphere that control movement. Therefore in general, each cerebral hemisphere perceives sensations from, and controls the movements of, the opposite (contralateral) side of the body.

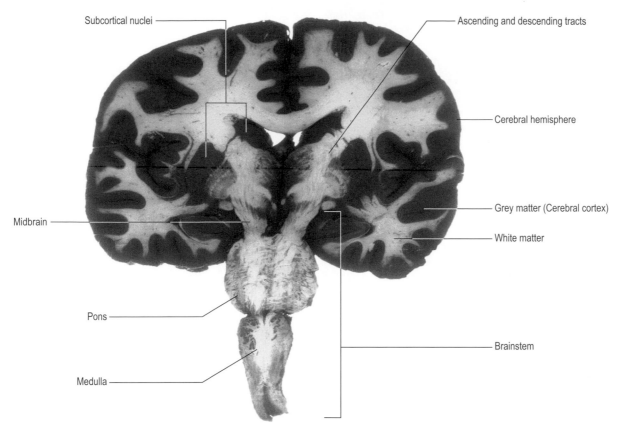

Subcortical nuclei

Ascending and descending tracts

Cerebral hemisphere

Grey matter (Cerebral cortex)

White matter

Midbrain

Pons

Brainstem

Medulla

Fig. 1.7 Coronal section through the brain illustrating the distribution of grey and white matter. The section has been stained by Mulligan's technique, which colours grey matter blue, leaving white matter relatively unstained.

Components and organisation of the nervous system

- The structural and functional unit of the nervous system is the nerve cell, or neurone. Neurones have a resting membrane potential of about –70 mV

- A neurone receives information primarily through its dendrites and passes this on by action potentials, which are carried away from the cell body by the axon.

- Information is passed between neurones at synapses by release of neurotransmitters from presynaptic terminals; these act upon receptors in the postsynaptic membrane to cause either depolarisation or hyperpolarisation of the postsynaptic cell.

- Neuroglial cells are more numerous than nerve cells and have roles other than information processing.

- The nervous system is divided into the central nervous system (CNS), which consists of the brain and spinal cord, and the peripheral nervous system (PNS), which consists of cranial and spinal nerves and their ramifications.

- The autonomic nervous system (ANS) innervates visceral structures and is important in homoeostasis of the internal environment.

- Individual neurones may be defined as either afferent or efferent with respect to the CNS, or as interneurones.

- Within the CNS, areas rich in either nerve cell bodies or nerve fibres constitute grey or white matter, respectively.

- Clusters of cell bodies with similar functions are known as nuclei.

- Tracts, or pathways, of nerve fibres link together distant regions.

- Generally, ascending sensory pathways and descending motor pathways in the CNS decussate along their course, so that each side of the brain is functionally associated with the contralateral half of the body.

Development of the central nervous system

By the beginning of the second week of human embryonic development, three germ cell layers become established: ectoderm, mesoderm and endoderm. Subsequently, these each give rise to particular tissues and organs in the adult. The ectoderm gives rise to the skin and the nervous system. The mesoderm forms skeletal, muscular and connective tissues. The endoderm gives rise to the alimentary, respiratory and genitourinary tracts.

The process of formation of the embryonic nervous system is referred to as **neurulation**. During the third week of embryonic development, the dorsal midline ectoderm undergoes thickening to form the **neural plate** (Figs 1.8, 1.9). The lateral margins of the neural plate become elevated, forming **neural folds** on either side of a longitudinal, midline depression, called the **neural groove**. The neural folds then become apposed and fuse together, thus sealing the neural groove and creating the **neural tube**. Some cells from the apices of the neural folds become separated to form groups lying dorsolateral to the neural tube. These are known as the **neural crests**. The formation of the neural tube is complete by about the middle of the fourth week of embryonic development.

Enormous growth, distortion and cellular differentiation occur during the subsequent transformation of the neural tube into the adult CNS. This is maximal in the rostral part, which develops into the brain, the caudal portion becoming the spinal cord. The central cavity within the neural tube becomes the central canal of the spinal cord and the ventricles of the brain. The neural crests form the sensory ganglia of spinal and cranial nerves, and also the autonomic ganglia.

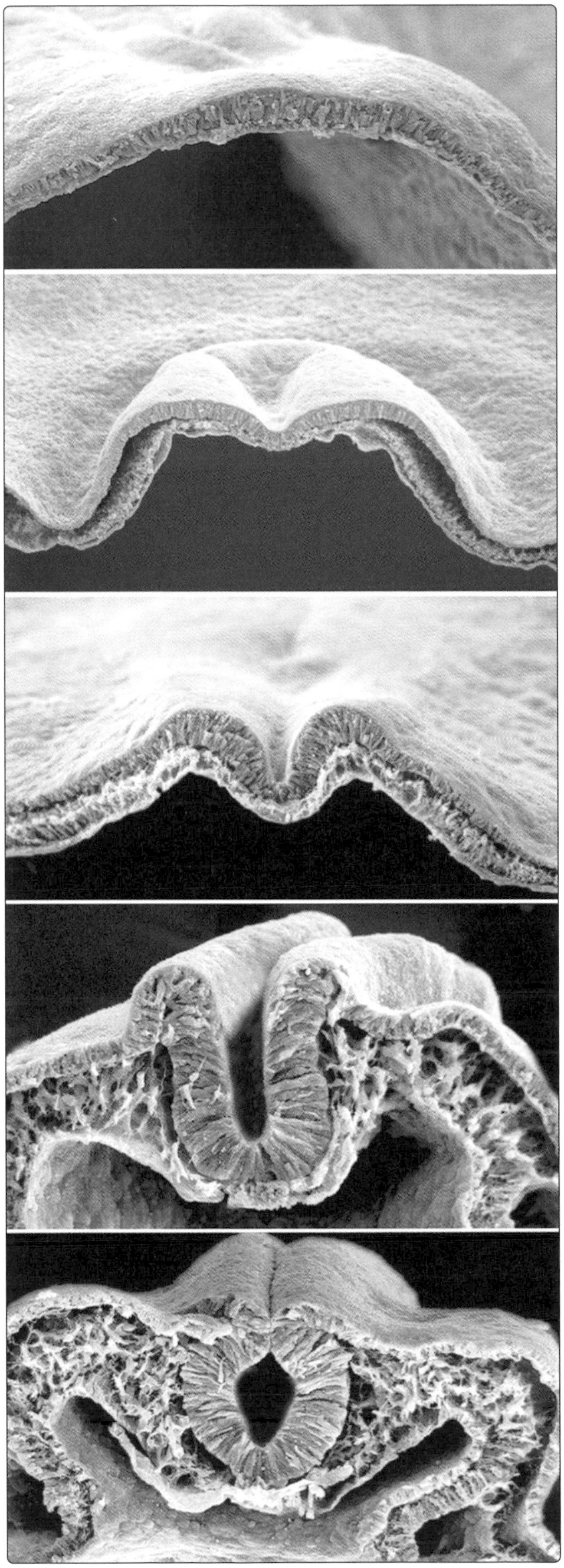

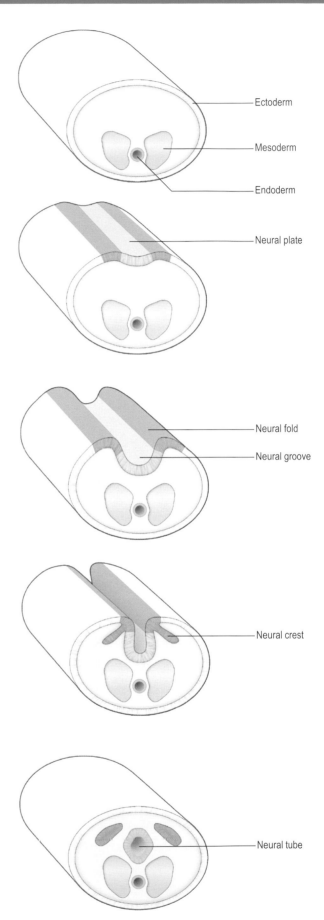

Fig. 1.8 Scanning electron micrographs of transverse sections through the dorsal ectoderm of the chick embryo illustrating the stages (from top to bottom) in formation of the neural tube (×140).
(Courtesy of Dr G C Schoenwolf, Dept. of Neurobiology and Anatomy, University of Utah School of Medicine, Salt Lake City, USA.)

Fig. 1.9 Schematic representation of the formation of the neural tube from the embryonic ectoderm.

Ectoderm

Mesoderm

Endoderm

Neural plate

Neural fold

Neural groove

Neural crest

Neural tube

As development continues, a longitudinal groove, the **sulcus limitans**, appears on the inner surface of the lateral walls of the embryonic spinal cord and caudal part of the brain (Fig. 1.10A). The dorsal and ventral cell groupings thus delineated are referred to as the **alar plate** and the **basal plate**, respectively. Nerve cells that develop within the alar plate have predominantly sensory functions, while those in the basal plate are predominantly motor.

Further development also brings about the differentiation of grey and white matter. The grey matter is located centrally around the central canal, with white matter forming an outer coat. This basic developmental pattern can still easily be recognised in the adult spinal cord (Fig. 1.10B).

Further differentiation distinguishes seven neuronal cell groupings within the alar and basal plates (Fig. 1.11). These are arranged in discontinuous longitudinal columns, based on their anatomical connections and physiological roles:

- Special somatic afferent: associated with the developing inner ear and ultimately receiving auditory and vestibular input.
- General somatic afferent: receiving general sensory input from the periphery.
- Special visceral afferent: subserving the sense of taste.
- General visceral afferent: receiving afferent input from the viscera.
- General visceral efferent: composed of preganglionic autonomic efferents.
- Branchial efferent: containing motor neurones to muscles derived from branchial (pharyngeal) arches.
- Somatic efferent: containing motor neurones to somatic muscles.

During embryonic development, the rostral portion of the neural tube undergoes massive differentiation and growth to form the brain (Fig. 1.12). By about the fifth week, three so-called **primary brain vesicles** can be identified: the **prosencephalon** (forebrain), **mesencephalon** (midbrain) and **rhombencephalon** (hindbrain). The longitudinal axis of the developing CNS (neuraxis) does not remain straight but is bent by a midbrain or cephalic flexure, occurring at the junction of midbrain and forebrain, and a cervical flexure between the brain and the spinal cord.

By the seventh week, further differentiation distinguishes five **secondary brain vesicles** produced by division of the prosencephalon into the **telencephalon** and **diencephalon** and division of the rhombencephalon into the **metencephalon** and **myelencephalon**. The junction between the latter is marked by an additional bend in the neuraxis, called the pontine flexure.

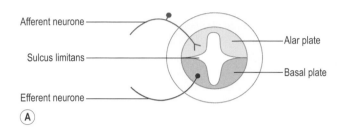

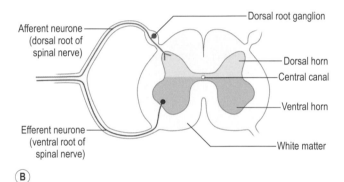

Fig. 1.10 Schematic representation of transverse sections through (A) the developing neural tube and (B) the adult spinal cord. Neuronal connections with peripheral structures are illustrated only on one side.

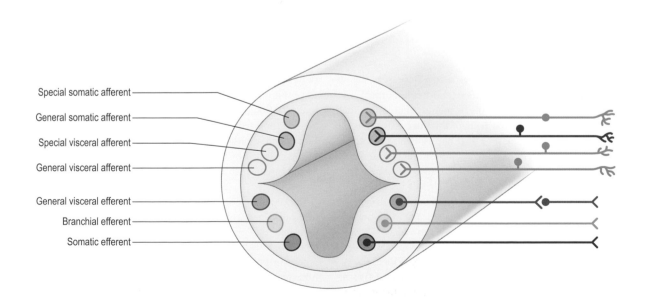

Fig. 1.11 Schematic transverse section through the developing nervous system showing the arrangement of afferent and efferent cell groupings. *The colour coding is recapitulated in Fig. 10.2, which illustrates the arrangement of cranial nerve nuclei in the adult brainstem, and in Table 10.1 which describes the components and functions of the cranial nerves..*

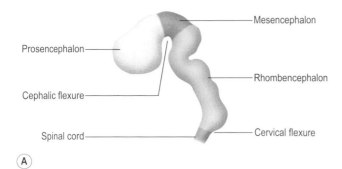

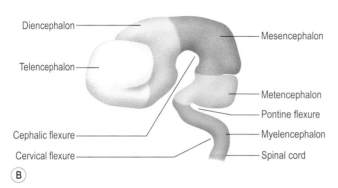

Fig. 1.12 The early development of the brain. (A) The primary brain vesicles at about 4 to 5 weeks and (B) the secondary brain vesicles at about 7 to 8 weeks.

 Developmental anomalies

Disorders of development disrupt the normal growth and structural organisation of the spinal cord and brain. Because the nervous system is derived from embryonic ectoderm, these developmental anomalies also involve the coverings of the nervous system (skin and bone). In **anencephaly**, the brain and skull are minute and the infant does not usually survive. In **spina bifida**, the lower spinal cord and nerve roots are underdeveloped and may lie uncovered by skin or the bony spine on the infant's back **(meningomyelocele)**. Such infants are left with withered, paralysed and anaesthetic lower limbs together with incontinence of the bowel and bladder.

As the brain develops, its central cavity also undergoes considerable changes in size and shape, forming a system of chambers or **ventricles** (Fig. 1.13 and see Fig. 1.23), which contain **cerebrospinal fluid**.

Parallels have been drawn between the embryological development of the brain and the major changes that the brain has undergone during ascent of the phylogenetic, or evolutionary, scale from simple to more complex animals. Although this is certainly an oversimplification, the concept does have the educational merit of introducing some of the principal parts of the brain, and their relationships to one another, in a graphic and memorable way (Fig. 1.13).

The simplest of chordate animals (e.g. amphioxus), from which the vertebrates evolved, possess a dorsal tubular nerve cord that is reminiscent of the neural tube of the developing mammalian embryo. During phylogeny, the rostral end of the tubular nervous system has undergone enormous modification and change; consequently, the adult human brain bears little obvious similarity to its evolutionary ancestors.

Regional specialisation has been an important theme in the evolution of the brain and this is especially obvious in relation to the senses and in movement control. Long ago in phylogeny, centres devoted to these functions developed as expansions or outgrowths from the dorsal aspect of the simple tubular brain (Fig. 1.13). In form, they consisted of an outer cortex of nerve cell bodies with an underlying core of nerve fibres. Bilaterally paired centres developed in relation to the senses of smell, vision and hearing, and a symmetrical, midline centre developed in association with vestibular function and the maintenance of equilibrium. Each of these centres underwent subsequent evolutionary change, but this was most evident in the rostral, 'olfactory', part of the brain, which developed into the massive cerebral hemispheres (Figs 1.14, 1.15). During this process, known as **prosencephalisation**, the cerebral hemispheres came to take on an executive role in many areas of brain function. For example, the highest level for the perception and interpretation of input from all sensory modalities eventually became localised in the cortical surface of the cerebral hemispheres, as did the highest level for voluntary motor control. This is reflected by the fact that only a small proportion of the adult human cerebral hemisphere remains devoted to olfactory function.

The process of prosencephalisation meant that the other integrative centres became progressively subservient to the cerebral hemispheres. For example, those for vision and hearing underwent relatively little further development and fulfil largely automatic, reflex functions in the human brain. They may still be identified, however, as four small swellings on the dorsal surface of the midbrain: the **corpora quadrigemina** or **superior** and **inferior colliculi** (Figs 1.13, 1.14, 1.15). The motor centre near the caudal end of the brain developed into the cerebellum (Figs 1.13, 1.14, 1.15), which retains a central role in the maintenance of equilibrium and the coordination of movement.

Table 1.1 **Embryonic development of the brain.**		
Primary brain vesicles	**Secondary brain vesicles**	**Derivatives in mature brain**
Prosencephalon (forebrain)	Telencephalon	Cerebral hemisphere
	Diencephalon	Thalamus
Mesencephalon (midbrain)	Mesencephalon	Midbrain
Rhombencephalon (hindbrain)	Metencephalon	Pons, cerebellum
	Myelencephalon	Medulla oblongata

Some of the names of the embryological subdivisions of the brain are commonly used for descriptive purposes and it is, therefore, useful to know the parts of the mature brain into which they subsequently develop (Table 1.1). Of the three basic divisions of the brain, the prosencephalon or forebrain is by far the largest. It is also referred to as the **cerebrum**. Within the cerebrum, the telencephalon undergoes the greatest further development and gives rise to the two **cerebral hemispheres**. These consist of an outer layer of grey matter (the cerebral cortex) and an inner mass of white matter, within which various groups of nuclei lie buried (the largest being the **corpus striatum**). The diencephalon consists largely of the **thalamus**, which contains numerous cell groupings and is intimately connected with the cerebral cortex. The mesencephalon, or midbrain, is relatively undifferentiated (it still retains a central tube-like cavity surrounded by grey matter). The metencephalon develops into the **pons** and overlying **cerebellum**, while the myelencephalon forms the **medulla oblongata** (medulla). The medulla, pons and midbrain are collectively referred to as the **brainstem** (Fig. 1.13).

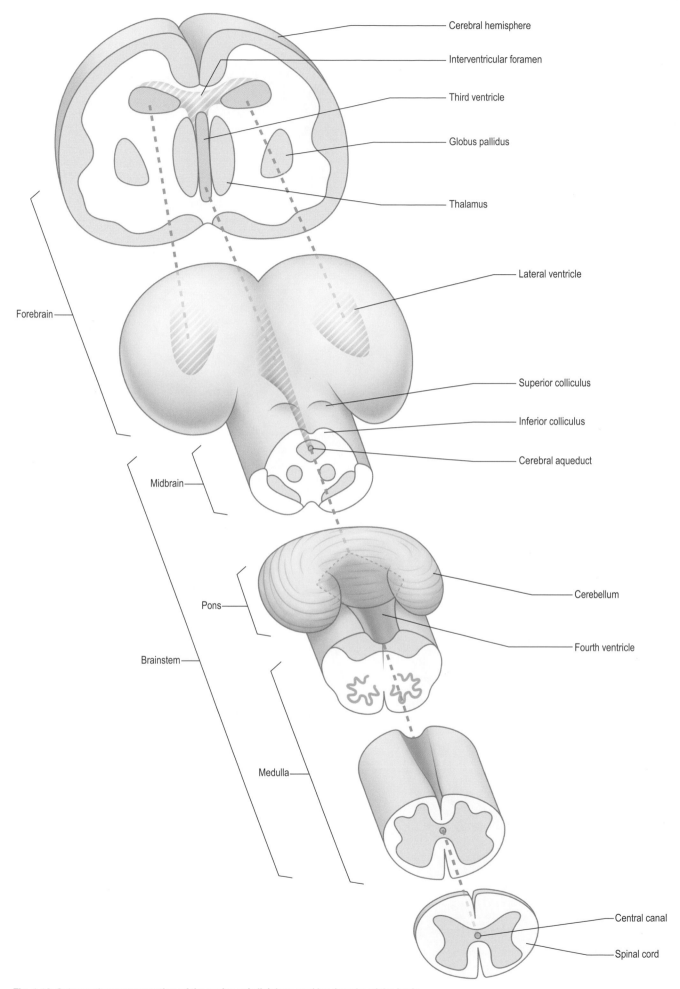

Fig. 1.13 Schematic representation of the major subdivisions and landmarks of the brain.

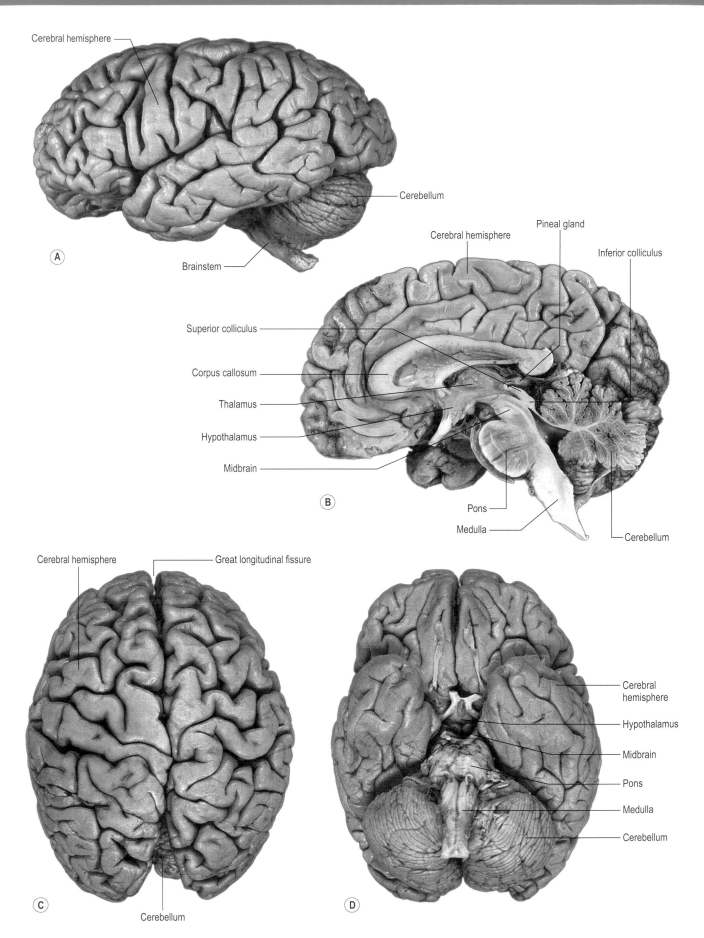

Fig. 1.14 Photographs of the brain. (A) Lateral aspect; (B) median sagittal section; (C) superior aspect; (D) inferior aspect.

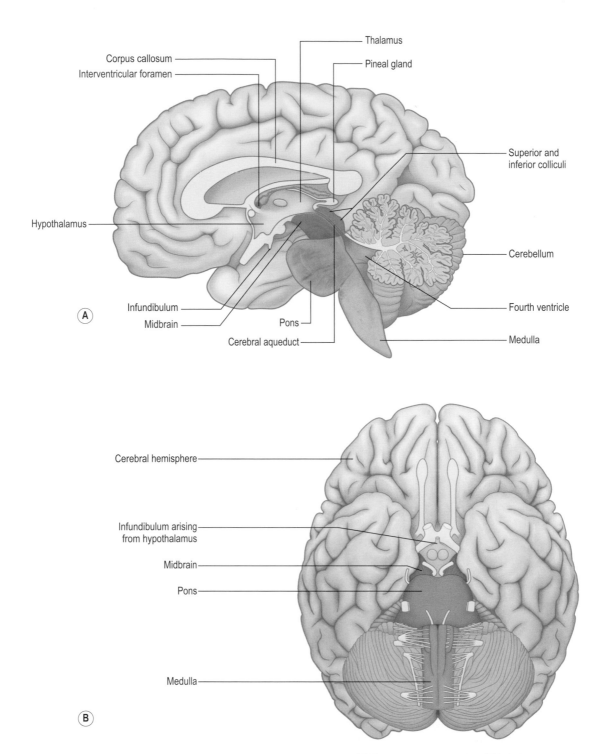

Fig. 1.15 Principal subdivisions and some important landmarks in the mature brain. (A) Median sagittal section; (B) inferior aspect. Cranial nerves are indicated in yellow.

Overview of the anatomy of the central nervous system

Coverings and blood supply

The brain and spinal cord are supported and protected by the bones of the skull and vertebral column, respectively. Within these bony coverings, the CNS is entirely ensheathed by three concentric layers of membranes, called the **meninges** (Fig. 1.16). The outermost membrane is the **dura mater**, a tough, fibrous coat that surrounds the brain and spinal cord like a loose-fitting bag (Fig. 1.17). The spinal dura and much of the cranial dura are separate from the periosteum, which forms the inner lining of the surrounding bones. At certain locations, however, such as on the floor of the cranial cavity, the dura and periosteum are fused and the cranial dura is tightly adherent to the interior surface of the skull. In addition, two large sheets (or reflections) of dura project into the cranial cavity, incompletely dividing it into compartments (Fig. 1.18). One of these, the **falx cerebri** lies in the sagittal plane

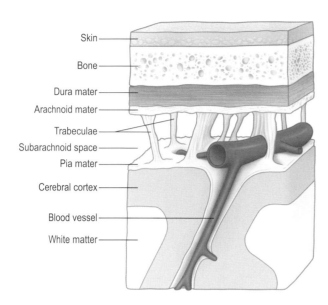

Fig. 1.16 A section through the skull, illustrating the relationships between the meninges and the CNS.

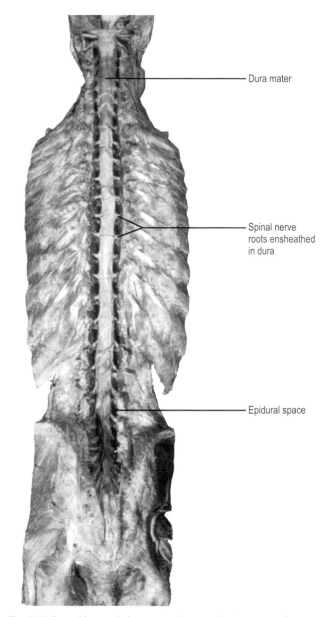

Fig. 1.17 Dorsal (posterior) aspect of the vertebral column after laminectomy to expose the vertebral canal and dura mater enclosing the spinal cord.

between the two cerebral hemispheres. Its free border lies just above the corpus callosum. The other dural sheet, the **tentorium cerebelli**, is oriented approximately horizontally, lying beneath the occipital lobes of the cerebral hemispheres and above the cerebellum. The tentorium cerebelli is continuous with the posterior part of the falx cerebri. The dura mater can be regarded as consisting of two layers. These are fused together except in certain locations, where they become separated to form spaces, the **dural venous sinuses**, which serve as channels for the venous drainage of the brain. Important dural sinuses occur:

- On the floor of the cranial cavity
- Along the lines of attachment of the falx cerebri and tentorium cerebelli to the interior of the skull (superior sagittal sinus, Fig. 1.18; transverse sinus, see Figs 7.9, 7.10)
- Along the line of attachment of the falx cerebri and tentorium cerebelli to one another (straight sinus, see Figs 7.9, 7.10)

Beneath the dura lies the **arachnoid mater**, the two being separated by a thin **subdural space**. The arachnoid is a translucent, collagenous membrane that, like the dura, loosely envelops the brain and spinal cord. The innermost of the meninges is the **pia mater**, a delicate membrane of microscopic thickness that is firmly adherent to the surface of the brain and spinal cord, closely following their surface contours. Between the arachnoid and pia is the **subarachnoid space** through which cerebrospinal fluid (CSF) circulates.

The brain is supplied with arterial blood by the **internal carotid** and **vertebral arteries**, which anastomose to form the **circulus arteriosus** (circle of Willis) on the base of the brain. The spinal cord is supplied by vessels arising from the vertebral arteries, reinforced by **radicular arteries** derived from segmental vessels. The arteries and veins serving the CNS run for part of their course within the subarachnoid space (Fig. 1.16). The meninges are supplied by a number of vessels, the most significant intracranial one being the **middle meningeal artery**, which ramifies extensively between the skull and dura mater overlying the lateral aspect of the cerebral hemisphere.

Coverings and blood supply of the central nervous system

- The brain and spinal cord are invested by three meningeal layers: the dura mater, arachnoid mater and pia mater.

- Two sheets of cranial dura mater, the falx cerebri and tentorium cerebelli, incompletely divide the cranial cavity into compartments.

- The cranial dura mater contains dural venous sinuses, which act as channels for the venous drainage of the brain.

- Beneath the arachnoid mater lies the subarachnoid space in which cerebrospinal fluid (CSF) circulates.

- The brain is supplied with blood by the internal carotid and vertebral arteries.

- The spinal cord is supplied with blood by vessels that arise from the vertebral arteries, reinforced by radicular arteries derived from segmental vessels.

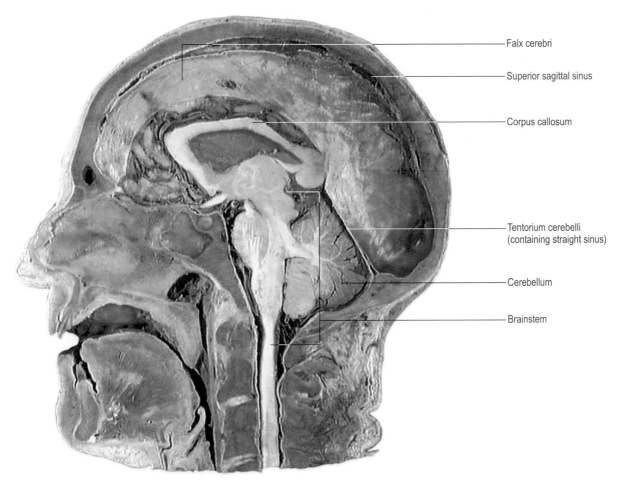

Fig. 1.18 Parasagittal section of the head showing the disposition of the falx cerebri and tentorium cerebelli.

Falx cerebri

Superior sagittal sinus

Corpus callosum

Tentorium cerebelli
(containing straight sinus)

Cerebellum

Brainstem

Anatomy of the spinal cord

The spinal cord lies within the **vertebral** (spinal) **canal** of the vertebral column and is continuous rostrally (superiorly) with the medulla oblongata of the brainstem (Fig. 1.19). The spinal cord receives information from, and controls, the trunk and limbs. This is achieved through 31 pairs of **spinal nerves** that are attached to the cord at intervals along its length and which contain afferent and efferent nerve fibres connecting with structures in the periphery. Near to the cord, the spinal nerves divide into **dorsal** (posterior) and **ventral** (anterior) **roots**, which attach to the cord along its dorsolateral and ventrolateral borders, respectively (Fig. 1.20). The dorsal roots carry afferent nerve fibres, the cell bodies of which are located in **dorsal root ganglia**. The ventral roots carry efferent nerve fibres, the parent cell bodies of which lie within the spinal grey matter. Spinal nerves leave the vertebral canal through small apertures, called **intervertebral foramina**, which are located between adjacent vertebrae. Because of the difference in the rates of growth of the spinal cord and vertebral column during development, the spinal cord in the adult does not extend for the full length of the vertebral canal, but ends at approximately the level of the intervertebral disc between L1 and L2 vertebrae. The lumbar and sacral spinal nerves, therefore, descend in a leash-like arrangement, called the **cauda equina** (Fig. 1.19), to reach their exit foramina.

The spinal cord is a relatively undifferentiated structure compared with the brain. Consequently, the basic principles of organisation, established early in embryonic development, can still be readily identified even in the adult human spinal cord (Fig. 1.20). The spinal cord is approximately cylindrical in shape, containing at its centre a vestigial **central canal**. The relative separation of cell bodies from nerve fibres confers a characteristic 'H' - or 'butterfly'- shape to the central core of grey matter that surrounds the central canal. Four projections of the central grey matter extend dorsolaterally and ventrolaterally towards the lines of attachment of the dorsal and ventral roots of the spinal nerves. These projections are known as the **dorsal (posterior) horns** and **ventral (anterior) horns**, respectively. The dorsal horn is the site of termination of numerous afferent neurones, conveying impulses from sensory receptors throughout the body, and is the site of origin of ascending pathways carrying sensory impulses to the brain. The ventral horn contains motor neurones that innervate skeletal muscle. In addition, at thoracic and upper lumbar levels of the cord only, another, smaller, collection of cell bodies comprises the **lateral horn**. This contains preganglionic neurones belonging to the sympathetic division of the autonomic nervous system (Chapter 4).

The periphery of the spinal cord consists of white matter that contains longitudinally running nerve fibres. These are organised into **ascending tracts** and **descending tracts**. Ascending tracts carry information derived from the trunk and limbs to the brain. Descending tracts are the means by which the brain controls the activities of neurones in the spinal cord (Fig. 1.21). The principal ascending tracts are the **dorsal columns** (fasciculus gracilis and fasciculus cuneatus), which carry fine touch and proprioception, the **spinothalamic tracts**, which carry pain, temperature, coarse touch and pressure, and the **spinocerebellar tracts**, which carry information from muscle and joint receptors to the cerebellum. Among the descending tracts, one of the most important is the **lateral corticospinal tract**, which controls skilled voluntary movements.

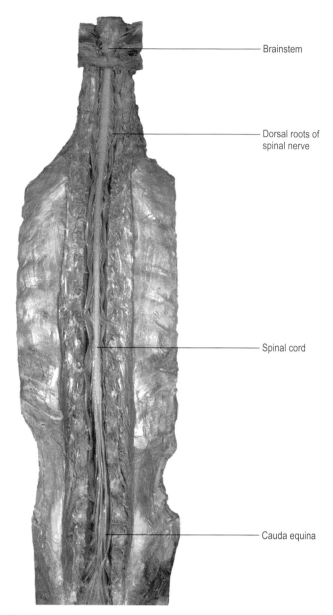

Fig. 1.19 Dorsal (posterior) aspect of the spinal cord in situ. This is the same specimen as shown in Fig. 1.17. The dura mater/arachnoid mater have been incised longitudinally to expose the spinal cord and spinal nerve roots lying within the subarachnoid space.

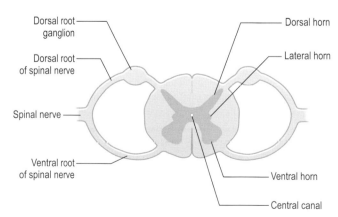

Fig. 1.20 Schematic diagram of a transverse section through the spinal cord, showing the attachment of spinal nerve roots and the arrangement of grey and white matter.

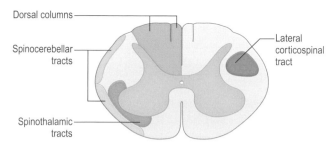

Fig. 1.21 Transverse section through the spinal cord showing the locations of the principal ascending and descending nerve fibre tracts. Ascending tracts are only depicted on the left side and descending only on the right, although both occur bilaterally.

Anatomy of the spinal cord

- The spinal cord lies within the vertebral canal. It bears 31 pairs of spinal nerves through which it receives fibres from, and sends fibres to, the periphery.

- Near the cord, spinal nerves divide to form dorsal and ventral roots; dorsal roots carry afferent fibres with cell bodies in dorsal root ganglia, and ventral roots carry efferent fibres.

- The spinal cord consists of a central core of grey matter, containing nerve cell bodies, and an outer layer of white matter containing nerve fibres.

- Within the grey matter, the dorsal horn contains sensory neurones, the ventral horn contains motor neurones and the lateral horn contains preganglionic sympathetic neurones.

- Within the white matter run ascending and descending nerve fibre tracts, which link the spinal cord with the brain.

- The principal ascending tracts are the dorsal columns, the spinothalamic tracts and the spinocerebellar tracts. The corticospinal tract is an important descending tract.

Anatomy of the brain
Major features and landmarks

The brain is dominated by the cerebral hemispheres (Figs 1.14, 1.15, 1.22). These have a highly convoluted outer mantle of grey matter, the **cerebral cortex**, and an inner core of white matter, within which are located further masses of grey matter. Certain of the surface convolutions of the cerebral hemisphere have specific sensory or motor functions, as described below. The two cerebral hemispheres are incompletely separated by a deep cleft, the **great longitudinal fissure**. The fissure is occupied by the falx cerebri and in its depths lies the **corpus callosum**, containing commissural nerve fibres that run between corresponding regions of the two hemispheres.

The brainstem can be seen clearly when the brain is viewed from its inferior aspect, although the relationships of the midbrain with other brain regions are best illustrated in sagittal section (Fig. 1.14B). The brainstem is the origin of 10 of the 12 pairs of cranial nerves (III–XII). Dorsal (posterior) to the brainstem is located the cerebellum. The tentorium cerebelli lies between the cerebellum and the posterior part of the cerebral hemispheres (occipital lobes).

Ventricular system

The highly simplified plan of the basic brain, described above (Fig. 1.13), is a useful one on which to consider the general disposition of the ventricular system (Figs 1.15, 1.23). As the central canal of the spinal cord is followed rostrally towards the brainstem, it moves progressively in a dorsal direction, eventually opening out to form a shallow, rhomboid-shaped depression on the dorsal surface of the medulla and pons (the hindbrain portion of the brainstem) beneath the cerebellum. The cavity thus formed is the **fourth ventricle**.

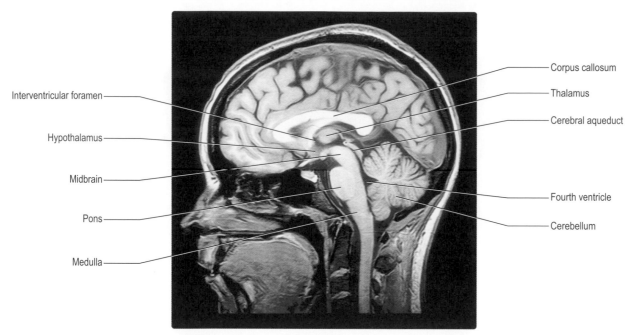

Fig. 1.22 Sagittal magnetic resonance image (MRI) of the head. The thalamus and hypothalamus form the upper and lower parts, respectively, of the lateral wall of the third ventricle. *(Courtesy of Professor A Jackson, Wolfson Molecular Imaging Centre, University of Manchester, Manchester, UK.)*

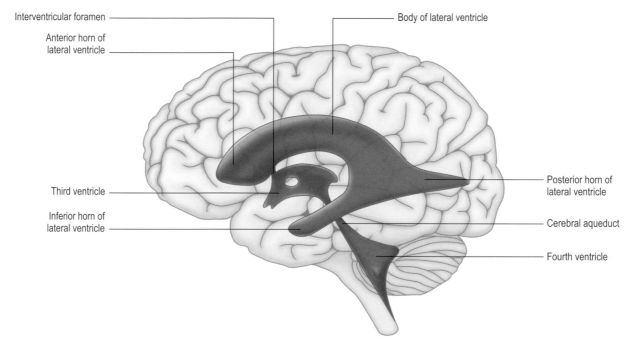

Fig. 1.23 The cerebral ventricular system.

At the rostral border of the pons, the walls of the fourth ventricle converge, forming once again a narrow tube, the **cerebral aqueduct**. The cerebral aqueduct dives into the substance of the brainstem, running the length of the midbrain beneath the inferior and superior colliculi. At the junction of midbrain and forebrain, the aqueduct opens into the **third ventricle**, a slit-like chamber, narrow from side to side but extensive in dorsoventral and rostrocaudal dimensions. The lateral walls of the third ventricle are formed by the thalamus and hypothalamus of the diencephalon. Near the rostral end of the third ventricle, a small aperture, the **interventricular foramen (foramen of Monro)**, communicates with an extensive chamber, the **lateral ventricle**, within each cerebral hemisphere. The ventricular system contains cerebrospinal fluid (CSF), which is secreted by the **choroid plexus** (Chapter 6).

Brainstem

The large cerebral hemispheres obscure many other structures from view, but the brainstem can be seen clearly on both a median sagittal section and an inferior view of the brain (Figs 1.14, 1.15). The brainstem consists of the medulla oblongata, pons and midbrain.

The brainstem forms only a small proportion of the entire brain but it is crucially important. Through it pass all of the ascending and descending nerve fibre tracts linking the brain and spinal cord (Fig. 1.24). These tracts carry sensory information from, and control the movement of, the trunk and limbs. The brainstem also contains the sites of origin and termination of most of the cranial nerves, through which the brain innervates the head. Moreover, within the brainstem lie centres that control the vital functions of breathing, the circulation of blood and the level of consciousness.

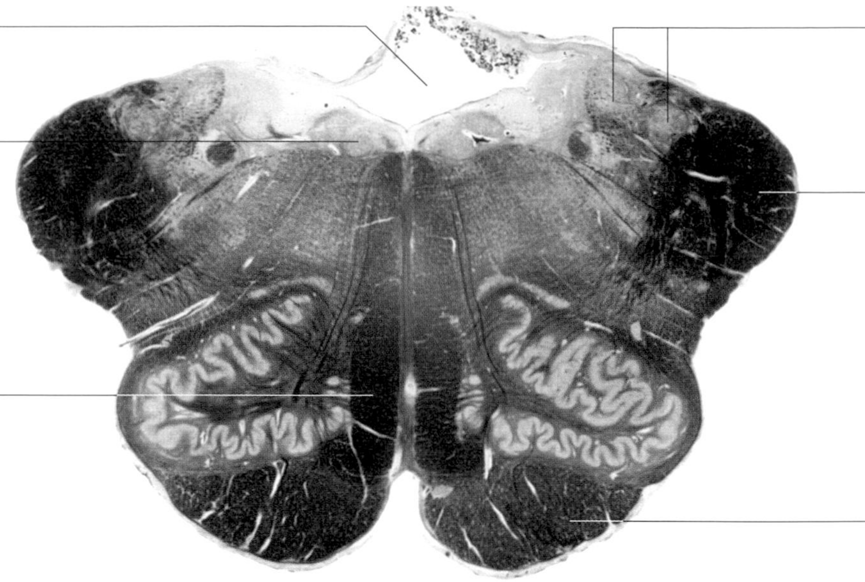

Fig. 1.24 Transverse section through the brainstem at the level of the medulla oblongata. The section has been stained by the Weigert–Pal method. Areas rich in nerve fibres stain darkly, while areas rich in cell bodies are relatively paler. The pyramid is a tract that contains descending motor fibres running from the cerebral cortex to the spinal cord. The medial lemniscus is a tract consisting of ascending axons carrying sensory information from the limbs to higher centres in the brain. The inferior cerebellar peduncle contains spinocerebellar fibres carrying information from joints and muscles to the cerebellum. The vestibular nuclei are the site of termination of the vestibular nerve, which carries information from the inner ear regarding the position and movement of the head. The hypoglossal nucleus is the site of origin of hypoglossal nerve fibres that innervate the muscles of the tongue.

The medulla oblongata is continuous caudally with the spinal cord and extends rostrally as far as the pons. The ponto-medullary junction can be seen clearly on inferior or sagittal views since the ventral part of the pons forms a prominent bulge on the surface of the brainstem. In sagittal section (Figs 1.14B, 1.15A), the lumen of the fourth ventricle is apparent between the pons and medulla ventrally and the cerebellum dorsally, into the latter of which its tent-shaped roof extends.

Cranial nerves

The brain directly receives sensory information from, and controls the activities of, peripheral structures, principally of the head and neck. Afferent and efferent nerve fibres run in 12 bilaterally paired cranial nerves, which are identified by individual names and by Roman numerals I–XII. Certain of the cranial nerves contain only sensory or only motor nerve fibres but the majority contain a mixture, as is the case with spinal nerves,. The first two cranial nerves (I olfactory, II optic) attach directly to the forebrain, whilst the others attach to the brainstem. Within the brainstem lie a number of nerve cell body groupings called the **cranial nerve nuclei**. These are the sites of termination of sensory fibres, and the origin of the motor fibres, that run in the cranial nerves (e.g. Figs 1.24, 10.2).

Cerebellum

The cerebellum is attached to the brainstem by a large mass of nerve fibres that lie lateral to the fourth ventricle on either side (see Fig. 9.1). The mass is split nominally into three parts: the **inferior**, **middle** and **superior cerebellar peduncles**. These carry nerve fibres between the medulla, pons and midbrain, respectively, and the cerebellum.

The cerebellum consists of an outer layer of grey matter, the cerebellar cortex, surrounding a central core of white matter (Fig. 1.14B). The cortical surface is highly convoluted to form a regular pattern of narrow, parallel folds, or **folia**. The cerebellar white matter consists of nerve fibres running to and from the cerebellar cortex. The white matter has a characteristic branching, tree-like arrangement in section, as its ramifications reach towards

the surface. The cerebellum is concerned with the coordination of movement and it operates at an entirely unconscious level.

Rostral to the pons is located the relatively small midbrain. On its dorsal surface can be seen the rounded eminences of the superior and inferior colliculi, beneath which runs the cerebral aqueduct (Figs 1.13, 1.14, 1.15).

Diencephalon and cerebral hemispheres

Rostral to the brainstem lies the forebrain, which consists of the diencephalon and the cerebral hemispheres. The diencephalon and cerebral hemisphere on each side of the brain are to a large extent physically separate from their counterparts on the other side, although important cross-connections do exist, as described below. The two sides of the diencephalon are separated by the lumen of the third ventricle, of which they constitute the lateral walls.

The diencephalon consists of four main divisions: in a dorsoventral direction, these are the **epithalamus**, **thalamus**, **subthalamus** and **hypothalamus**. The epithalamus is small and its most notable component is the **pineal gland**, which lies in the midline, immediately rostral to the superior colliculi of the midbrain (Figs 1.14B, 1.15A). The thalamus is by far the largest part of the diencephalon and it forms much of the lateral wall of the third ventricle. The thalamus plays an important part in sensory, motor and cognitive functions and it has extensive reciprocal connections with the cerebral cortex. The subthalamus is a small region lying deep to the ventricular wall. It contains the **subthalamic nucleus**, which is closely related functionally to the basal ganglia (Chapter 14). The hypothalamus forms the lower part of the walls, and the floor, of the third ventricle. It is a complex and highly important region because of its involvement in the autonomic nervous system (Chapter 4), the limbic system and the neuroendocrine system (Chapter 16). From the ventral aspect of the hypothalamus in the midline arises the **infundibulum** or pituitary stalk (Fig. 1.15A), to which is attached the **pituitary gland**.

The cerebral hemisphere is by far the largest part of the brain. Like the cerebellum, it consists of an outer layer, or cortex, of grey

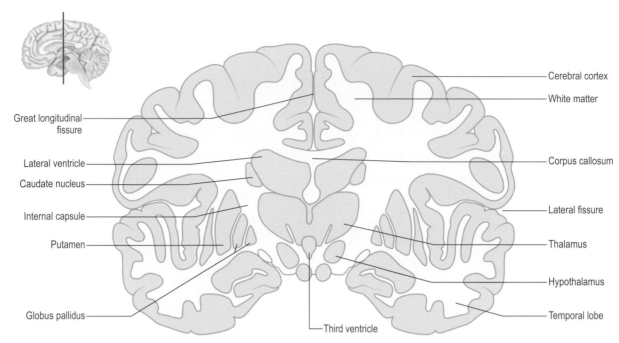

Fig. 1.25 Coronal section through the cerebral hemisphere.

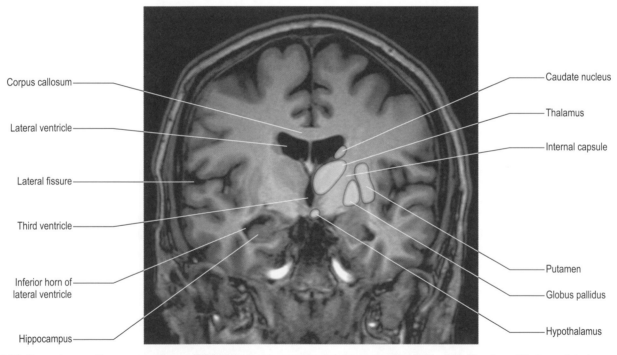

Fig. 1.26 Coronal magnetic resonance image (MRI) of the head, approximately corresponding to Fig. 1.25. *(Courtesy of Professor A Jackson, Wolfson Molecular Imaging Centre, University of Manchester, Manchester, UK.)*

matter and an inner mass of white matter (Figs 1.25, 1.26, 1.27, 1.28). In addition, partly buried within the subcortical white matter lie several masses of cell bodies, collectively referred to as the basal ganglia. The two cerebral hemispheres are separated in the sagittal plane by a deep midline cleft, the great longitudinal fissure (Figs 1.25, 1.26), which accommodates the falx cerebri, a sheet of dura mater reflected from the internal surface of the cranium. In the depths of the fissure lies the corpus callosum (Figs 1.15A, 1.25, 1.26), a large sheet of transversely running nerve fibres (commissural fibres) that link corresponding areas of the two cerebral cortices.

The cerebral cortex is highly convoluted. This has the effect of maximising the cortical surface area, which is about 1 m² for each hemisphere. The convolutions are called **gyri** (singular: gyrus) and the furrows between them are **sulci** (singular: sulcus). Some gyri and sulci have a relatively consistent configuration between individuals and they mark the location of important functional areas.

On the lateral surface of the hemisphere, a deep cleft, the **lateral fissure** (Figs 1.25, 1.29), is an important landmark. This, together with certain sulci, forms boundaries that divide the hemisphere into four **lobes** (Fig. 1.29). The lobes bear the names of the bones of the skull beneath which they lie.

The most anterior part of the cerebral hemisphere is called the **frontal lobe**, the most anterior convexity of which is the frontal pole. The posterior boundary of the frontal lobe is the **central sulcus**, which sometimes occurs as a single, continuous furrow running over the entire lateral surface of the hemisphere from the

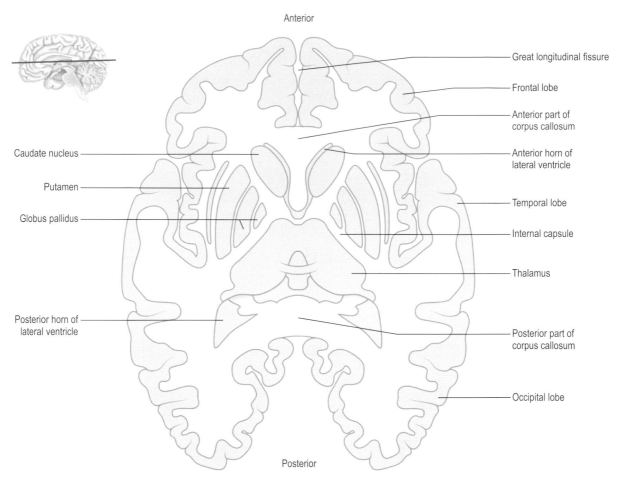

Anterior

Great longitudinal fissure

Frontal lobe

Anterior part of corpus callosum

Caudate nucleus

Anterior horn of lateral ventricle

Putamen

Temporal lobe

Globus pallidus

Internal capsule

Thalamus

Posterior horn of lateral ventricle

Posterior part of corpus callosum

Occipital lobe

Posterior

Fig. 1.27 Horizontal section through the cerebral hemisphere.

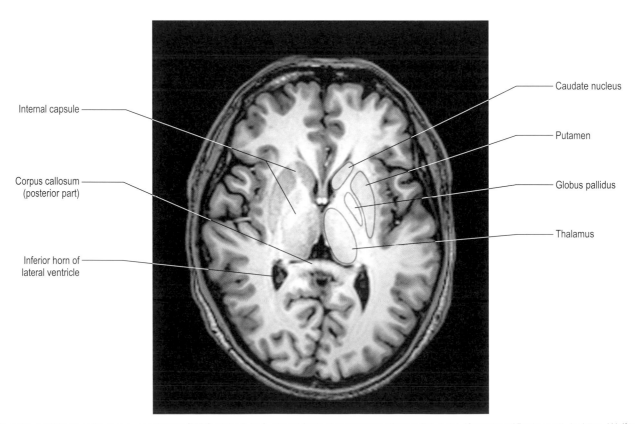

Internal capsule

Caudate nucleus

Putamen

Corpus callosum (posterior part)

Globus pallidus

Thalamus

Inferior horn of lateral ventricle

Fig. 1.28 Axial magnetic resonance image (MRI) of the head, approximately corresponding to Fig. 1.27. *(Courtesy of Professor A Jackson, Wolfson Molecular Imaging Centre, University of Manchester, Manchester, UK.)*

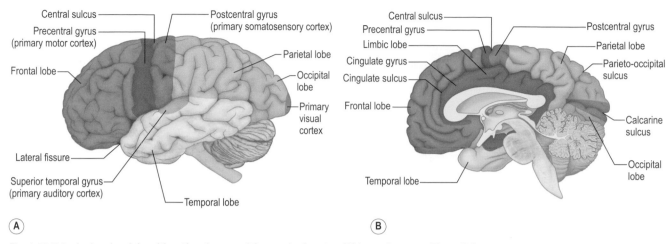

Fig. 1.29 Principal gyri, sulci and functional areas of the cerebral cortex. (A) Lateral aspect; (B) medial aspect.

great longitudinal fissure to the lateral fissure. Posterior to the central sulcus lies the **parietal lobe**, which is separated from the **temporal lobe** below by the lateral fissure. The tip of the **temporal lobe** is called the temporal pole. The posterior part of the hemisphere is the **occipital lobe**, ending in the occipital pole. The boundaries between parietal and temporal lobes and the occipital lobe are indistinct on the lateral surface of the hemisphere, since they do not correspond to any particular sulci. On the medial surface, however, the parietal and occipital lobes are separated by a deep **parieto-occipital sulcus**. On the medial aspect of the cerebral hemisphere, the **cingulate sulcus** runs parallel to the upper margin of the corpus callosum. This delineates a region of cortex that, together with parts of the medial aspect of the temporal cortex, is sometimes referred to as the **limbic lobe**.

The functions of the cerebral cortex are described in more detail in Chapter 13. It will be useful at the outset, however, to identify four important functional areas of cortex, one in each lobe (Fig. 1.29).

- In the frontal lobe, the gyrus immediately in front of the central sulcus is referred to anatomically as the **precentral gyrus**. Functionally, this comprises the **primary motor cortex**, which is the highest level in the brain for the control of voluntary movement. Here, in each hemisphere, the opposite half of the body is represented in a highly precise fashion. The opposite half of the body is represented because the neurones situated here that control movement have axons that cross over (decussate) to the opposite side of the brainstem and spinal cord, to control the motor neurones located there. The highly precise representation of the body is called 'somatotopic', which means that parts of the body that are close together are represented in parts of the cortex that are close together (see Fig. 13.20).
- In the parietal lobe, facing the primary motor cortex across the central sulcus, lies the **postcentral gyrus** or **primary somatosensory cortex**. This is the site of termination of pathways carrying the modalities of touch, pressure, pain and temperature from the opposite half of the body and it is the region where they are consciously perceived. Analogous to the arrangement in the primary motor cortex, the opposite half of the body is represented in the primary somatosensory cortex because the ascending pathways cross over at some point during their course. The representation of the body is, once again, somatotopic in a fashion that broadly mirrors that of the primary motor cortex (Fig. 13.20). The special senses of vision

and hearing have their highest level of representation in other areas.

- In the occipital lobe is located the **primary visual cortex**. It is mostly situated on the medial aspect of the hemisphere, in the gyri immediately above and below the horizontally orientated **calcarine sulcus**.
- In the temporal lobe lies the **primary auditory cortex**. It is localised to the **superior temporal gyrus**, which lies beneath, and parallel to, the lateral fissure.
- The limbic lobe is comprised primarily of the **cingulate gyrus**, lying on the medial aspect of the hemisphere parallel to the corpus callosum, and the **hippocampal formation** and **amygdala** which lie within the temporal lobe. These complex structures are concerned with the emotional aspects of behaviour and with memory.

During development, the cerebral hemisphere takes on a C-shaped configuration as a result of the forward migration of the temporal lobe, such that the temporal pole comes to lie adjacent to the frontal lobe, separated from it by the lateral fissure. The lateral ventricle within the hemisphere is, therefore, also basically C-shaped with 'horns' extending into the frontal, occipital and temporal lobes (Fig. 1.23).

The basic structure of the cerebral hemisphere is an outer mantle of grey matter, the cerebral cortex, beneath which lies a large and complex mass of white matter consisting of nerve fibres running to and from the cortex (Figs 1.25, 1.26, 1.27, 1.28).

Cortical afferent and efferent fibres that pass between the cerebral cortex and subcortical structures, such as the basal ganglia, thalamus, brainstem and spinal cord, are arranged in a characteristic radiating pattern, the **corona radiata**, which reaches out to the convolutions of the cortical surface (Fig. 1.30). Deeper inside the hemisphere, the fibres are concentrated into a dense sheet of white matter, known as the **internal capsule** (Figs 1.25, 1.26, 1.27, 1.28).

Within the hemisphere, both medial and lateral to the internal capsule, lie masses of grey matter, collectively referred to as the **basal ganglia**, **basal nuclei** or **corpus striatum**. The principal components of the basal ganglia are the **caudate nucleus**, the **putamen** (collectively referred to as the neostriatum, or simply the striatum) and the **globus pallidus** (Figs 1.25, 1.26, 1.27, 1.28). The caudate nucleus lies in the wall of the lateral ventricle throughout its extent and, like the ventricle, it is C-shaped. The basal ganglia are principally concerned with the control of movement, posture and muscle tone (Chapter 14).

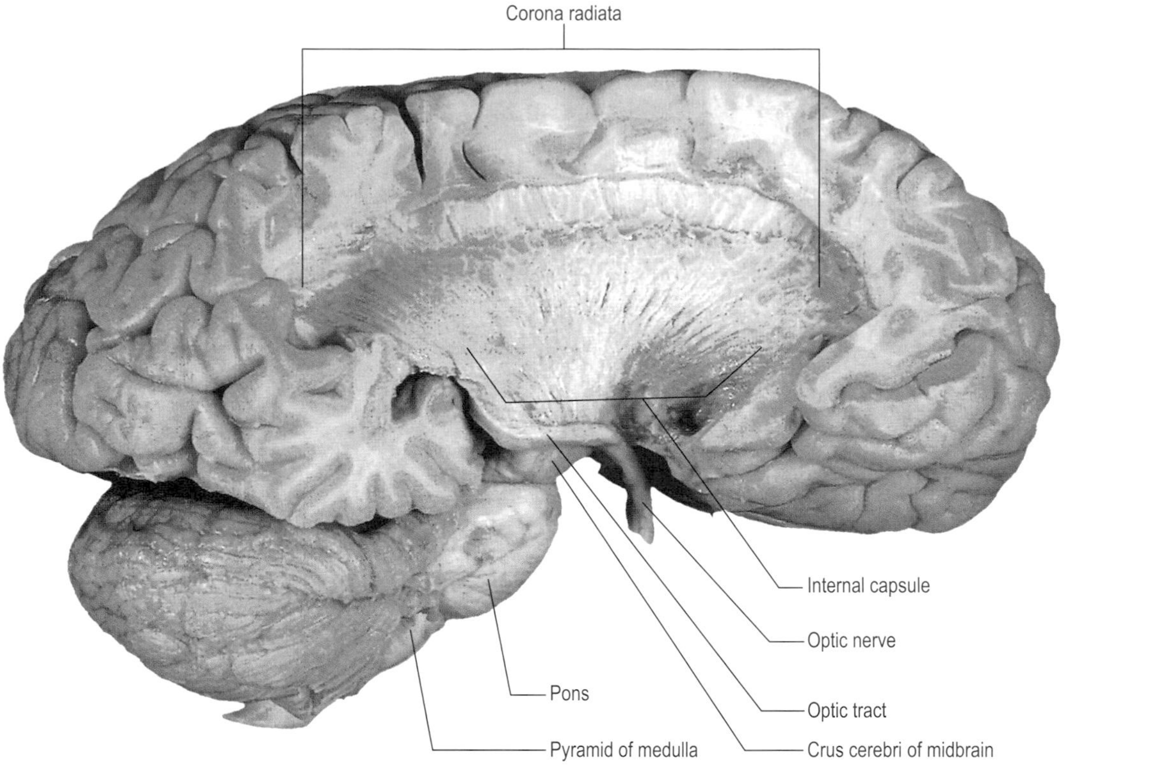

Corona radiata

Internal capsule

Optic nerve

Optic tract

Crus cerebri of midbrain

Pyramid of medulla

Pons

Fig. 1.30 Dissection of the right side of the brain from its lateral aspect, illustrating the corona radiata and the internal capsule.

Basic organisation of the brain

- The brain is conventionally divided into hindbrain, midbrain and forebrain.

- The hindbrain is further subdivided into the medulla oblongata, pons and cerebellum.

- The medulla, pons and midbrain constitute the brainstem.

- The forebrain consists of the diencephalon (principally the thalamus and hypothalamus) and the cerebral hemisphere.

- Within the cerebral hemisphere lie several large nuclei called the basal ganglia.

- The brain contains a system of cavities or ventricles containing CSF, which is produced by the choroid plexus.

- The brain possesses 12 pairs of cranial nerves, which carry afferent and efferent fibres, principally to and from structures of the head.

- The two cerebral hemispheres are linked by the commissural fibres of the corpus callosum.

- The surface of the cerebral hemisphere consists of cortical grey matter, which is folded to form gyri and sulci. Beneath the surface lie the dense fibre masses of the corona radiata and the internal capsule. The surface is divided into lobes:

  - Frontal lobe containing the primary motor cortex
  - Parietal lobe containing the primary somatosensory cortex
  - Temporal lobe containing the primary auditory cortex
  - Occipital lobe containing the primary visual cortex
  - Limbic lobe containing regions for memory and emotional aspects of behaviour

Major sensory pathways

Sensory information about the internal and external environments is carried to the CNS in afferent nerve fibres running in cranial and spinal nerves. Sensory information can be classified under the headings of 'special senses' and 'general senses'. The special senses are all carried in cranial nerves and are comprised of olfaction (cranial nerve I), vision (II), taste (VII and IX) and hearing and

vestibular function (VIII). The special senses are dealt with in more detail elsewhere.

The general senses include the modalities of touch, pressure, pain and temperature (relayed from exteroceptors in the skin and interoceptors in the viscera), and awareness of posture and movement (from proprioceptors in joints, tendons and muscles). General sensory information from the trunk and limbs is carried in spinal nerves; from the head, it is carried in the trigeminal nerve (cranial nerve V).

For all modalities in the category of general sensation, there is a sequence of three neurones between the sensory receptor located in the periphery and the perception of sensation at the level of the cerebral cortex (Fig. 1.31). The first neurone (**first-order neurone** or **primary afferent neurone**) enters the spinal cord through a spinal nerve, or the brainstem through the trigeminal nerve, on the same side of the body as its peripheral receptor is located. The cell body of the first-order neurone is located outside the CNS, either in the dorsal root ganglion of a spinal nerve, or in the trigeminal ganglion. Within the CNS, the axon of the first-order neurone remains on the same side (ipsilateral) and synapses upon the second neurone (**second-order neurone**). The second-order neurone has its cell body in the spinal cord or brainstem, the exact location depending on the modality concerned. Its axon crosses over (decussates) to the other side of the CNS and ascends to the thalamus, where it terminates. The third neurone in the sequence (**third-order neurone**) has its cell body in the thalamus and its axon projects to the somatosensory cortex, located in the postcentral gyrus of the parietal lobe of the cerebral hemisphere.

More specifically, primary spinal afferents carrying coarse touch/pressure, pain and temperature information from the limbs and trunk terminate near their level of entry into the spinal cord. They synapse with second-order neurones, the axons of which decussate within a few segments and thereafter form the **spinothalamic tract**. In contrast, primary spinal afferents carrying proprioceptive information and discriminative (fine) touch ascend uninterrupted on the same side of the cord as their entry, forming the **dorsal**

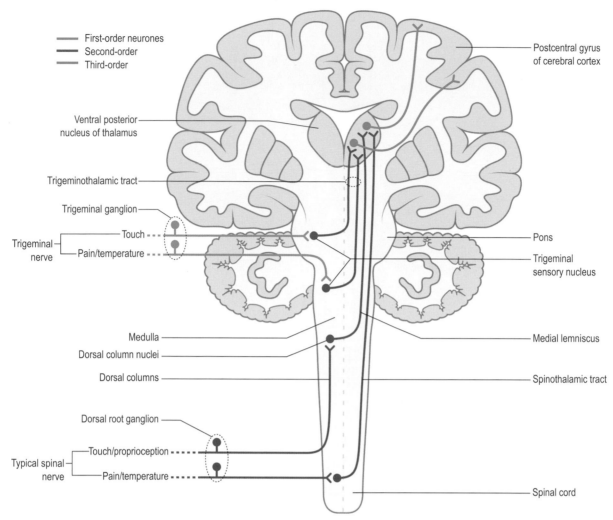

Fig. 1.31 Overview of the major pathways for general sensation.

columns (fasciculus gracilis and fasciculus cuneatus). They terminate in the **dorsal column nuclei** (nuclei gracilis and cuneatus) located in the medulla. From here, second-order neurones decussate and ascend to the thalamus as a fibre tract known as the **medial lemniscus**. Primary afferent neurones that enter the brainstem in the trigeminal nerve terminate ipsilaterally in the **trigeminal sensory nucleus**, one of the cranial nerve nuclei. From here, second-order neurones decussate and ascend to the thalamus as the **trigeminothalamic tract**. Second-order sensory neurones, of either spinal cord or brainstem origin, converge upon the same region of the thalamus (the ventral posterior nucleus), synapsing upon third-order neurones that project to the somatosensory cortex in the postcentral gyrus of the parietal lobe. Throughout the central projections of the somatosensory system, there is a high degree of spatial segregation of the neurones representing different parts of the body (so-called somatotopic organisation). This is most dramatically demonstrated at the level of the cerebral cortex (see Fig. 13.20). Here, the somatosensory area occupies a strip of cortex that extends from the medial aspect of the hemisphere (leg area) to the inferolateral aspect of the parietal lobe (head area).

Major motor pathways

The motor neurones that directly innervate skeletal muscle have cell bodies lying in the grey matter of the spinal cord and brainstem and are often referred to as **lower motor neurones**. They constitute the so-called 'final common pathway' by which the nervous system controls movement. In contrast, the neurones that control the activity of lower motor neurones are themselves collectively referred to as **upper motor neurones**. The latter form a number of **descending tracts** that run through the brainstem and spinal cord. Among the most important of these are the **corticospinal** and **corticobulbar** (or corticonuclear) **tracts** (Fig. 1.32). These tracts originate partly from neurones in the motor area of the cerebral cortex, where the whole body is represented in a precisely organised, or somatotopic, fashion (see Fig. 13.20). The descending axons pass through the internal capsule and into the brainstem, where most of them decussate to the other side. This means that movements of one side of the body are controlled by the opposite cerebral cortex. Corticobulbar, or corticonuclear, fibres control the activity of motor neurones located in cranial nerve nuclei of the brainstem, which innervate skeletal muscles of the head and neck through the cranial nerves ('bulb' is an archaic and little-used term for the medulla, in which some of the motor neurones lie). Corticospinal fibres control the activity of motor neurones in the spinal cord, which innervate trunk and limb muscles. Descending corticospinal fibres form a prominent ridge on the ventral surface of the medulla. This is called the **pyramid** and, hence, the corticospinal tract is also known as the **pyramidal tract**. The place where these fibres cross over to the other side is called the **decussation of the pyramids** (see Fig. 9.4).

The main function of the corticobulbar and corticospinal pathways is the control of skilled, voluntary movements. A large proportion of the motor cortex and its descending pathways are, therefore, devoted to those parts of the body capable of delicate, so-called 'fractionated', movements such as the muscles of speech and facial expression and the muscles controlling the hand.

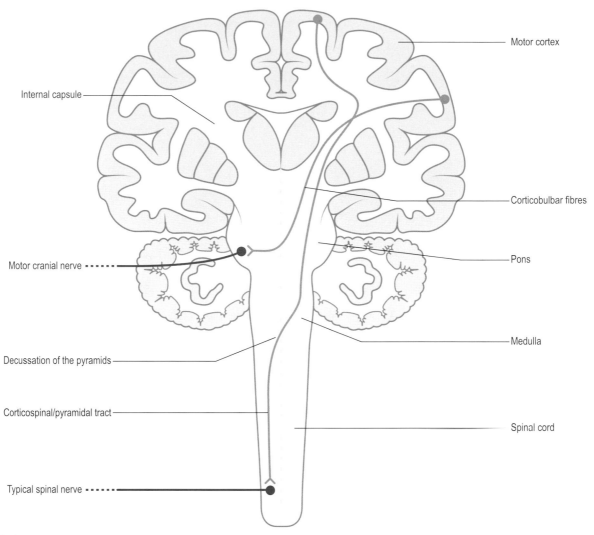

Internal capsule

Motor cranial nerve

Decussation of the pyramids

Corticospinal/pyramidal tract

Typical spinal nerve

Motor cortex

Corticobulbar fibres

Pons

Medulla

Spinal cord

Fig. 1.32 Overview of the major motor pathways.

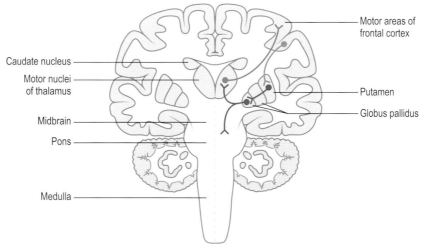

Caudate nucleus

Motor nuclei of thalamus

Midbrain

Pons

Medulla

Motor areas of frontal cortex

Putamen

Globus pallidus

Fig. 1.33 Overview of the connections of the basal ganglia.

Numerous brain structures, apart from the corticospinal, or pyramidal, system are involved in the control of movement, posture and muscle tone. These are sometimes collectively referred to as the **extrapyramidal** system and their descending projections as extrapyramidal pathways. Included in this definition are certain nuclei in the brainstem, such as the **vestibular nuclei**, the **reticular nuclei (reticular formation)**, the **red nucleus** and also the basal ganglia and related subcortical nuclei located in the forebrain. The vestibular, reticular and red nuclei influence spinal motor neurones partly through descending connections in the **vestibulospinal**,

reticulospinal and **rubrospinal** tracts. They are important in the control of muscle tone and the posture of the body. The basal ganglia exert their actions on the lower motor neurones of the brainstem and spinal cord of the contralateral side through complex, indirect pathways (Fig. 1.33). These include projections via the thalamus to the motor areas of the cerebral cortex and projections to the reticular formation of the brainstem. The basal ganglia are important in the control of muscle tone and posture and, importantly, the facilitation of appropriate motor behaviour and the inhibition of unwanted movements (Chapter 14).

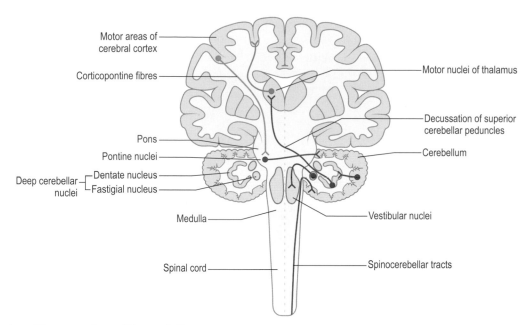

Fig. 1.34 Overview of the connections of the cerebellum.

The cerebellum is an important centre in which programmes of movement, generated in the motor region of the cerebral cortex, are compared with sensory feedback concerning the speed and direction of active movements of the limbs, head and neck in space. This is essential for accurate, coordinated, purposeful movement. The cerebellum receives afferent connections from the spinal cord via the **spinocerebellar tracts**. It also receives input from the vestibular system and from the motor cortex (the latter indirectly via nuclei in the pons). The efferent connections of the cerebellum are complex but are primarily in the form of feedback to the motor cortex via the thalamus (Fig. 1.34). Afferents to each side of the cerebellum come from the ipsilateral half of the spinal cord and brainstem and from the contralateral cerebral cortex. Efferent cerebellar projections are directed to the contralateral thalamus and cerebral cortex through a decussation in the midbrain. Because of this, and the decussation of cortical descending motor pathways, each side of the cerebellum coordinates the movements of the ipsilateral side of the body (Chapter 11).

Basic clinical diagnostic principles

A knowledge of neuroanatomy is an essential prerequisite for the clinical diagnosis of disorders of the nervous system. The process of reaching a diagnosis proceeds by history-taking, then neurological examination and, finally, by confirmatory investigations (Fig. 1.35). History-taking provides clues to the aetiology or cause of disease, whereas the clinical examination pinpoints the site of the lesion (Fig. 1.36). A pathological lesion acting at a specific location within the neuromuscular axis forms a recognisable syndrome, investigation of which leads to establishing the aetiology or diagnosis.

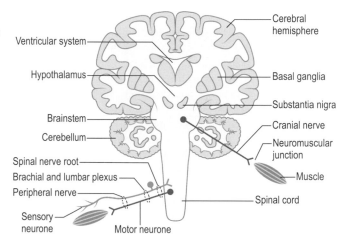

Fig. 1.36 The central and peripheral nervous systems and possible sites of pathological lesion.

Aetiology of neurological disease

The disorders of the neuromuscular system are of four major types (Fig. 1.37) in relation to causation or aetiology.

For each major cause of disease there are appropriate types of investigation, leading to specific forms of treatment. The four causes are ranked in order of clinical priority so that conditions that are common, potentially life-threatening and reversible with prompt treatment are either established or excluded first. Conditions that are rare, chronic and incurable can be considered later.

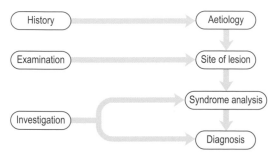

Fig. 1.35 The process of clinical diagnosis.

Cause	Investigation/treatment
Extrinsic	Neurosurgery
Systemic	Medicine
Vascular	Cardiovascular
Intrinsic	Neurology

Fig. 1.37 The four major categories of disorders of the neuromuscular system.

Extrinsic disorders

Extrinsic disorders lead to compression of the brain, spinal cord, nerve roots and peripheral nerves (Fig. 1.38) and are, therefore, surgically remediable. Investigations, such as radiological imaging of the CNS, must be promptly carried out prior to neurosurgical intervention. Delay in decompressive neurosurgery can lead to permanent paralysis, sensory loss and incontinence.

The brain, spinal cord and peripheral nerves can be compressed by disease of adjacent structures. The brain may be compressed on its outer surface by blood clots (**haematomas**), abscesses and tumours arising within the skull and coverings of the cerebrum. Alternatively, the fluid-filled ventricles may compress the brain from within when blockage to the flow of CSF leads to a rise in pressure and expansion of the ventricles (**hydrocephalus**).

The spinal cord may be compressed by disease of the spine, such as arthritis (**spondylosis**), prolapsed intervertebral discs and bone tumours, as well as by tumours of the meninges (**meningiomas**). The central canal of the spinal cord, normally a minute vestigial space, may expand into a cavity (**syrinx**), compressing the nerve fibres in the centre of the cord (**syringomyelia**).

The cranial nerves emerging from the brainstem may be compressed, as they course through the cranium and leave the foramina of the skull, by tumours and swollen arteries (**aneurysms**). The spinal nerve roots leaving the spinal cord in the neck and back may be trapped by tumours and prolapsed intervertebral discs, causing pain, weakness and sensory loss in their region of distribution (**radiculopathy**). The peripheral nerves may become trapped at vulnerable pressure sites in the limbs by ribs and tough fibrous bands, leading to pain, weakness and sensory loss in their distribution (**entrapment neuropathy**).

Investigations for extrinsic disorders are chiefly neuroradiological (e.g. computed tomographic (CT) brain scan and magnetic resonance imaging (MRI)) to delineate the disorders (lesions) for neurosurgical decompression. Surgery may be required urgently to prevent permanent disability and that is why extrinsic disorders should be the first diagnostic consideration.

Systemic disorders

Systemic disorders are primarily disorders of organs other than the nervous system that disrupt neuromuscular function by abnormal metabolism (Fig. 1.39). The patient presents with a neurological condition or syndrome, but the cause lies primarily elsewhere. It may be intoxication with drugs (e.g. alcohol), dietary deficiency (e.g. of vitamin B), failure of the cardiorespiratory system, liver or kidneys, or hormonal (endocrine) disorders such as thyroid disease, diabetes mellitus and abnormalities in calcium and potassium balance. Investigations for systemic disease are chiefly haematological, biochemical tests and specific measures of cardiorespiratory, liver, renal and endocrine function. Treatment of the systemic disease by the appropriate specialist can lead to cure of the neurological disorder.

Vascular disorders

Vascular disorders (Fig. 1.40) damage the circulation to the nervous system in a number of ways:

- Occlusion of the vessels (**thrombosis**)
- Restriction of the blood and oxygen supply (**infarction**)
- Bleeding into the nervous tissues (**haemorrhage**)

The rapid development of a vascular lesion is called a **stroke**. Congenital swellings of arteries (**aneurysms**) or tumours of blood vessels (**angiomas**) can compress cranial nerves and the brain itself. Investigations for vascular disorders are aimed at excluding abnormal clotting disorders of the circulating blood, testing the valves and muscles of the heart (echocardiography, electrocardiography and cardiac angiography), and displaying the vessels of the neck and brain by angiography. The treatment of vascular disorders may be haematological or cardiological and may require surgery to the heart or arteries in the neck and skull.

Intrinsic disorders

Intrinsic disorders (Fig. 1.41) are primary disorders of the nervous system itself. Intrinsic, primary neurological disorders are uncommon, but when they occur they are often chronic and

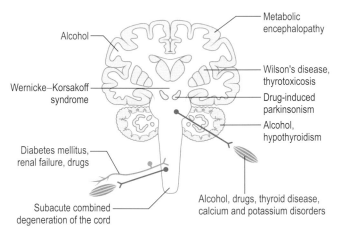

Fig. 1.39 Systemic disorders of the neuromuscular system.

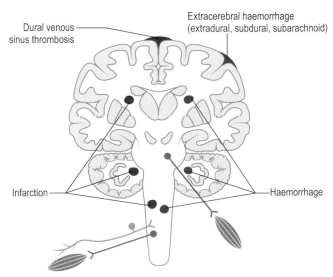

Fig. 1.40 Vascular disorders of the neuromuscular system.

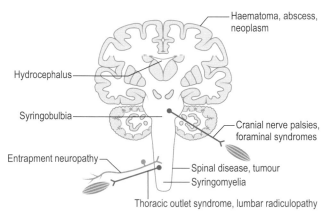

Fig. 1.38 Extrinsic disorders of the neuromuscular system.

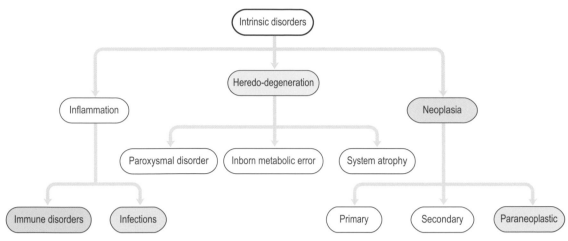

Fig. 1.41 Intrinsic disorders of the neuromuscular system. Colours refer to Figs 1.42–46.

irreversible. Many nervous system disorders are under genetic influences (**heredo-degeneration**). **Inborn errors of metabolism** lead to mental subnormality and disability in children and are usually caused by deficiencies of specific enzymes. **Paroxysmal disorders** consist of episodic loss of consciousness (**epilepsy**), excessive sleep (narcolepsy) and headache (**migraine**). **System degenerations** (Fig. 1.42) occur in youth and old age and lead to the premature death (**atrophy**) of certain neuromuscular components, with sparing of others. When system degenerations occur in youth, they often have an obvious hereditary or genetic cause, for example the **muscular dystrophies**, the **hereditary sensorimotor neuropathies**, **hereditary spastic paraparesis**, **cerebellar ataxias** and **Huntington's disease**. When they occur later in life, they are more often sporadic: e.g. **motor neurone disease**, **Parkinson's disease** and **Alzheimer's disease**. The system degenerations are remarkably selective as to the nerve cells that are affected. For example, in motor neurone disease there is paralysis of muscle but no abnormalities of sensation, whereas in Alzheimer's disease, there is severe amnesia but no paralysis.

Neoplasia refers to excessive, uncontrolled growth of tissues forming a benign or malignant tumour. Primary neoplasms arise in the neuromuscular tissues themselves (Fig. 1.43); secondary neoplasms spread in the circulation from other primary organ sites (e.g. lung or breast). Rarely, tumours at distant sites damage the nervous system by humoral or immune mechanisms and the resulting disorders are termed non-metastatic or paraneoplastic, syndromes (Fig. 1.44).

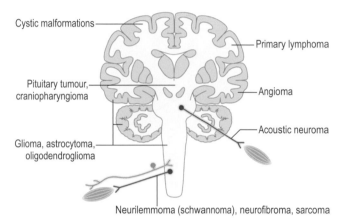

Fig. 1.43 Neoplasia of the neuromuscular system.

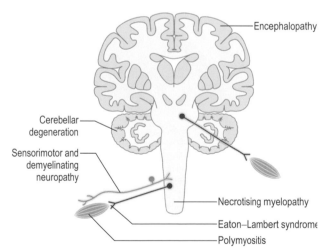

Fig. 1.44 Paraneoplastic syndromes of the neuromuscular system.

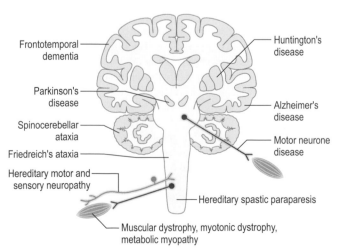

Fig. 1.42 Degenerative disorders of the neuromuscular system.

Inflammation of neuromuscular tissue may result from **infection** by microorganisms (Fig. 1.45) and can affect a variety of structures, for example the meninges (**meningococcal meningitis**), the brain (**viral encephalitis**, **neurosyphilis**) or peripheral nerves (**leprosy**). Alternatively, inflammation can occur in **immune disorders** (Fig. 1.46), in the absence of infection. The most common immune disorder of the CNS is **multiple sclerosis**. Immune disorders may also strike peripheral nerves (**acute inflammatory neuropathy** or **Guillain–Barré syndrome**), the neuromuscular junction (**myasthenia gravis**) or muscle

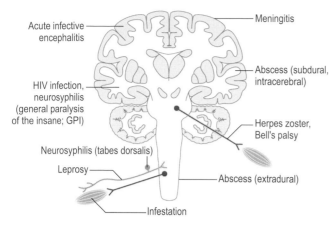

Fig. 1.45 Infections of the neuromuscular system.

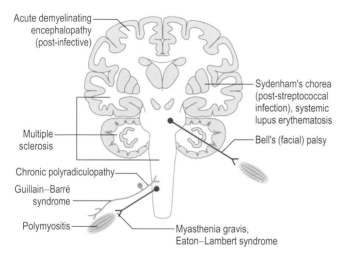

Fig. 1.46 Immune disorders of the neuromuscular system.

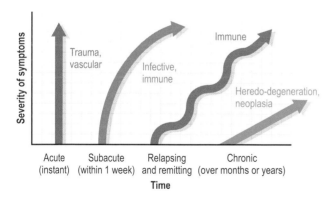

Fig. 1.47 History (onset) limits possible aetiologies.

(polymyositis). Inflammatory disorders are investigated by microbiological and serological tests of the blood and CSF. Treatment of infection with antimicrobial agents and suppression of immune responses by drugs such as corticosteroids may cure or control these infective or immune diseases.

Time-course of disease

History-taking can be valuable for suggesting the likely cause of illness, by determining the rate of evolution of the disorder, which is often characteristic of the different aetiologies (Fig. 1.47). Disorders of sudden (acute), dramatic onset are caused by external injury (trauma) or a vascular accident (stroke). When the condition develops over days (subacute) to become maximal in about one week, this is strongly suggestive of an inflammatory disorder, which may be infective (e.g. meningitis) or immune (e.g.

multiple sclerosis). Recovery from immune disorders takes weeks or months, or it is incomplete. Moreover, immune disorders often run a relapsing and remitting course, with acute events superimposed on chronic decline over months and years. This paroxysmal course is highly characteristic of multiple sclerosis - hence the name of the disease. System degenerations, by contrast, take many years to develop (chronic) and the onset is often difficult to date, especially since patients accommodate slowly to their accumulating disability. In muscular dystrophy, hereditary sensorimotor neuropathies, Parkinson's and Alzheimer's diseases, the disorders may last from 5 to 30 years. Neoplasms (tumours) usually develop over months or years, with symptoms such as epileptic seizures and headache. Only rarely do highly malignant tumours (gliomas and secondary tumours) declare themselves over days or weeks.

Basic clinical diagnostic principles

- History-taking, clinical examination and investigations lead to the diagnosis of the cause (aetiology) of disease.
- The site of the lesion(s) determines the clinical syndrome revealed by the neurological examination.
- Disorders of the nervous system can be classified as extrinsic, systemic, vascular or intrinsic.
- Intrinsic disorders consist of system degenerations (atrophy), inborn errors of metabolism, paroxysmal disorders, neoplasms, infections and immune disorders.

Site of the lesion and clinical syndromes

Whatever the cause of a lesion may be, its site in the neuromuscular system leads to a characteristic syndrome. This is defined clinically by careful examination of the cranial nerves, the motor system, reflexes, sensation and coordination. In this book, the functional status of these systems is depicted diagrammatically (Fig. 1.48) so that the syndromes produced by particular types of lesion can be illustrated pictorially in a way that links neuroanatomy with clinical signs. In appropriate chapters, the description of the anatomy and basic functions of the nervous system is accompanied by figures, based upon the prototypical Fig. 1.48, that summarise the principal clinical syndromes in terms of sensory and motor deficits. In order to understand fully the relationship between neuroanatomy and clinical signs, it is necessary to know the routes of the major sensory and motor pathways, the significance of lesions of the 'lower motor neurone' and 'upper motor neurone' and the general functions of the cerebellum, basal ganglia and cerebral cortex.

The neuroanatomical information contained in this chapter represents the minimal and essential knowledge required before the clinical approach to the neurological patient. Without this knowledge, it is impossible to interpret the significance of the signs elicited on examination of the nervous system as described in the standard texts on 'clinical methods'. The continual practice of the examination of the nervous system through experience, and the development of clinical acumen, permit the highly accurate localisation of lesions within the central and peripheral nervous systems. The site of the lesion may be strictly focal, for example a tumour in the left cerebral hemisphere; or may represent localisation within a functional neuroanatomical system, for example the upper and lower motor neurones in motor neurone disease; or the peripheral nerves in sensorimotor polyneuropathy. A further delineation of focal lesions is to determine whether they lie within the nervous system (intrinsic lesions) or whether they lie outside and compress the nervous system (extrinsic lesions). This is an important distinction, since extrinsic lesions represent disorders that are potentially remediable by neurosurgery.

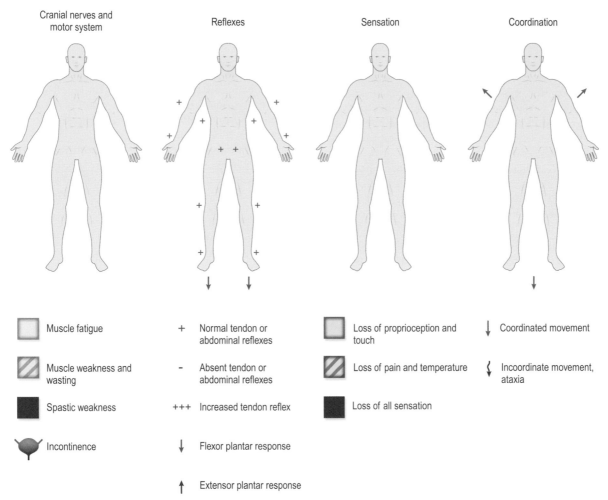

Fig. 1.48 Prototypical figure for illustration of major syndromes of the neuromuscular system. Throughout the text, simplified outlines of the major anatomical–clinical syndromes are presented diagrammatically, following the conventional neurological examination of cranial nerves, motor function, reflexes, sensation, coordination and mental state described in textbooks of clinical methods.

There are certain principles that can be drawn from the organisation of the neuroanatomical structures described, which are of high explanatory value to the clinician in determining the site of the lesion.

Major sensory pathways

Sensation in the trunk and limbs is conducted from sensory receptors in the periphery, by the peripheral nerves and spinal nerve roots, to the dorsal root ganglia and then into the spinal cord. Within the spinal cord there is a divergence of sensory pathways carrying different sensory modalities (see Fig. 1.31). The sensory pathways for pain and temperature decussate within the spinal cord and ascend in the contralateral spinothalamic tract to reach the thalamus and thence the contralateral sensory cortex of the cerebral hemisphere. In contrast, tactile and proprioceptive pathways ascend ipsilaterally in the dorsal (posterior) columns of the spinal cord before decussating in the lower brainstem and passing, via the thalamus, to the contralateral sensory cortex.

This divergent arrangement permits lesions of the spinal cord and brainstem to damage one pathway preferentially and spare the other. The term **dissociated sensory loss** refers to the clinical finding of selective loss of the modalities of touch and proprioception, with preservation of pain and temperature modalities or vice versa. This selective loss of sensory modalities results from the selective involvement by lesions of the functionally specific pathways for touch/proprioception or pain/temperature. Lesion of the dorsal columns of the spinal cord leads to an ipsilateral loss of touch/proprioception below the level of the lesion. In contrast, lesion of the spinothalamic tract leads to

contralateral loss of pain/temperature below the level of the lesion.

A unilateral lesion of the thoracic spinal cord, for example, leads to an ipsilateral loss of touch sensation and proprioception and a contralateral loss of pain and temperature sensation in the trunk and lower limbs below the level of the lesion. In addition, as described below, there is an ipsilateral 'pyramidal weakness' of the lower limb. Collectively, these are known as a hemicord or **Brown–Séquard syndrome** (see Fig. 8.25C).

Selective lesion in the brainstem of the medial lemniscus leads to loss of touch sensation, whereas lesion of the trigeminothalamic tract leads to loss of pain and temperature sensation in the face. Therefore, the clinical finding of dissociated sensory loss implies the presence of an intrinsic, focal lesion within the spinal cord or brainstem.

Because of the decussation of all ascending sensory pathways in either the spinal cord or lower brainstem, lesions of the upper brainstem or cerebral hemisphere lead to loss of all sensation on the opposite (contralateral) side of the body. (See also spinal cord lesions in Fig. 8.25A, brainstem lesions in Fig. 9.17 and unilateral cerebral hemisphere lesions in Fig. 13.18.).

Patterns of sensory loss in disease

- Unilateral lesions of the spinal cord or lower brainstem lead to dissociated sensory loss.
- Lesions of the upper brainstem or cerebral hemisphere lead to loss of all sensation on the contralateral side of the body.

Major motor pathways

Motor neurones that originate in cranial nerve nuclei of the brainstem or the ventral horn of the spinal cord are called lower motor neurones and they innervate specific groups of skeletal muscle fibres. Damage to lower motor neurones leads, therefore, to weakness (**paresis**) or **paralysis** and **wasting** of individual muscles. The muscles show depressed stretch (tendon) reflexes (**hyporeflexia**) and they lose their tone (**hypotonia**). Spontaneous contractions of the muscle fibres associated with a single motor nerve (motor unit) occur when the muscle fibres are denervated and are seen as **fasciculations**, i.e. ripple-like movements of muscle beneath the skin. Since all lower motor neurones innervate muscles on the same side of the body as the location of the nerve cell body, the effects of lower motor neurone lesions are seen ipsilateral to the lesion.

The descending motor pathways that control the activity of lower motor neurones are referred to as upper motor neurones. They arise from the cerebral cortex and brainstem. The corticospinal (pyramidal) and corticonuclear/corticobulbar pathways are particularly important (Fig. 1.32). These descending motor pathways are highly organised somatotopically but are also concerned with concerted movements of the limbs. Damage to the corticospinal pathway (upper motor neurone lesion) leads to loss of individual movements of the digits and a breakdown in movements of extension and abduction of the upper limb and of flexion of the lower limb. This characteristic weakness of movements is clinically referred to as a **pyramidal weakness**.

Lower and upper motor neurone lesions

Damage to lower motor neurones is associated with a number of motor signs and symptoms that distinguish it from upper motor neurone lesions. The distinction is critical in neurological examination and diagnosis.

Lower motor neurone syndrome

- Weakness (paresis) or paralysis (plegia) of individual muscles.
- Wasting of muscles.
- Visible spontaneous contractions of motor units (fasciculation).
- Reduced resistance to passive stretching (hypotonia).
- Diminution or loss of stretch (tendon) reflexes (hyporeflexia or areflexia).

Upper motor neurone syndrome

- Weakness of specific muscles ('pyramidal weakness').
- No wasting of muscles.
- Hyperreflexia.
- Spasticity.
- Positive Babinski (extensor plantar) response.
- Absent abdominal reflexes.

Pyramidal weakness is also associated clinically with overactive tendon stretch reflexes (**hyperreflexia**) and with increased muscle tone (**hypertonia**), i.e. resistance to passive limb movement, this combination being termed **spasticity**. The increase in tone occurs at the initial stretch of the limb muscles and is then followed by sudden relaxation of tone (**clasp-knife response**). Spasticity manifests in the flexor muscles of the upper limbs and extensor muscles of the lower limbs. These are the stronger muscle groups in the respective limbs, and the combination of spasticity and greater power contributes to the development of an abnormal posture in which the arm is relatively fixed in flexion and the leg in extension (see Fig. 13.18). The lower limb also demonstrates the positive **Babinski reflex** (dorsiflexion of the great toe on stimulation of the sole of the foot), which is considered as pathognomonic of corticospinal tract damage.

The fact that the descending motor pathways in the corticonuclear/corticobulbar and corticospinal tracts decussate in the lower brainstem means that a unilateral lesion in the cerebral hemisphere (see Fig. 13.18) or brainstem (see Fig. 9.17) leads to contralateral paralysis of the limbs.

The use of the term 'pyramidal' to describe the effects of upper motor neurone lesions implies that these clinical features result solely from damage to the pyramidal or corticospinal tract. However, individual tracts are rarely damaged in isolation and, therefore, it is often difficult to attribute clinical deficits to involvement of particular pathways. Damage to the pyramidal tract itself probably accounts for the loss of discrete movements and the appearance of the Babinski reflex. Hyperreflexia and spasticity are due to the additional involvement of other pathways.

Cerebellum

The current concept of cerebellar function is that, as movement is initiated by the motor parts of the cerebral cortex, the pattern of intended movement is transmitted simultaneously to the cerebellum via the pons (Fig. 1.34). At the same time, afferent impulses from sensory receptors in muscles, joints and tendons, convey information about the ongoing movement through peripheral nerves into the spinal cord and ascend in the spinocerebellar tracts to the cerebellum. The cerebellum, therefore, is in a unique position to compare the intended movement with the actual movement. When there is a discrepancy between these, the cerebellum is able to correct deviant movements. This is achieved by ascending cerebellar efferent pathways travelling via the thalamus to the motor cortex and, thence, through descending fibres passing to the brainstem and spinal cord. There are also direct cerebellar connections to the vestibular and reticular nuclei of the brainstem, which themselves give rise to descending pathways influencing tone, posture and balance.

Lesions of the cerebellum or its connections lead to a cerebellar syndrome comprised of incoordination of eye movements (**nystagmus**), speech (**dysarthria**), the upper limbs (**intention tremor**) and gait (**ataxia**), in the absence of weakness or loss of sensation. The symptoms and signs occur on the same side as (ipsilateral to) the lesion in the cerebellum.

A lesion interrupting cerebellar connections may lie in the cerebellum itself, in the brainstem or in the ascending spinocerebellar tracts. Unilateral lesions of the cerebellum lead to ipsilateral loss of coordination. Similarly, a unilateral lesion of the brainstem inevitably destroys the cerebellar connections to the cerebral hemisphere and spinal cord and leads to ipsilateral incoordination and, as described above, a contralateral pyramidal weakness of the limbs.

Disorders of the cerebellum

Cerebellar lesions cause:

- Nystagmus.
- Dysarthria (scanning speech).
- Intention tremor.
- Ataxia.

The signs and symptoms occur ipsilateral to the lesion.

It is sometimes mistakenly thought that incoordination of the limbs is synonymous with a disorder of the cerebellum. This is not the case, whereas it is true that lesions of the cerebellum do lead to incoordination. A patient with a short leg and an arthritic hip joint, for example, will have an incoordinate gait. Moreover, weakness of the limbs due to disease of the central or peripheral nervous system will cause incoordination. Damage to the peripheral sensory nerves or to the dorsal columns of the spinal cord deprives the brain of proprioceptive information from the limbs, thus causing lack of coordination of the arms and an ataxic gait. This is known as 'sensory ataxia'. When patients with sensory ataxia close their eyes, they readily lose their balance and this is known as **Romberg's sign**. This does not happen with lesions of the cerebellar pathways.

Because of these problems of interpretation, it is conventional to carry out tasks of coordination at the end of the neurological examination, in order to assess the contribution of orthopaedic deformities, neurological weakness and sensory loss to the degree of incoordination. If these prior deficits can be excluded on examination, then incoordination can reliably be blamed on lesions of the cerebellar pathways themselves. This can sometimes be a difficult exercise; for example, in diseases such as multiple sclerosis, there are multiple lesions in the cerebellum, brainstem and spinal cord, each making a contribution to the nature and degree of neurological disability.

Basal ganglia

The basal ganglia, lying deep within the cerebral hemisphere, receive sensory and motor information from widespread regions of the cerebral cortex (Fig. 1.33) and also input from the brainstem. They are involved in the control of movement, posture and muscular tone (Chapter 14). Lesions or disorders of the basal ganglia do not lead to loss of sensation, power or coordination. Instead, there is a loss of control of voluntary movement and posture, increase in muscular tone (**rigidity**) and the emergence of involuntary movements (**dyskinesia**). Unilateral lesions of the basal ganglia lead to a contralateral motor disorder.

Impaired motor control manifests as delayed initiation and slowness of movement (**akinesia/bradykinesia**), episodic hurrying (**festinant gait**) and sudden stops, causing falls. Posture is flexed or, less commonly, extended and there is an absence of arm-swinging when walking. The face lacks expression.

Rigidity is an increase in muscular tone that manifests as resistance to passive movement throughout the extent of the movement. It may be smooth (lead pipe) or jerky (cog-wheel) in type. This contrasts with spasticity, where there is an initial resistance to passive movement at the onset of muscular stretch, followed by relaxation.

Tremor is a to-and-fro, alternating, sinusoidal movement of the limbs. It may be rapid and present while maintaining posture (postural tremor) – for example, in the outstretched arms as in thyrotoxicosis – or slow and present at rest (resting tremor), as in Parkinson's disease.

Chorea consists of rapid, irregular, unpredictable, 'fidgety'-like movements. It is usually most marked in the head, neck and distal limbs and often resembles attenuated fragments of purposeful movements. Chorea manifests in Huntington's disease and also as a long-term complication of the treatment of Parkinson's disease with L-DOPA, when it may coexist with dystonia (L-DOPA-induced dyskinesia).

Dystonia consists of relatively fixed abnormal postures and slow twisting movements that may occur in the face and mouth (orofacial dystonia), the neck (torticollis), the trunk or the limbs. In the latter case, it tends to be most marked proximally. Dystonia manifests in hereditary neurodegenerative disease (hereditary dystonia) and in L-DOPA-induced dystonia as a complication of the treatment of Parkinson's disease.

Tics are brief involuntary movements, which may be simple or complex and which remain stereotyped in the otherwise normal individual. They usually commence in childhood or adolescence and remain characteristic of the adult, emerging at times of stress and anxiety. In children with Tourette's syndrome, a repertoire of different complex tics develops serially over time in individuals who often display obsessional behaviours and sometimes utter involuntary obscenities (coprolalia).

Disorders of the basal ganglia

Basal ganglia disorders cause:

- Slow initiation and execution of movement (bradykinesia, akinesia).
- Increased muscular tone (rigidity).
- Abnormal involuntary movements (dyskinesia, tremor) and postures (dystonia).
- A unilateral lesion leads to signs and symptoms on the contralateral side.

Neuropsychological functions

The neuropsychological functions of language, perception, spatial analysis, learned skilled movements, memory and problem-solving (or executive functions) are organised within the cerebral hemispheres (Fig. 1.49). Accordingly, lesions of the spinal cord, brainstem or cerebellum are not accompanied by psychological deficits. The organisation of neuropsychological functions within the cerebral hemisphere is highly localised, as with the sensory and motor systems.

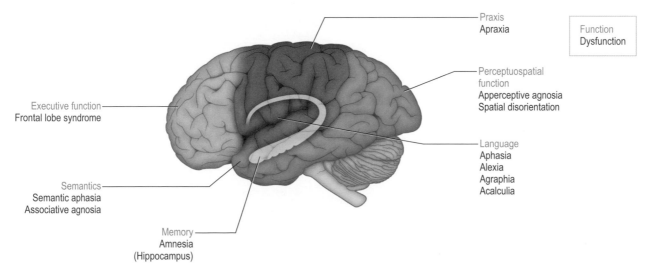

Fig. 1.49 Regional localisation of neuropsychological functions in the cerebral hemisphere and the syndromes associated with dysfunction.

Language functions (speech, reading, writing and calculation) are organised in the left hemisphere in regions of the frontal, parietal and temporal lobes adjacent to the lateral fissure, the so-called **language area**. Although primary visual processes are organised in the occipital lobes, the perception or **recognition of objects** and human faces is organised in projections to the temporal lobes. The ability to navigate the limbs and body in space (**visuospatial function**) is organised through projections to the parietal lobes. The premotor areas of the frontal lobes, including the supplementary motor area, which lies on the medial aspect of the hemisphere, govern the enactment of learned, skilled movements of the head, neck and limbs (**praxis**). Structures in the medial aspects of the temporal lobes, part of the limbic system, are responsible for **learning** new information and recollecting from experience (**memory**) whereas temporal neocortices are critical for understanding the meaning of words, objects and other sensory stimuli (semantic memory). The organisation of behaviour involving problem-solving and the achievement of goal-directed behaviour (**executive function**) is organised within the prefrontal areas of the frontal lobes.

It can be deduced from these neuropsychological and anatomical correlations that lesions of the language area will lead to loss of speech (**aphasia**), reading (**alexia**), writing (**agraphia**) and calculation (**acalculia**), whereas lesions of the temporoparietal cortex lead to loss of perception (**agnosia**) and spatial orientation (**visuospatial disorientation**). Loss of the knowledge of learned skilled movements (**apraxia**) follows lesions of the premotor cortex. Bilateral disorders of the medial temporal lobes and limbic system lead to loss of memory function (**amnesia**). Damage to the prefrontal cortex leads to marked behavioural disturbance with loss of forethought, planning and appropriate affect, manifest in a marked change of personality and behaviour (**frontal lobe** or **dysexecutive syndrome**).

Investigation of neuromuscular disease

The clinical definition of a particular syndrome permits the choice of appropriate investigations to confirm the diagnosis. The major focus of investigations involves:

- CSF analysis
- Neuroradiology
- Neurophysiology
- Neuropathology (biopsy)

Lumbar puncture enables the measurement of CSF pressure and the collection of CSF for bacteriological, biochemical, serological and cytological analyses. These may reveal the presence of blood (**subarachnoid haemorrhage**), infection, immune disease such as multiple sclerosis or the presence of tumour cells.

Neuroradiology encompasses a number of techniques that can be used to obtain both structural and functional images of the central nervous system and surrounding structures. Conventional **x-ray imaging** is applied to the skull and vertebral column, while structural images of the brain and spinal cord are obtained using **computed tomography** (**CT**; Fig. 1.50) and **magnetic resonance imaging** (**MRI**; Figs 1.22, 1.26, 1.28, 1.51). Functional images of regional cerebral blood flow, cerebral metabolism and the binding of ligands such as drugs to the brain can be obtained using **single photon emission computed tomography** (**SPECT**; Fig. 1.52) and **positron emission tomography** (**PET**; see Fig. 14.11). In contrast radiology an opaque medium is injected into the arteries or veins (**angiography**) to delineate the blood vessels (Fig. 1.53).

Neurophysiology enables the study of the electrical activity of the CNS by **electroencephalography** (**EEG**) and the detection and measurement of **evoked responses** to visual, auditory and

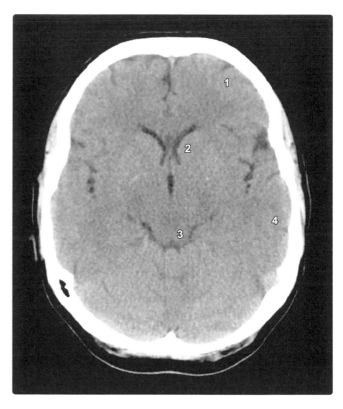

| 1 | Frontal lobe | 3 | Brainstem |
| 2 | Caudate nucleus | 4 | Temporal lobe |

Fig. 1.50 Axial computed tomography (CT) scan of the head. *(Courtesy of Professor P D Griffiths, Academic Unit of Radiology, University of Sheffield, Sheffield, UK.)*

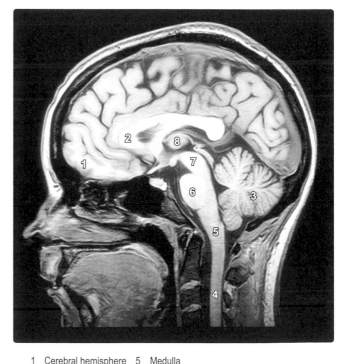

1	Cerebral hemisphere	5	Medulla
2	Corpus callosum	6	Pons
3	Cerebellum	7	Midbrain
4	Spinal cord	8	Thalamus

Fig. 1.51 Sagittal magnetic resonance image (MRI) of the head. *(Courtesy of Professor A Jackson, Wolfson Molecular Imaging Centre, University of Manchester, Manchester, UK.)*

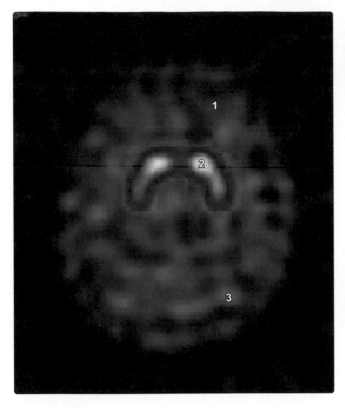

1   Frontal lobe
2   Striatum
3   Occipital lobe

Fig. 1.52 Axial single photon emission computed tomography (SPECT) scan of the head in a normal subject. The radiolabelled ligand 123I-FP-CIT has been used to label the dopamine transporter (DAT) in the striatum. *(Courtesy of Professor D J Brooks, Faculty of Medicine, Imperial College, London, UK.)*

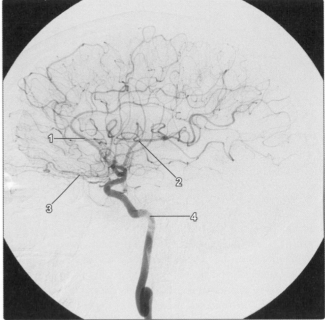

1   Anterior cerebral artery
2   Middle cerebral artery
3   Ophthalmic artery
4   Left internal carotid artery

Fig. 1.53 Lateral view of a carotid angiogram. This image was obtained by injecting an iodine-containing contrast agent selectively into the left internal carotid artery. This was done via a catheter that was introduced into the femoral artery and then guided into the aortic arch and carotid artery under fluoroscopic control. *(Courtesy of Professor P D Griffiths, Academic Unit of Radiology, University of Sheffield, Sheffield, UK.)*

somatosensory stimuli. **Central** (transcranial) **magnetic stimulation** of the brain enables measurement of the motor conduction time to the spinal cord and limb muscles. In the peripheral nervous system, measures of sensory and motor **nerve conduction velocity** and **evoked sensory action potentials** are combined with measurement of individual muscle responses to voluntary and electrically evoked contraction (**electromyography**).

The **biopsy** of nerve, muscle and brain tissue sheds light on the pathophysiological process (e.g. axonal degeneration, demyelination, muscular degeneration) and on the aetiology (e.g. inflammation, neoplasia).

2 | Cells of the nervous system

The functional unit of the nervous system is the nerve cell or neurone. These cells are highly specialised for the encoding, conduction and transmission of information. Neuroglial cells, or glia, are present in the nervous system in even larger numbers than neurones. Glia do not take part directly in information processing but are, nonetheless, crucial for normal neural function. Other cells are also present in the nervous system, such as those forming the walls of blood vessels but, unlike neurones and neuroglia, these are not unique to the nervous system.

The neurone

Neuronal structure

The main structural features common to all neurones have been described briefly in Chapter 1. There are, however, numerous variations on the basic plan. The size of the cell body (soma) varies considerably, depending upon its location and function. For example, some interneurones in the CNS have cell bodies as small as 5 μm in diameter, while the cell bodies of motor neurones innervating striated muscle may exceed 100 μm. The size of the cell body is usually correlated with the length of the axon. Therefore small interneurones usually have short axons, perhaps only a fraction of a millimetre in length. At the other extreme, large motor neurones possess long axons (e.g. those passing from the spinal cord to the muscles of the foot have axons about 1 m in length).

The **dendritic arborisation** of neurones also shows great variation in the number, size and density of branches, which reflects the complexity of afferent inputs to the cell. For example, pyramidal cells in the cerebral cortex have one or two apical dendrites which course towards the pial surface (Fig. 2.1A), while Purkinje cells in the cerebellar cortex have highly complex, tree-like dendritic arborisations (Fig. 2.1B).

The configuration of the cell body in relation to the dendrites and axon follows one of three basic patterns (Fig. 2.2). **Multipolar** neurones are by far the most common. Typically, they possess an axon and a number of dendrites that arise directly from the cell body. Motor neurones are a good example. **Bipolar** neurones have a centrally placed cell body, from which extend a single dendrite and a single axon. Bipolar neurones occur in the afferent pathways of the visual, auditory and vestibular systems. **Unipolar** neurones possess a single process emerging from the cell body. This divides into dendritic and axonal branches. Neurones of this type constitute the primary afferents of spinal and some cranial nerves, having their cell bodies in the dorsal root ganglia and sensory ganglia of cranial nerves.

Like most other cells, neurones possess a nucleus. This is usually located in the centre of the cell body and contains the chromosomal DNA. The rest of the intracellular space is occupied by cytoplasm, which contains numerous organelles and inclusions (Fig. 2.3). Many of these are common to cells other than neurones, but some have particular prominence or significance in

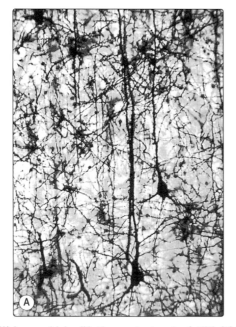
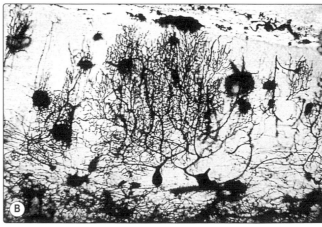

Fig. 2.1 (A) A pyramidal cell in the cerebral cortex (×100). (B) A Purkinje cell in the cerebellar cortex (×90) showing the diversity of dendritic arborisations. (Golgi–Cox stain.)

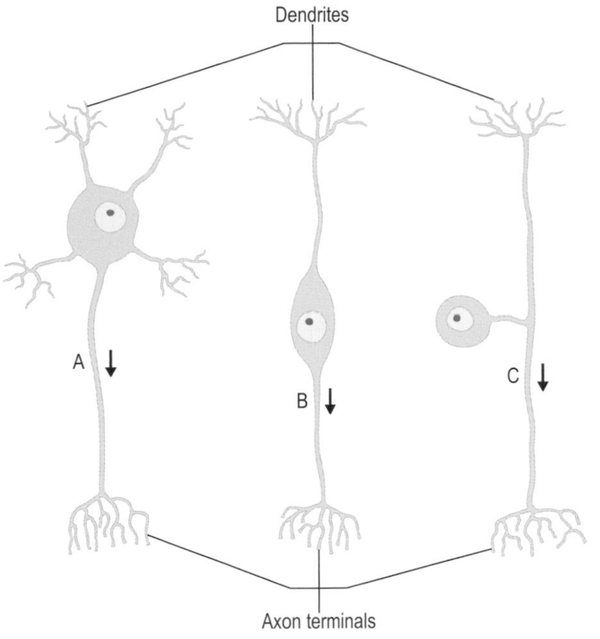

Dendrites

A Multipolar
B Bipolar
C Unipolar

Fig. 2.2 Unipolar, bipolar and multipolar neurones. Arrows indicate the direction of impulse conduction.

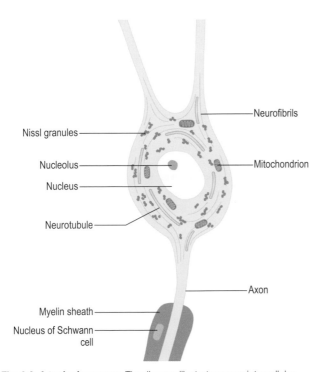

Axon terminals

Fig. 2.3 A typical neurone. The diagram illustrates some intracellular organelles. See also Fig. 1.3.

Dendrites   Nissl granules

Nucleolus

Nucleus

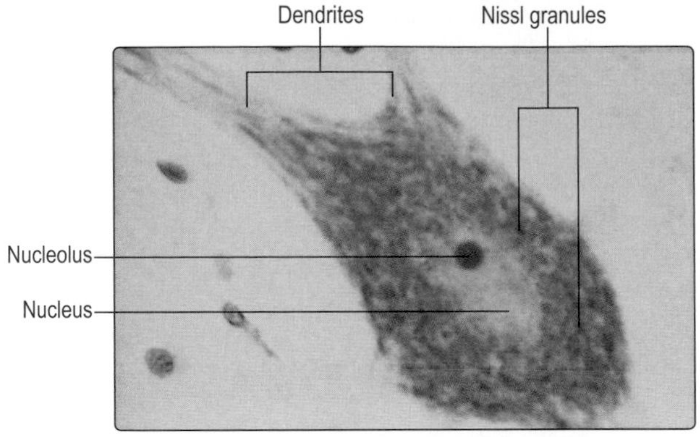

Fig. 2.4 A spinal motor neurone cell body. Cresyl violet (a basophilic dye) stain shows prominent Nissl granules (×600).

neurofibrils (Fig. 2.3). They also possess a system of **neurotubules** that are involved in the transport of materials throughout the cell. Transport of materials occurs both away from and towards the cell body (**anterograde** and **retrograde transport**, respectively). This phenomenon is exploited in experimental neuroanatomical tracing techniques used to elucidate neuronal connectivity.

Some neurones contain pigment granules. **Neuromelanin** is a brown-black pigment produced as a by-product of the synthesis of catecholamines. Neuromelanin thus occurs most abundantly in cell groups that utilise catecholamines as their neurotransmitter, notably the pars compacta of the substantia nigra in the midbrain and the locus coeruleus in the pons. **Lipofuscin** is a yellow-brown pigment that accumulates in some neurones with age.

Each nerve cell is a separate physical entity with a limiting cell membrane. In order for information processing to occur in networks of neurones, therefore, information has to pass between neurones. This occurs at synapses. The basic structure of the synapse has been outlined in Chapter 1. The most common location for synapse formation is between the terminal axonal arborisation of one neurone and the dendrite of another (**axodendritic** synapse). Other locations are also possible and they give **axosomatic**, **axoaxonal** and **dendrodendritic** synapses. Neurotransmission between neurones occurs by release of specific chemical agents from the presynaptic ending that act upon receptors in the postsynaptic membrane.

Neurotransmitters

Neurotransmitter (transmitter) chemicals are stored in vesicles within the presynaptic ending. A single neurone is thought to release the same transmitter at all its synapses, and all neurones of a particular type, in terms of origin, termination and function, utilise the same transmitter. Numerous transmitter substances have been identified at various sites in the nervous system. It has long been known that, in the periphery, **acetylcholine** (ACh) is the transmitter between motor neurones and striated muscle. It is also an important transmitter in the autonomic nervous system (Chapter 4), being released by preganglionic neurones of both the sympathetic and parasympathetic divisions, and by postganglionic parasympathetic neurones. Furthermore, ACh is a transmitter at numerous, widespread sites within the CNS. Synapses that use ACh as their transmitter are called cholinergic. Some simple amino acids act as neurotransmitters. The most important are **glutamic acid (glutamate)** and **gamma-aminobutyric acid (GABA)**, which occur widely (forming glutamatergic and GABAergic synapses) and are the principal excitatory and inhibitory transmitters, respectively, in the CNS. Glycine is an inhibitory transmitter in the spinal cord. Several monoamines are

neurones. Numerous microscopic clumps of **Nissl granules** (Nissl bodies, Nissl substance) can usually be seen in nerve cell bodies stained with basophilic dyes. Nissl granules consist of rough endoplasmic reticulum and associated ribosomes. The ribosomes contain RNA (which accounts for the basophilic staining properties) and are the sites of protein synthesis. Nerve cells are highly metabolically active and, therefore, the Nissl granules are often very prominent (Fig. 2.4).

Neurones contain a complex meshwork of structural protein strands called **neurofilaments**, which are assembled into larger important transmitters. **Noradrenaline (norepinephrine)** is released by postganglionic sympathetic neurones peripherally as well as at some sites within the CNS. **Dopamine** and **serotonin** (**5-hydroxytryptamine, 5-HT**) also act as transmitters in the brain and spinal cord. Most neurones that utilise monoamines as their neurotransmitter have their cell bodies located in nuclei within the brainstem, e.g. the locus coeruleus (noradrenaline), the substantia nigra (dopamine) and the raphé nuclei (5-HT).

Some small molecule transmitter substances, particularly the amino acids and ACh, are often referred to as fast transmitters because they bring about rapid changes in postsynaptic membrane permeability to certain ions (notably Na^+, K^+, Ca^{2+} and Cl^-), resulting in changes to the postsynaptic membrane potential. Other transmitters have a slower action because they act through the intermediary of a so-called second messenger, such as cyclic adenosine monophosphate (cAMP). Dopamine falls into this category.

A number of peptides (neuropeptides) are stored and released at synapses. These include **enkephalin**, **substance P**, **cholecystokinin**, **somatostatin**, **dynorphin** and others. These peptides are often found co-localised in the same neurones as ACh, amino acid or monoamine neurotransmitters and are sometimes called co-transmitters. In many instances, their precise functions are poorly understood. It is believed that some neuropeptides modulate the release, re-uptake and postsynaptic effects of other transmitters and they are, therefore, often referred to as **neuromodulators**.

In order for there to be efficient transmission of information between neurones, the effect of a neurotransmitter must be terminated once it has acted upon the postsynaptic membrane. This is achieved either by enzymic destruction of the transmitter or by its active re-uptake into nerve endings and glia. For example, at the neuromuscular junction (see Fig. 3.6) and at cholinergic synapses, the action of ACh is terminated through hydrolysis by the enzyme **acetylcholinesterase (AChE)**. In contrast, monoamine- and amino acid–mediated transmission is usually terminated by a re-uptake mechanism, although degrading enzymes also exist. Neuropeptides are degraded by peptidases.

The neurone

- The neurone is the principal functional unit of the nervous system, specialised for the receipt, processing and transmission of information.

- Great variability exists in the size and shape of nerve cell bodies, their dendritic arborisations and axons, which reflects their functional specialisation.

- Nerve cells contain a number of organelles and inclusions. Among these are Nissl granules, neurofilaments and neurotubules, and pigment granules.

- A large number of neurotransmitter substances are known that mediate transmission between neurones. These include primarily acetylcholine, various amino acids (GABA, glutamate) and monoamines (dopamine, noradrenaline (norepinephrine) and serotonin).

- Peptide neuromodulators are co-localised with other transmitters in many neurones.

Neuroglia

Neuroglia are the predominant cell types within the nervous system but they are not directly involved in information processing. They are, however, crucial for normal functioning of the nervous system, providing an appropriate structural matrix and chemical environment for neurones. Various types of neuroglial cell are recognised: principally astrocytes, oligodendrocytes (oligodendroglia) and microglia.

Astrocytes

Astrocytes (literally, 'star-shaped' cells) possess numerous processes. Some of these form so-called 'perivascular end-feet' upon the walls of blood capillaries (Fig. 2.5). In this way, they line the capillaries of the brain and are involved in controlling the exchange of chemicals between the circulatory system and nervous tissue. Thus they are a physical constituent of the so-called **blood–brain barrier**, which selectively restricts the access of circulating chemicals to the CNS. The blood–brain barrier is an important phenomenon, since it can prevent both some harmful substances and some potentially therapeutic drugs from entering the CNS.

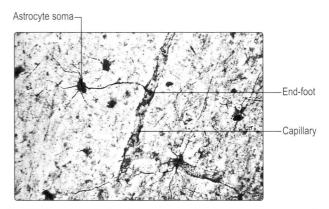

Astrocyte soma — End-foot — Capillary

Fig. 2.5 An astrocyte showing a process forming a perivascular end-foot on a blood capillary. Cajal's gold chloride stain (×180).

Oligodendrocytes

Oligodendrocytes (literally, 'cells with few processes') have, as their main role, the production of the myelin sheath that surrounds many axons in the CNS. **Schwann cells** perform this function in the peripheral nervous system. At any point along the length of a myelinated axon, the myelin sheath is comprised of numerous concentric layers of the cell membrane of a single oligodendrocyte or Schwann cell (Fig. 2.6A). Each glial cell produces the myelin sheath over only a short segment of axon (up to about 1 mm). A long axon is, therefore, enveloped by the membranes of many glial cells. Adjacent segments of myelin, derived from different glial cells, are separated by a small gap, called the **node of Ranvier** (see Fig. 1.3). Unmyelinated axons also have a close physical association with glial cells, but several axons usually share a single glial cell (Fig. 2.6B).

In myelinated axons, ionic fluxes across the axonal membrane, which mediate generation of the action potential, occur only at the nodes of Ranvier where the axon is exposed to the extracellular space. Between nodes, where the axon is insulated by myelin, depolarisation spreads by passive means (electrotonus). This mode of propagation of action potentials in myelinated axons is known as **saltatory conduction** (Latin: *saltare*, to jump), since the action potential may be thought of as 'jumping' from node to node. It is considerably faster than conduction in unmyelinated axons.

Microglia

Microglia are small cells with few processes. They are quiescent in health but, in response to damage to the CNS, they proliferate and migrate to the site of injury. There, they have a phagocytic

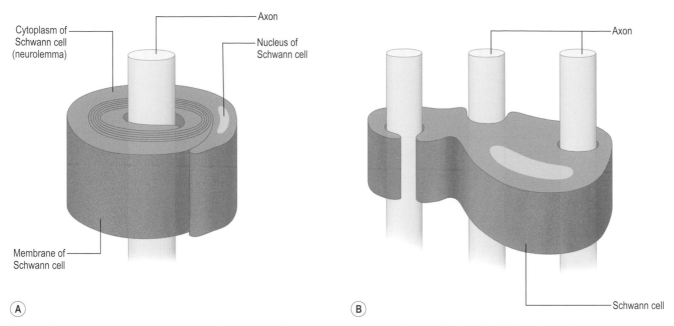

Cytoplasm of
Schwann cell
(neurolemma)

Axon

Nucleus of
Schwann cell

Membrane of
Schwann cell

(A)

Axon

(B)

Schwann cell

Fig. 2.6 (A) Transverse section through a myelinated axon, illustrating the structure of the myelin sheath. (B) Unmyelinated axons.

role, similar to macrophages elsewhere, removing tissue debris.

Ependyma

The **ependyma** (ependymal cells) are epithelial cells that line the ventricles and cover the choroid plexus. They are sometimes considered to be a fourth type of glial cell. Their ventricular surface is ciliated and this is said to aid the circulation of CSF.

Neuroglia

- Neuroglia are important for normal neural function because of their ancillary, or supporting, roles.

- Astrocytes possess long processes that form perivascular end-feet around blood capillaries. They are involved in the transfer of materials between the vascular system and neural tissue.

- Oligodendroglia give rise to the myelin sheath surrounding axons in the CNS. Schwann cells form myelin in the peripheral nervous system.

- Microglia have a phagocytic role in injury to the nervous system.

Neuronal and glial disorders

Once development has been completed, individual neurones no longer replicate, but they do undergo continual repair to maintain their integrity. Hence, they are prone to **neurodegenerative diseases**, which in childhood and youth are often genetically determined and in the elderly are sporadic. Glia, unlike neurones, are capable of replication and they are, therefore, susceptible to neoplasia. Consequently, most brain tumours are gliomas and not tumours of neurones themselves. According to the cell of origin, they may become either **oligodendrogliomas** or **astrocytomas**. Microglia form part of the immune system and may proliferate to become cerebral **lymphomas**.

Multiple sclerosis

The myelin sheath of neuronal axons can be the seat of inflammatory diseases. In Europe and North America, the most common immune disorder of the CNS is multiple sclerosis, which leads to episodes of **demyelination** and **remyelination** of axons, corresponding to relapses and remission of neurological signs and symptoms. Since the disorder is chiefly of axons, not cell bodies, magnetic resonance (MR) brain imaging can detect abnormal signals from demyelinating foci in the cerebral white matter.

3 | Peripheral nervous system

The peripheral nervous system consists of sensory and motor nerve endings, peripheral nerve trunks, plexuses and ganglia, which link the CNS with other parts of the body. Most of the neurones in the peripheral nervous system are, therefore, either afferent or efferent with respect to the CNS.

- Nerve endings include sensory receptors, that detect changes in the internal and external environments, and efferent endings, which control the contraction of muscles and the activity of secretory glands.
- Peripheral nerves consist of spinal and cranial nerves and their branches, and the numerous named nerves to which these give rise.
- Plexuses (e.g. the brachial plexus and lumbosacral plexus) are structures in which the nerve fibres within certain spinal and cranial nerves are redistributed, without synapse, to form other peripheral nerves.
- Peripheral ganglia (e.g. dorsal root ganglia and autonomic ganglia) are structures outside the CNS, where some nerve cell bodies are located.

Muscle

All behaviour depends upon the ability to control the activity of skeletal muscles, which maintain posture and permit movement. Such control is subserved by a rich innervation of muscle with both motor and sensory neurones. Individual muscle cells (fibres) run parallel to the main axis of the muscle and fall into two main functional groups: namely **extrafusal** and **intrafusal** muscle fibres (Fig. 3.1).

Extrafusal muscle fibres are by far the more numerous, constituting the bulk of the muscle and conferring its contractile strength. Extrafusal muscle fibres are innervated by **alpha motor neurones**, the cell bodies of which lie in the ventral horn of the spinal cord grey matter and in the motor cranial nerve nuclei of the brainstem. The axon of an individual alpha motor neurone typically branches within the target muscle to innervate a number of muscle fibres and these fibres contract simultaneously when activated by the motor neurone. The combination of a single motor neurone and the muscle fibres that it innervates is known as a **motor unit**. In those muscles capable of controlling delicate, precise movements, such as the muscles of the hand, the muscles of facial expression and the extraocular muscles, individual motor units are comprised of relatively small numbers of muscle fibres. In contrast, the motor units of large postural muscles such as the quadriceps, for example, are comprised of relatively large numbers of muscle fibres.

Intrafusal muscle fibres are specialised muscle cells that act as sensory receptors. They occur in groups known as **muscle spindles**, interspersed amongst the extrafusal fibres (Fig. 3.1). Intrafusal muscle fibres bear sensory endings that signal muscle stretch and tension to the CNS. Their function is fundamental to the monosynaptic stretch reflex and the control of muscle tone (pp. 75–76), to the coordination of movement by the cerebellum (p. 121) and to the conscious perception and control of movement of the body in space (praxis). Intrafusal muscle fibres receive a motor innervation from **gamma motor neurones**, whose cells of origin, like those of alpha motor neurones, lie in the ventral horn of the spinal cord and the motor cranial nerve nuclei

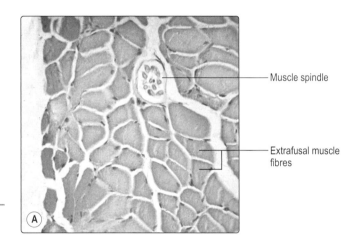

Muscle spindle

Extrafusal muscle fibres

A

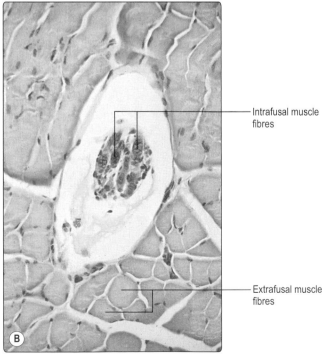

Intrafusal muscle fibres

Extrafusal muscle fibres

B

Fig. 3.1 (A,B) Transverse sections through striated muscles showing extrafusal muscle fibres and intrafusal muscle fibres (within muscle spindles).

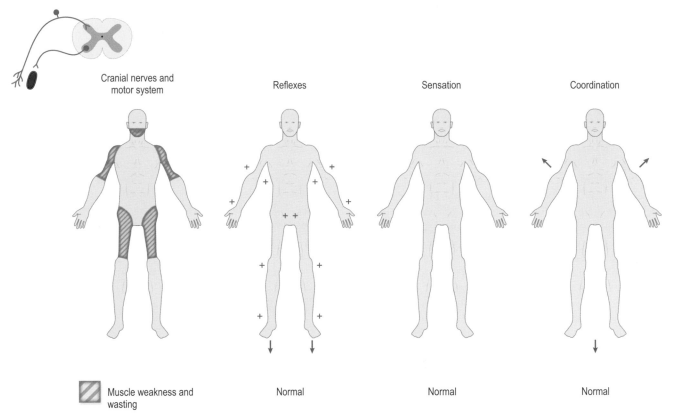

Fig. 3.2 **Myopathy.** Refer also to Fig. 1.48.

of the brainstem. Gamma motor neurones function to control the sensitivity of the sensory endings on intrafusal muscle fibres. Various disorders of the CNS can affect gamma motor neurone activity and, thus, cause abnormalities of the stretch reflex and muscle tone (pp. 75–76).

Myopathies

- **Myopathy** is characterised by weakness and muscle wasting (of facial, bulbar and proximal limb muscles) with preservation of tendon reflexes and sensation (Fig. 3.2).
- **Polymyositis** is an immune disorder of muscle causing a painful or painless myopathy. When it occurs in the elderly, there is often a primary neoplasm elsewhere (paraneoplastic syndrome). In children, the skin is also inflamed, causing a rash. This is referred to as dermatomyositis.
- **Duchenne muscular dystrophy** is an inherited degenerative disorder of male children (X-linked inheritance). After 2 to 3 years of age, the child develops progressive weakness of the arms and legs with muscular contractures, is wheelchair-bound by the age of 10 years and dies in youth.

Nerve endings

There are various overlapping conventions for the classification of nerve endings. Overall, they may be classified as either afferent or efferent. Afferent nerve endings respond to mechanical, thermal or chemical stimulation (mechanoreceptors, thermoreceptors or chemoreceptors, respectively). The nerve fibres to which they belong conduct action potentials to the CNS. If the afferent information reaches a conscious level, then the pathway is termed sensory. Efferent nerve endings innervate muscle or secretory cells and, under control from the CNS, influence muscular contraction or cellular secretion. Nerve endings that induce movement are called motor; those that induce secretion are sometimes called secretomotor.

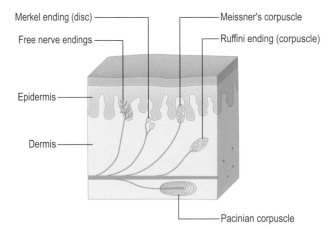

Fig. 3.3 **Sensory nerve endings in skin.**

Afferent nerve endings

The sensory systems, or modalities, are broadly divided into the general and the special senses. The special senses are olfaction, vision, hearing, balance and taste and these are considered elsewhere (see Chapters 10, 15 and 16).

Regarding general sensory endings, there are three functional types:

- **Exteroceptors.** These occur superficially in the skin and respond to nociceptive (painful) stimuli, temperature, touch and pressure.
- **Interoceptors.** These occur in viscera and respond principally to mechanical and chemical stimuli.
- **Proprioceptors.** These occur in muscles, joints and tendons and provide awareness of posture and movement (kinaesthesia).

Structurally, sensory nerve endings may be either unencapsulated or encapsulated (Fig. 3.3). Unencapsulated endings, or **free nerve endings**, consist of the terminal branches of sensory nerve fibres lying freely in the innervated tissue. These are the most abundant type of sensory ending, occurring widely in the integument and also within muscles, joints, viscera and other structures. In the skin, they mediate thermal and painful sensations. The parent nerve fibres are designated physiologically as group Aδ (III) finely myelinated and group C unmyelinated fibres. These are of relatively small diameter and slow conducting. **Merkel endings** (discs) are located near the border of the epidermis. These are slowly adapting receptors that respond to touch/pressure. The axons of origin are large and myelinated.

Encapsulated nerve endings are surrounded by a structural specialisation of non-neural tissue, the combination of nerve and its encapsulation often being referred to as a corpuscle. **Meissner's corpuscles** occur in the dermal papillae of the skin and are especially numerous in the fingertips. They respond with great sensitivity to touch. They are rapidly adapting receptors and are responsible for fine, or discriminative, touch. **Pacinian corpuscles** occur in skin and in deep tissues, e.g. surrounding joints and in mesentery. The largest are a few millimetres long and they are associated with group Aα (I) large diameter, myelinated axons. Pacinian corpuscles are rapidly adapting and respond to mechanical distortion, especially vibration. **Ruffini endings** (corpuscles) are slowly adapting mechanoreceptors occurring in the dermis of the skin.

Within skeletal muscles, intrafusal muscle fibres, which in small groups constitute muscle spindles, act as stretch receptors (Fig. 3.4). There are two types of intrafusal muscle fibre, referred to as **nuclear bag** and **nuclear chain** fibres. Intrafusal muscle fibres bear two types of sensory ending, which become activated when the muscle in which they lie is stretched. **Annulospiral** endings (Fig. 3.5) are associated with fast conducting group Ia afferent fibres and **flower-spray** endings are associated with slower conducting group II afferents. Muscle spindles are particularly abundant in muscles capable of fine, skilled movements. They are important in kinaesthesia and in the control of muscle tone, posture and movement. Their functional importance in motor control is considered in more detail in Chapter 8.

Golgi tendon organs occur in tendons and respond to relatively high levels of tension. They are associated with group Ib afferent fibres.

Efferent nerve endings

Efferent endings occur in association with muscle and secretory cells. The endings resemble the synapses that occur between neurones. Transmission is by chemical means, depolarisation of the endings causing release of a neurotransmitter that acts upon receptors in the target cell membrane. In striated muscle, both alpha motor neurones (innervating extrafusal muscle fibres) and gamma motor neurones (innervating intrafusal muscle fibres) end upon muscle cells in synaptic specialisations called **neuromuscular junctions** or **motor end-plates** (Figs 3.6, 3.7). The neurotransmitter at all neuromuscular junctions in striated muscle is acetylcholine.

Nerve endings

- The peripheral nervous system consists of nerve endings, peripheral nerves, plexuses and ganglia.

- Nerve endings are broadly classified as afferent (sensory) or efferent (motor).

- Sensory endings function as mechanoreceptors, thermoreceptors or chemoreceptors.

- In terms of location, they can be subdivided into exteroceptors, interoceptors and proprioceptors.

- Structurally, they may consist of unencapsulated (free) nerve endings, or encapsulated endings (such as Meissner's and Pacinian corpuscles).

- Skeletal muscles contain muscle spindles, which are composed of intrafusal muscle fibres. These consist of nuclear bag and nuclear chain types. They possess annulospiral and flower-spray sensory endings.

- Efferent nerve endings are either motor end-plates in muscle or endings in association with secretory cells (secretomotor).

- Alpha motor neurones innervate extrafusal muscle fibres and gamma motor neurones innervate intrafusal muscle fibres.

Nuclear bag muscle fibre

Nuclear chain muscle fibre

Muscle spindle

Flower-spray sensory nerve ending

Group Ia afferent fibre

Gamma motor neurones

Group II afferent fibre

Motor end-plate

Annulospiral sensory nerve ending

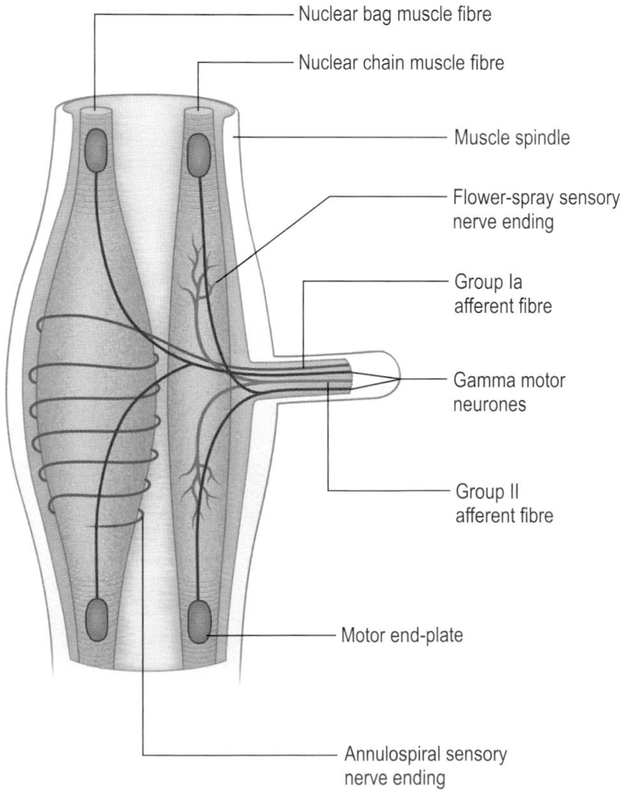

Fig. 3.4 Innervation of intrafusal muscle fibres. For clarity, only an annulospiral ending is shown on the nuclear bag fibre and only a flower-spray ending on the nuclear chain fibre although, in reality, both types of ending are found on both types of intrafusal fibre.

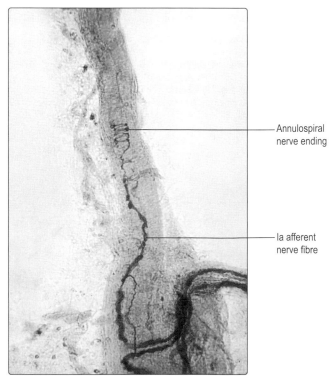

Annulospiral nerve ending

Ia afferent nerve fibre

Fig. 3.5 An annulospiral nerve ending on an intrafusal muscle fibre.

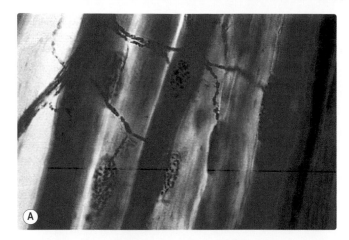

Myasthenia gravis is an immune disorder; it is the most common disorder of the peripheral neuromuscular junction. It causes weakness and fatigue of cranial muscles (e.g. extraocular, facial and bulbar muscles) and limb (especially proximal) muscles. This occurs without muscular wasting, changes in reflexes or sensation (Fig. 3.8). Treatment with drugs that inhibit acetylcholine esterase (anticholinesterases) potentiates neuromuscular transmission, with relief of symptoms. The **Lambert–Eaton syndrome** causes similar fatigue and is an immune and paraneoplastic syndrome. It does not respond to anticholinesterases.

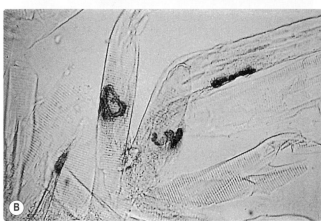

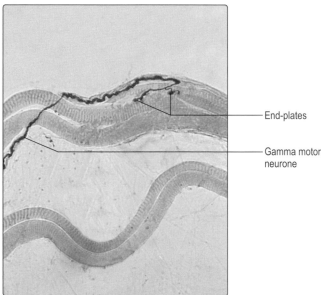

Fig. 3.6 Motor end-plates on extrafusal muscle fibres in striated muscle. (A) Ranvier's gold chloride stain showing efferent nerve fibres terminating in neuromuscular junctions (×600). (B) Acetylcholinesterase stain. The neurotransmitter at the neuromuscular junction is acetylcholine. The action of the transmitter is terminated by the enzyme acetylcholinesterase. The brown stain shows the specific localisation of the enzyme at the neuromuscular junction (×500).

Fig. 3.7 A gamma motor neurone ending in motor end-plates on intrafusal muscle fibres.

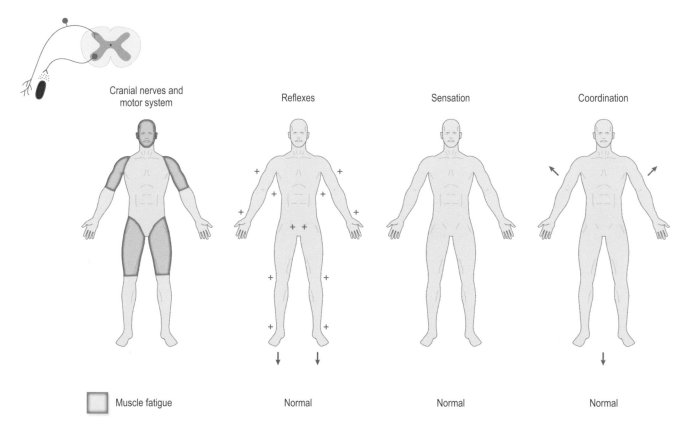

Fig. 3.8 Neuromuscular junction syndrome. Refer also to Fig. 1.48.

Peripheral nerves

The term 'peripheral nerve' applies to all the nerve trunks and branches that lie outside the CNS. They are the principal route through which the brain and spinal cord communicate with the rest of the body. A typical peripheral nerve consists of numerous nerve fibres, which may be either afferent or efferent with respect to the CNS.

Some peripheral nerve fibres are myelinated and others are unmyelinated. Within peripheral nerves, the nerve fibres are arranged in bundles and surrounded by sheaths of connective tissue (Fig. 3.9). Between individual fibres is a delicate connective tissue known as **endoneurium**. Bundles of fibres are surrounded by **perineurium** and the whole nerve is ensheathed by a tough coat known as **epineurium**. This configuration provides strength and support for the nerve. The cranial and spinal meninges are continuous with the connective tissue sheaths of spinal and cranial nerves. Thus, the dura mater is continuous with the epineurium, while the arachnoid and pia are continuous with the perineurium and endoneurium.

Degeneration and regeneration

When a peripheral nerve fibre is transected or otherwise seriously damaged, the portion distal to the transection (furthest from the cell body) undergoes degeneration and dies. This is known as **anterograde** or **Wallerian degeneration**. The proximal portion of the neurone, which remains attached to the cell body, may, however, survive and eventually undergo recovery or **regeneration**. The further from the cell body that transection occurs, the more likely it is that the cell body will survive. Initially, it too usually shows degenerative changes, known as **retrograde degeneration**. This is characterised by dispersal and loss of staining of Nissl granules (chromatolysis), swelling of the cell body and movement of the normally central nucleus to a peripheral location. If the cell recovers, the distal end of the surviving nerve fibre undergoes sprouting. If the two ends of the peripheral nerve are physically aligned (e.g. by surgery following traumatic injury), the new regenerating fibres may enter the endoneurial tubes that have lost their nerve fibres. Continued growth of the new fibres, at a rate of 1 to 2 mm/day, may eventually lead to re-innervation of the original structure and recovery of function. Many factors influence the degree to which successful re-innervation and functional recovery take place.

The degenerative processes that follow nerve cell injury are essentially similar in the CNS. Sprouting of surviving neurones also occurs in the CNS, but the re-establishment of previous connections does not, unfortunately, take place to any significant extent.

🔎 Peripheral sensorimotor neuropathies

Peripheral sensorimotor neuropathies are characterised by muscular weakness and wasting (especially of distal muscles), distal areflexia and a 'glove and stocking' distribution of sensory loss (Fig. 3.10). Peripheral neuropathies may be caused by systemic disease, vascular disease, heredo-degenerative disorders, infection, immune disorders and paraneoplastic syndromes.

In general, there are two pathological types. **Demyelinating neuropathies** predominantly damage Schwann cells and myelin sheaths. **Axonal neuropathies** primarily cause axonal degeneration. Recovery from neuropathy requires remyelination and regeneration of axons.

Distribution of spinal and peripheral nerves

At the roots of the upper and lower limbs are located the brachial plexus (Figs 3.11, 3.12) and the lumbosacral plexus (Fig. 3.13), respectively. Here, the nerve fibres present in spinal nerves become redistributed to form named peripheral nerves, which then run distally to their targets. Because of the redistribution of nerve fibres within the plexuses, the territories supplied by peripheral nerves are different from those of spinal nerves.

Each spinal nerve carries the sensory innervation for a particular part of the body surface. The area of skin that is supplied by a particular spinal nerve is known as a **dermatome**. Dermatome maps are given in Fig. 3.14. These are only approximate since, in reality, the cutaneous territories of adjacent spinal nerves overlap

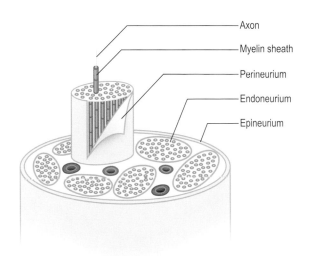

Fig. 3.9 The structure of a peripheral nerve.

Axon
Myelin sheath
Perineurium
Endoneurium
Epineurium

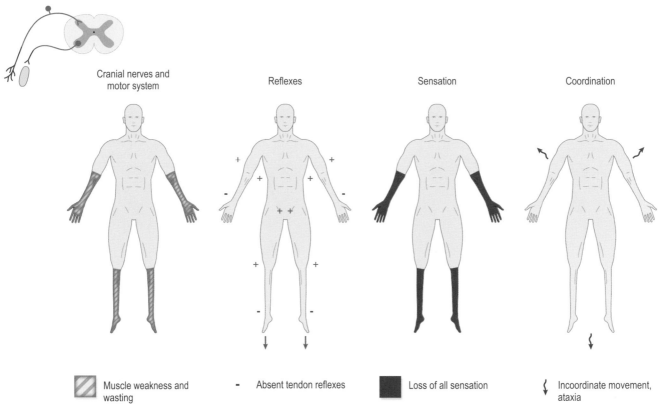

Fig. 3.10 **Peripheral sensorimotor neuropathy.** Refer also to Fig. 1.48.

Muscle weakness and wasting	− Absent tendon reflexes
Loss of all sensation	⟨ Incoordinate movement, ataxia

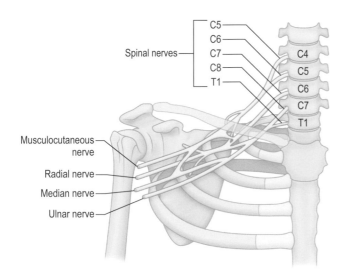

Fig. 3.11 **The right brachial plexus.**

considerably. There is, however, little overlap where adjacent areas of skin are served by non-contiguous spinal nerves, such boundaries being referred to as **axial lines**. The cutaneous distribution of important peripheral nerves is also illustrated in Fig. 3.14.

The group of skeletal muscles innervated by a particular spinal nerve is collectively known as a **myotome**. These muscles are usually functionally related and are responsible for particular patterns of movement. The segmental spinal nerve values of some important movements are shown in Fig. 3.15.

Brachial plexus lesions

In motorcycle accidents, trauma to the shoulder and neck may cause **avulsion of the brachial plexus** (Fig. 3.12), causing immediate weakness and loss of feeling in one upper limb. Later, the arm wastes and becomes painful.

A tumour of the apex of the lung may infiltrate the lower part of the brachial plexus, producing severe pain in the arm, weakness and wasting of the hand and sensory loss on the inner aspect of the forearm and hand (**Pancoast's syndrome**).

An acute immune inflammation of the brachial plexus (brachial plexus neuropathy) causes severe pain, weakness and sensory loss in one arm, which usually recovers after a year.

Lumbosacral plexus lesions

Malignant disease and surgical procedures for cancer can damage the lumbosacral plexus in its course through the pelvis, causing pain, weakness and wasting of the muscles and numbness of the leg(s), with bladder and bowel incontinence.

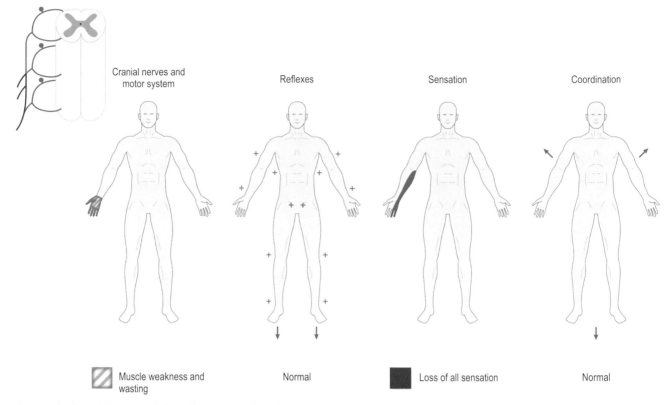

Cranial nerves and motor system	Reflexes	Sensation	Coordination

Muscle weakness and wasting — Normal — Loss of all sensation — Normal

Fig. 3.12 Lesion of the brachial plexus (lower cord; C8–T1). Refer also to Fig. 1.48.

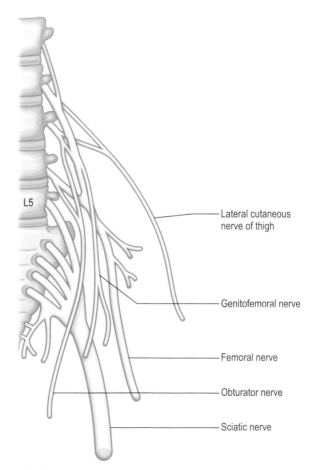

L5

Lateral cutaneous nerve of thigh

Genitofemoral nerve

Femoral nerve

Obturator nerve

Sciatic nerve

Fig. 3.13 The left lumbosacral plexus.

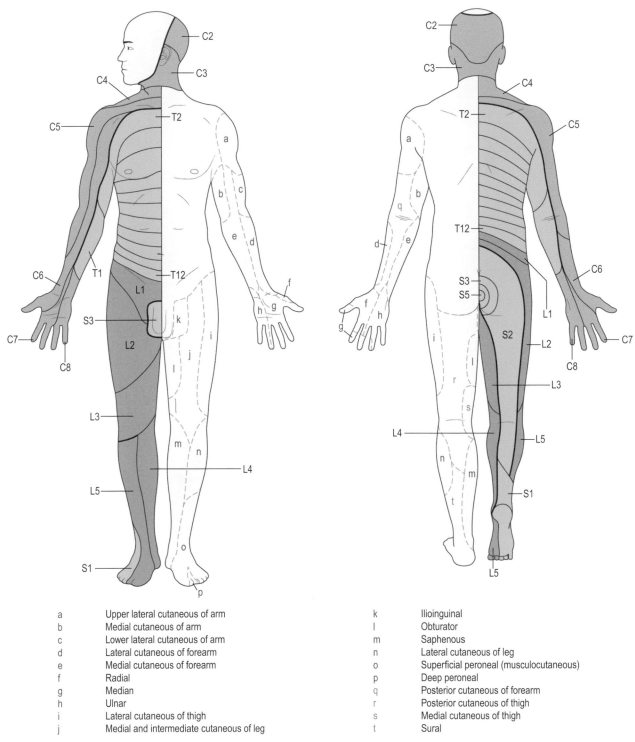

a	Upper lateral cutaneous of arm	k	Ilioinguinal
b	Medial cutaneous of arm	l	Obturator
c	Lower lateral cutaneous of arm	m	Saphenous
d	Lateral cutaneous of forearm	n	Lateral cutaneous of leg
e	Medial cutaneous of forearm	o	Superficial peroneal (musculocutaneous)
f	Radial	p	Deep peroneal
g	Median	q	Posterior cutaneous of forearm
h	Ulnar	r	Posterior cutaneous of thigh
i	Lateral cutaneous of thigh	s	Medial cutaneous of thigh
j	Medial and intermediate cutaneous of leg	t	Sural

Fig. 3.14 The cutaneous distribution of spinal nerves (dermatomes) and named peripheral nerves. Axial lines are in bold.

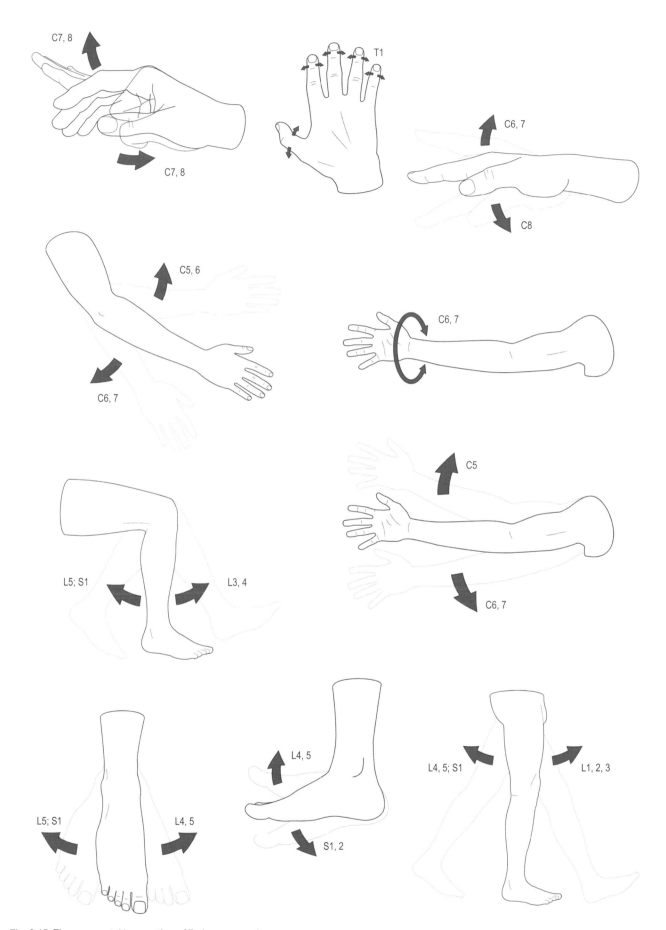

Fig. 3.15 The segmental innervation of limb movements.

Ulnar nerve	
Sensory	Motor
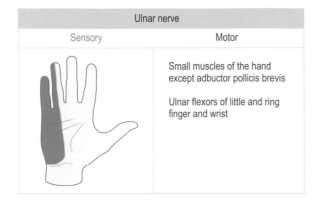	Small muscles of the hand except adbuctor pollicis brevis Ulnar flexors of little and ring finger and wrist

Lateral cutaneous nerve of the thigh	
Sensory	Motor
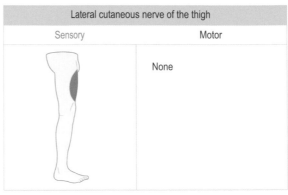	None

Median nerve	
Sensory	Motor
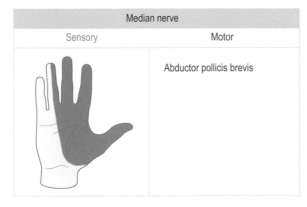	Abductor pollicis brevis

Common peroneal nerve	
Sensory	Motor
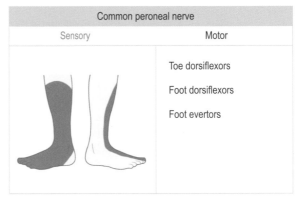	Toe dorsiflexors Foot dorsiflexors Foot evertors

Radial nerve	
Sensory	Motor
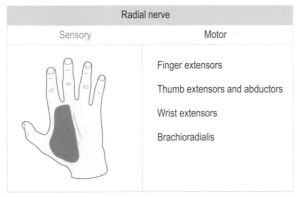	Finger extensors Thumb extensors and abductors Wrist extensors Brachioradialis

Fig. 3.16 **Sensory and motor deficits associated with peripheral nerve lesions.**

Peripheral nerves

- Nerve fibres in some spinal nerves become rearranged as they course peripherally, passing through the brachial or lumbosacral plexuses, to emerge as named peripheral nerves.

- Peripheral nerves consist of variable numbers of bundles, or fascicles, of nerve fibres.

- The nerve fibres are ensheathed in three connective tissue coverings: endoneurium, perineurium and epineurium.

- The endoneurial tubes within which individual axons lie are important for successful regeneration and re-innervation following nerve injury.

- The area of skin supplied by a spinal nerve is called a dermatome.

- The group of muscles innervated by a spinal nerve is called a myotome.

Compression and entrapment neuropathies

Peripheral nerves are vulnerable to acute extrinsic compression (e.g. excessive pressure on a recumbent limb) and to chronic entrapment by normal or diseased anatomical structures adjacent to them. The most common examples are acute **radial nerve** compression in the spiral groove of the humerus and chronic entrapment of the **ulnar nerve** at the elbow and of the **median nerve** at the wrist (carpal tunnel syndrome) in the upper limb. Chronic entrapment of the **lateral cutaneous nerve of the thigh** and acute compression of the **common peroneal nerve** at the head of the fibula occur in the lower limb (Fig. 3.16).

The term 'autonomic nervous system' is used to describe those nerve cells, located within either the central or peripheral nervous systems, that are concerned with the innervation and control of visceral organs, smooth muscle and secretory glands. The principal function of the autonomic nervous system can broadly be described as the maintenance of the internal environment, or **homeostasis**. This is achieved by regulation of cardiovascular, respiratory, digestive, excretory and thermoregulatory mechanisms, which occurs automatically and with relatively little volitional control.

Autonomic afferent and efferent nerve fibres enter and leave the CNS through spinal and cranial nerves. Within the spinal cord and brainstem, they establish connections through which autonomic reflexes are mediated. Afferent fibres also establish connections with ascending neurones through which conscious awareness of visceral functions is achieved. Changes in the internal and external environments, and emotional factors, profoundly influence autonomic activity, most notably via descending connections from the **hypothalamus** (Chapter 16). Autonomic efferent neurones differ from those of the somatic nervous system in that, in the autonomic nervous system, there is a sequence of two neurones between the CNS and the innervated structure (Fig. 4.1). The synaptic connection between the two neurones is located peripherally in an **autonomic ganglion**. The first neurone is, thus, called the **preganglionic neurone** and its cell body is located in the spinal cord or brainstem. The second neurone is referred to as the **postganglionic neurone** and its cell body is located peripherally in an autonomic ganglion.

The efferent neurones of the autonomic nervous system fall into two distinct anatomical and functional divisions or systems: **sympathetic** and **parasympathetic**. Many, although not all, structures that receive autonomic innervation are dually innervated by both sympathetic and parasympathetic systems. These exercise opposite effects upon the innervated structure (Table 4.1).

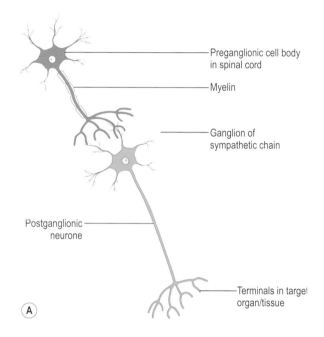

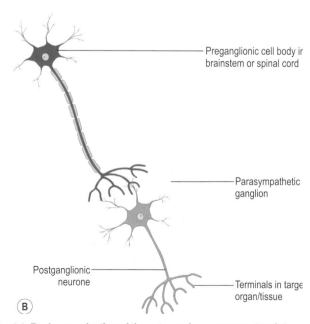

Fig. 4.1 Basic organisation of the autonomic nervous system into preganglionic and postganglionic neurones. In the sympathetic division **(A)**, ganglia constitute the sympathetic chain, lying near the vertebral column. Preganglionic neurones, therefore, have relatively short axons, while postganglionic fibres are relatively long. In the parasympathetic division **(B)**, ganglia are located close to the target organ. Consequently, preganglionic axons are long and postganglionic axons are short.

Table 4.1 **Functions of the autonomic nervous system**		
Structure	**Sympathetic effect**	**Parasympathetic effect**
Iris of eye	Dilates pupil	Constricts pupil
Ciliary muscle of eye	Relaxes	Contracts
Salivary glands	Reduces secretion	Increases secretion
Lacrimal gland	Reduces secretion	Increases secretion
Heart	Increases rate and force of contraction	Decreases rate and force of contraction
Bronchi	Dilates	Constricts
Gastrointestinal tract	Decreases motility	Increases motility
Sweat glands	Increases secretion	
Erector pili muscles	Contracts	

Sympathetic division

Preganglionic sympathetic neurones are located exclusively in the thoracic and upper two or three lumbar segments of the spinal cord (Fig. 4.2). They lie in the **lateral horn** of the spinal grey matter which is, therefore, only present at these levels (see Figs 8.8, 8.9B). Preganglionic axons leave the cord in the ventral nerve roots and join the spinal nerve. Postganglionic sympathetic neurones have their cell bodies in one of two locations: either the **sympathetic chain** of ganglia that lies either side of the vertebral column, or the plexuses (coeliac, superior mesenteric, inferior mesenteric) that surround the main branches of the abdominal aorta. In order to reach any of these locations, preganglionic axons in the spinal nerve enter the sympathetic chain. Those spinal nerves that contain sympathetic outflow are linked to ganglia of the sympathetic chain by two small nerves, the **rami communicantes** (Fig. 4.3). Preganglionic fibres pass into the chain via the white ramus communicans, so called because the constituent fibres are myelinated.

Those fibres concerned with innervation of structures in the head and thorax terminate in synaptic contact with postganglionic cell bodies in the sympathetic chain. The postganglionic fibres return to the spinal nerve via the grey ramus communicans, so called because the constituent fibres are unmyelinated. Those preganglionic sympathetic fibres concerned with innervation of pelvic and abdominal viscera pass uninterrupted through the sympathetic chain and travel to the plexuses where their corresponding postganglionic cell bodies are located. The neurotransmitter released by preganglionic sympathetic neurones is acetylcholine. The transmitter of postganglionic sympathetic cells is generally noradrenaline (norepinephrine), although the cells innervating sweat glands are cholinergic. The adrenal medulla is an exceptional organ, in that it is directly innervated by preganglionic sympathetic neurones.

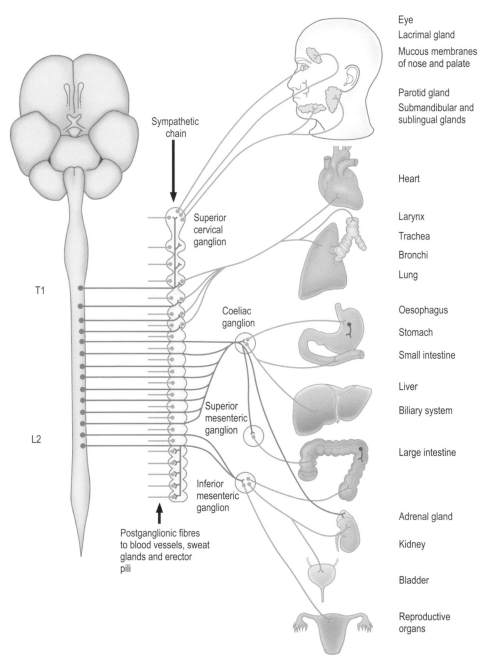

Fig. 4.2 Organisation of the sympathetic division of the autonomic nervous system.

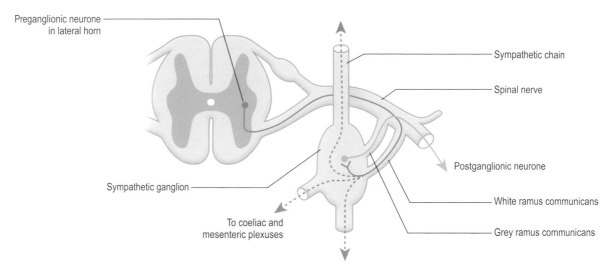

Preganglionic neurone
in lateral horn

Sympathetic chain

Spinal nerve

Postganglionic neurone

Sympathetic ganglion

White ramus communicans

To coeliac and
mesenteric plexuses

Grey ramus communicans

Fig. 4.3 Relationships between a typical thoracic spinal nerve and the sympathetic chain.

The effects of sympathetic nervous system activity are most apparent under conditions of stress, excitement or fear and are classically referred to as the 'fight or flight' response. The heart rate and blood pressure are increased. The bronchi are dilated to increase airflow to and from the lungs. Vasodilatation in skeletal muscles allows the increased blood flow required for energetic activity, while gastrointestinal blood flow and motility are decreased. Metabolic changes occur, such as an increase in blood glucose, to support high energy utilisation and sweating occurs to increase heat loss.

Lesions of the sympathetic nervous system

Peripheral autonomic failure leads to fainting through failure to control the heart rate and blood pressure (**postural syncope**), urinary and bowel incontinence and impotence.

Autonomic neuropathies often complicate acute and chronic sensory motor neuropathies, but rarely manifest as chronic familial neurodegenerative disorders of the peripheral autonomic nerves.

Horner's syndrome refers to drooping of the eyelid (ptosis) and constriction of the pupil (miosis) caused by damage to the sympathetic innervation of the levator palpebrae superioris muscle and the radial (pupillodilator) fibres of the iris. The sympathetic neurones, or the descending pathways controlling them, may be damaged at a number of levels: as they descend in the brainstem (by stroke or tumour) and the spinal cord (by an expanded cavity or syrinx), as they emerge in the first thoracic nerve root (by tumour of the apical lung) and as they ascend in the sympathetic plexus around the carotid arteries (by swelling of the arteries in a migrainous attack).

Parasympathetic division

Preganglionic parasympathetic neurones are located in the brainstem and the spinal cord (Fig. 4.4). Within the brainstem, such cells lie in cranial nerve nuclei associated with the oculomotor, facial, glossopharyngeal and vagus nerves and provide innervation for structures of the head, thorax and abdomen. The parasympathetic components of these nerves are described in Chapter 10. Within the cord, preganglionic parasympathetic neurones lie in the second, third and fourth sacral segments and provide innervation for pelvic viscera. The cell bodies of postganglionic parasympathetic neurones lie in ganglia that are located close to the structures which they innervate. Within the alimentary canal, these neurones contribute to the myenteric (Auerbach's) and submucosal (Meissner's) plexuses.

These plexuses are also referred to as the 'enteric nervous system'. Such a concept has arisen because the plexuses additionally contain afferent neurones and interneurones. The rich local interconnections of these cells are capable of sustaining the motility of the gastrointestinal tract in the absence of input from the CNS. Furthermore, these cells cannot simply be equated with the parasympathetic nervous system as traditionally defined, since they are known also to receive synaptic input from postganglionic sympathetic neurones. The neurotransmitter released by both preganglionic and postganglionic parasympathetic neurones is acetylcholine.

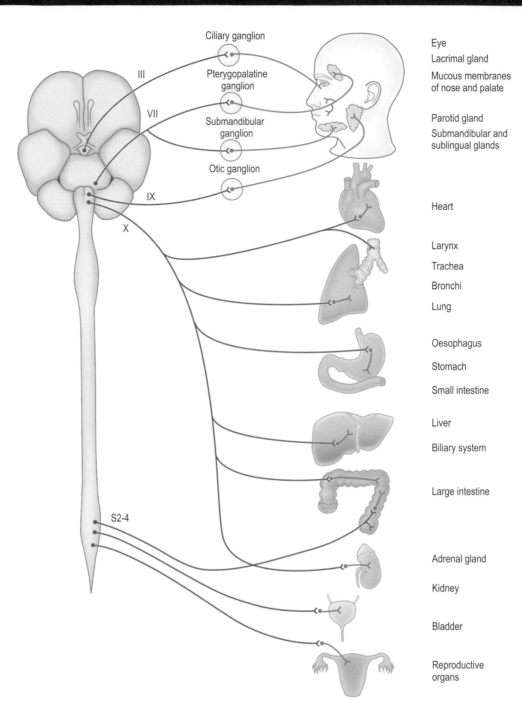

Fig. 4.4 Organisation of the parasympathetic division of the autonomic nervous system.

5 | Coverings of the central nervous system

The central nervous system (CNS) is supported and protected by bone and membranous coverings. The brain is located within the cranial cavity of the skull and the spinal cord lies in the vertebral, or spinal, canal within the vertebral column, or spine. Within their bony coverings, the brain and spinal cord are invested by three concentric membranous envelopes. The outermost membrane is the dura mater, the middle layer is the arachnoid mater and the innermost layer is the pia mater. The vertebral column and spinal meninges are described in Chapter 8; consequently, only the skull and cranial meninges are considered here.

Skull

The brain lies on the floor of the cranial cavity, which, together with the bones of the cranial vault, provides support and protection from physical injury. The floor of the cranial cavity consists of three **fossae**. Each of these accommodates particular parts of the brain and possesses **foramina** through which cranial nerves and blood vessels enter and leave the cranial cavity (Fig. 5.1).

Anterior cranial fossa

The anterior cranial fossa is formed by the frontal, ethmoid and sphenoid bones. It accommodates the frontal lobes of the brain. The greater part of the floor of the anterior cranial fossa consists of the frontal bone and it also forms the roof of the orbit. The part of the frontal bone that forms the anterior wall of the fossa contains the **frontal air sinus**. The medial part of the floor of the anterior cranial fossa is composed of the ethmoid bone. In the midline, a sharp ridge, the crista galli, is the anterior point of attachment of the dural falx cerebri. In a narrow, elongated depression on either side of the crista galli lies the **cribriform plate** of the ethmoid bone, upon which lies the **olfactory bulb**. The bone of the cribriform plate is peppered with small perforations through which the fascicles of the olfactory nerve enter the cranial cavity from the nasal cavity to attach to the olfactory bulb.

Middle cranial fossa

The middle cranial fossa is formed by the sphenoid and temporal bones. In the midline, the body of the sphenoid forms a deep depression, the **hypophyseal fossa**, encompassed by four spurs of bone, the anterior and posterior clinoid processes. The hypophyseal fossa accommodates the **hypophysis**, or **pituitary gland**. Lateral to the body of the sphenoid, the rest of the middle cranial fossa holds the temporal lobes of the cerebral hemisphere. The middle cranial fossa contains numerous points of entry to, and exit from, the cranial cavity for cranial nerves and blood vessels. In particular:

- The **optic canal** is located medial to the anterior clinoid process and communicates with the orbit. Through it pass the optic (II) nerve and the ophthalmic artery (a branch of the internal carotid artery).
- The **superior orbital fissure** lies between the greater and lesser wings of the sphenoid bone and also communicates with the orbit. It carries the oculomotor (III), trochlear (IV) and abducens (VI) nerves and the ophthalmic division of the trigeminal (V) nerve.
- The **foramen rotundum** opens into the pterygopalatine fossa and carries the maxillary division of the trigeminal nerve.
- The **foramen ovale** carries the large mandibular division of the trigeminal nerve.
- The **foramen spinosum** is the point of entry of the middle meningeal artery.

Posterior cranial fossa

The posterior cranial fossa is formed by the occipital and petrous temporal bones. Anteriorly, in the midline, it forms a steep, smooth slope (the **clivus**) that is continuous with the body of the sphenoid bone, posterior to the hypophyseal fossa. The brainstem rests upon the clivus, the medulla passing through the **foramen magnum** to become continuous with the spinal cord. The foramen magnum also admits the vertebral arteries and the spinal root of the accessory (XI) nerve. In the lateral wall of the foramen magnum lies the **hypoglossal canal** through which the hypoglossal (XII) nerve leaves the cranial cavity. Between the occipital and petrous temporal bones lies the large **jugular foramen** through which pass the internal jugular vein and the glossopharyngeal (IX), vagus (X) and accessory (XI) nerves. In the vertical wall of the petrous temporal bone is located the **internal auditory** (acoustic) **meatus**, which transmits the vestibulocochlear (VIII) and facial (VII) nerves. The cerebellum rests on the floor of the posterior cranial fossa.

 Raised intracranial pressure

A **space-occupying lesion** is an expanding focal lesion such as a tumour, haematoma or abscess. Since the cranial cavity is closed and unyielding, the brain is distorted and displaced downwards, towards the foramen magnum, as the intracranial pressure rises (Fig. 5.2). The patient complains of headache, vomiting, blurring of vision and drowsiness. The optic discs are swollen (**papilloedema**) and signs of brainstem dysfunction are found. Coma and death supervene if the pressure is not relieved by neurosurgery (craniotomy). **Benign intracranial hypertension** is caused by generalised swelling of the brain in the absence of a focal space-occupying lesion. It often occurs in obese young women; the syndrome of raised intracranial pressure mimics a brain tumour - hence the old designation, 'pseudo tumour cerebri'.

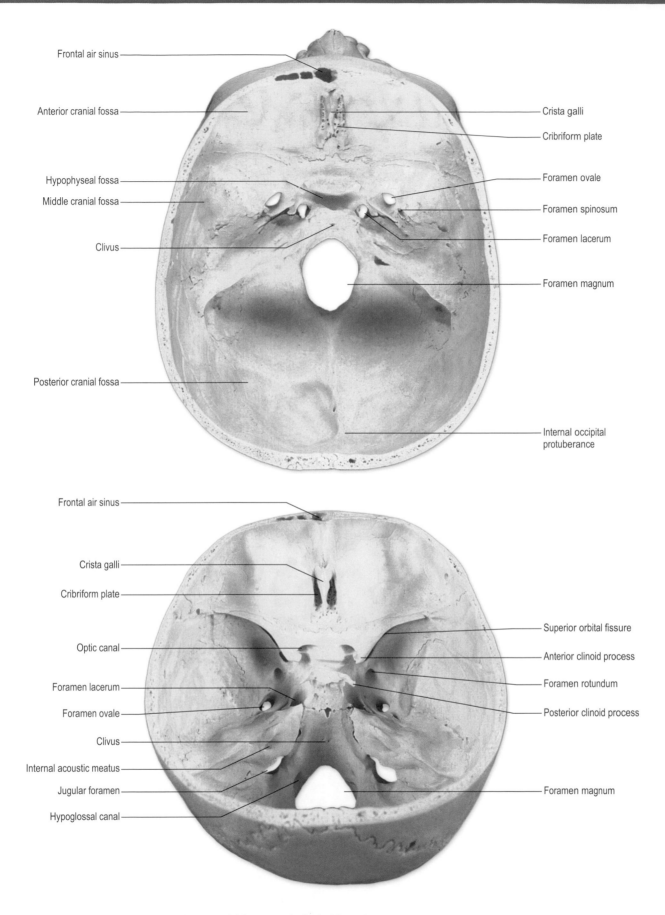

Frontal air sinus

Anterior cranial fossa

Hypophyseal fossa

Middle cranial fossa

Clivus

Posterior cranial fossa

Crista galli

Cribriform plate

Foramen ovale

Foramen spinosum

Foramen lacerum

Foramen magnum

Internal occipital protuberance

Frontal air sinus

Crista galli

Cribriform plate

Optic canal

Foramen lacerum

Foramen ovale

Clivus

Internal acoustic meatus

Jugular foramen

Hypoglossal canal

Superior orbital fissure

Anterior clinoid process

Foramen rotundum

Posterior clinoid process

Foramen magnum

Fig. 5.1 Floor of the skull showing the three cranial fossae and principal foramina.

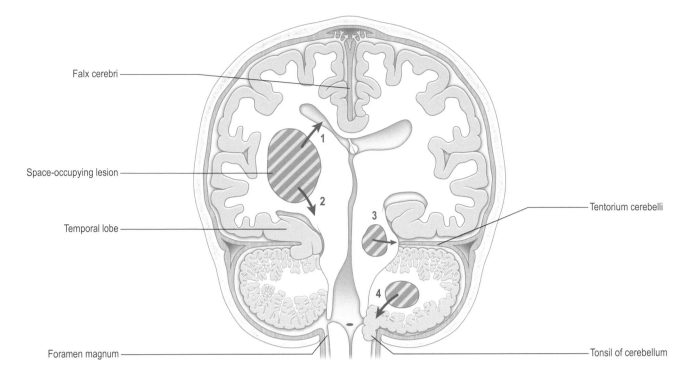

Falx cerebri

Space-occupying lesion

Temporal lobe

Foramen magnum

Tentorium cerebelli

Tonsil of cerebellum

Fig. 5.2 A space-occupying lesion leads to displacement of the brain and raised intracranial pressure. 1: Herniation of cortex beneath falx cerebri. 2: Herniation of temporal lobe into posterior cranial fossa. 3: Compression of midbrain against tentorium cerebelli. 4: Herniation of cerebellar tonsils through foramen magnum.

 Foraminal syndromes

The exit foramina of the skull represent sites of potential extrinsic compression of structures running through them, by disorders such as bony deformity and tumours of bone, meninges or blood vessels. The particular cranial nerves damaged at the exit site lead to 'foraminal syndromes', e.g. of the **superior orbital fissure** or **jugular foramen**. In the **foramen magnum syndrome** the spinal cord, lower brainstem and tonsils of the cerebellum are compromised.

Skull

- The bones of the skull and the meninges provide protection for the brain.

- The brain lies on the floor of the cranial cavity, which consists of three fossae.

- The anterior cranial fossa contains the frontal lobes of the cerebral hemispheres. It forms the roof of the orbit and is closely associated with the frontal air sinus.

- The cribriform plate admits the olfactory nerves to the cranial cavity and accommodates the olfactory bulb.

- The middle cranial fossa contains the temporal lobe. In the midline, the hypophyseal fossa holds the pituitary gland.

- A number of foramina provide entry and exit for important blood vessels and cranial nerves (indicated in parentheses):

  - Optic canal (optic nerve, ophthalmic artery)

  - Superior orbital fissure (oculomotor, trochlear, abducens and ophthalmic division of trigeminal nerves)
  - Foramen rotundum (maxillary division of trigeminal nerve)
  - Foramen ovale (mandibular division of trigeminal nerve)
  - Foramen spinosum (middle meningeal artery)
  - The posterior cranial fossa accommodates the brainstem and cerebellum.
  - A number of important structures pass through the foramina of the posterior fossa:
  - Foramen magnum (medulla oblongata, vertebral arteries, spinal root of the accessory nerve)
  - Hypoglossal canal (hypoglossal nerve)
  - Jugular foramen (internal jugular vein, glossopharyngeal, vagus and accessory nerves)
  - Internal auditory meatus (facial and vestibulocochlear nerves)

Cranial meninges

Dura mater

The cranial dura mater is a tough, fibrous membrane that ensheathes the brain like a loose-fitting bag. In some regions, such as the floor of the cranial cavity and the midline of the cranial roof, the dura is tightly adherent to the interior surface of the skull, while elsewhere, such as the frontoparietal area, the two are separated by a narrow extradural space. Two large folds, or reflections, of dura extend into the cranial cavity and occupy the fissures between major components of the brain (Figs 5.3, 5.4). In the midline, a vertical sheet of dura, the **falx cerebri**, extends from the cranial roof into the great longitudinal fissure between the cerebral hemispheres. The falx, therefore, has an attached border that adheres to the inner surface of the skull and a free border that lies above the corpus callosum. Anteriorly, the falx is attached to the bony ridge of the crista galli. Posteriorly, it becomes continuous with a horizontal shelf of dura, the **tentorium cerebelli**, which extends inwards from the occipitotemporal region of the skull to lie in the transverse cerebral fissure, between the posterior part of the cerebral hemispheres and the cerebellum. The tentorium has a free border that encircles the midbrain, as the brainstem communicates between the posterior and middle cranial fossae. In the midline, the tentorium becomes continuous superiorly with the falx cerebri (Fig. 5.3).

The dura mater is considered to be comprised of two layers. These are normally closely adherent to one another but, in certain locations, they become separated to enclose blood-filled spaces, the dural venous sinuses. Major venous sinuses lie in the attached borders of the falx cerebri (superior sagittal sinus; Fig. 5.4) and tentorium cerebelli (straight sinus, transverse sinuses; see Figs 7.9, 7.10) and also on the floor of the cranial cavity (e.g. cavernous sinus; see Fig. 7.11). Venous blood from the brain flows into the sinuses through a series of venous channels and in turn the sinuses drain principally into the internal jugular vein, through which blood is returned to the general extracranial circulation. The dural venous sinuses are described further in Chapter 7, which deals with the vasculature of the CNS.

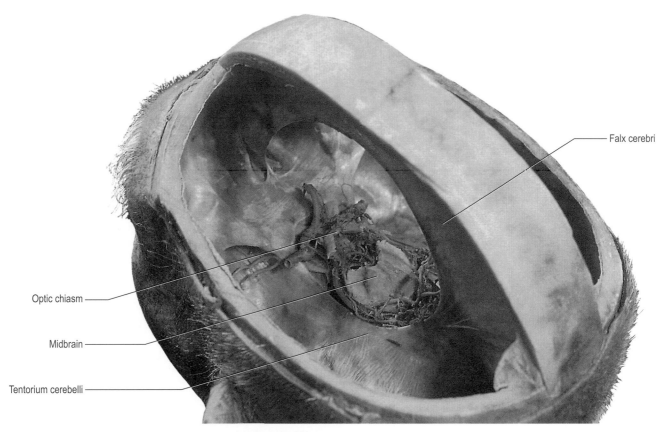

Falx cerebri

Optic chiasm

Midbrain

Tentorium cerebelli

Fig. 5.3 Cranial cavity showing the arrangement of the dura mater.

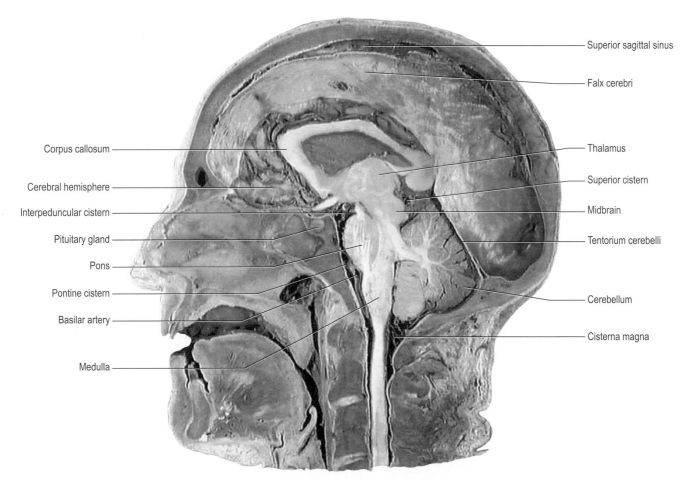

Superior sagittal sinus

Falx cerebri

Corpus callosum

Cerebral hemisphere

Interpeduncular cistern

Pituitary gland

Pons

Pontine cistern

Basilar artery

Medulla

Thalamus

Superior cistern

Midbrain

Tentorium cerebelli

Cerebellum

Cisterna magna

Fig. 5.4 Paramedian sagittal section of the head, showing the disposition of the brain and meninges.

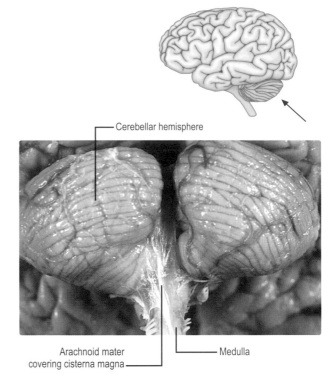

Head trauma

Head trauma, especially resulting from road traffic accidents, is the most common cause of death and disability in youth. The injury may be blunt ('closed') or caused by a penetrating missile. The skull may be fractured and depressed, tearing brain coverings and the brain itself. Displacement and torsion of the brain lead to contusion, tearing of white matter and bleeding into the brain (**intracerebral haematoma**), causing unconsciousness (concussion), neurological and psychological deficits and post-traumatic epilepsy.

Tearing of the middle meningeal artery causes bleeding into the extradural space (**extradural haematoma**). As the blood clot expands, the brain is compressed; as a result, coma supervenes a delayed period of hours after the blow. Without neurosurgical evacuation, the rising intracranial pressure causes brain displacement and death.

Tearing of the veins stretching across the subdural space causes gradual seepage of blood, collecting to form a chronic **subdural haematoma** with eventual coma. The delay between the blow and the development of symptoms may be of weeks or months. The elderly are particularly vulnerable and the head injury may be slight and forgotten. Again, surgical removal of the clot is life-saving.

— Cerebellar hemisphere

Arachnoid mater covering cisterna magna —

— Medulla

Fig. 5.5 Cisterna magna.

Arachnoid mater and pia mater

The arachnoid mater is a soft, translucent membrane that, like the dura mater, loosely envelops the brain (see Figs 1.16, 6.10). It is separated from the dura by a narrow subdural space, through which pass veins en route to the dural venous sinuses (Chapter 7).

The pia mater is a microscopically thin, delicate and highly vascular membrane which is closely adherent to the surface of the brain, following all its concavities and convexities. Between the pia and arachnoid mater lies the **subarachnoid space**. This contains a filamentous network of connective tissue sheets and strands (trabeculae) and is traversed by numerous arteries and veins (see Fig. 1.16). It also contains cerebrospinal fluid (CSF), which is produced by the choroid plexus within the cerebral ventricles (Chapter 6). Since the arachnoid mater fits loosely round the brain while the pia closely follows its surface contours, the subarachnoid space is of greatly varying depth in different regions. Where significant depressions or fissures in the brain are spanned by the arachnoid mater, **subarachnoid cisterns** are formed. Two of these are particularly large:

- The **cisterna magna** (cerebellomedullary cistern) lies between the cerebellum and the dorsal surface of the medulla (Figs 5.4, 5.5). CSF flows into this cistern from the fourth ventricle.
- The **interpeduncular cistern** is located at the base of the brain (Fig. 5.4) where the arachnoid spans the space between the two temporal lobes. This cistern contains the optic chiasm. The cistern is deepest between the two cerebral peduncles of the midbrain.
- Other cisterns include the **superior cistern** lying between the posterior portion (splenium) of the corpus callosum and the cerebellum and the **pontine cistern** through which runs the basilar artery (Fig. 5.4).

Cranial meninges

- The dura mater is the outermost meningeal membrane. Two dural sheets, or reflections, extend into the cranial cavity:
  - The falx cerebri, lying between the two cerebral hemispheres
  - The tentorium cerebelli, lying between the cerebellum and the occipital lobes of the cerebrum and encircling the midbrain
- The dura contains a number of venous sinuses, which are important in the venous drainage of the brain.
- Important sinuses lie within the falx cerebri, tentorium cerebelli and on the floor of the cranial cavity.
- The middle meningeal layer is the arachnoid mater. Both the dura and arachnoid surround the brain loosely.
- The innermost meningeal layer is the pia mater, which adheres to the surface of the brain, closely following its contours. This creates a subarachnoid space of variable depth.
- The subarachnoid space contains CSF, which is secreted by the choroid plexus within the cerebral ventricles.

Meningitis

Inflammation of the meninges may result from infection with viruses (e.g. lymphocytic choriomeningitis), bacteria (meningococcus, pneumococcus, haemophilus influenzae and tuberculosis), fungi (cryptococcus) and protozoa (toxoplasma). The patient complains of headache, photophobia and vomiting, is febrile and has neck stiffness on attempting to move the head. Viral meningitis is normally mild and self-limiting. Bacterial or fungal meningitis, however, leads to damage to cranial nerves and the brain itself; if untreated, it proceeds to raised intracranial pressure, brain displacement and death.

Ventricular system 6

The central nervous system (CNS) contains an interconnecting series of chambers and channels which are derived from the lumen of the embryonic neural tube. In the spinal cord, this is represented by the vestigial and insignificant central canal. Within the brain, however, the enormous growth and distortion of the original tube-like structure is paralleled by the development of an elaborate series of chambers, the cerebral ventricles (Figs 6.1, 6.2; see also Fig. 1.23).

Topographical anatomy of the ventricular system

Passing rostrally from the spinal cord to the brainstem, the central canal of the spinal cord moves progressively more dorsal until, in the rostral (open) medulla, it opens out into a wide and shallow depression, the **fourth ventricle** (Fig. 6.3), which lies on the dorsal surface of the brainstem beneath the cerebellum. The fourth ventricle is rhomboid or diamond-shaped. On each side, a **lateral recess** extends towards the lateral margin of the brainstem and is in continuity, through a small **lateral aperture** (the **foramen of Luschka**), with the subarachnoid space of the cerebellopontine angle (Fig. 6.4). For the most part, the roof of the fourth ventricle is formed by the cerebellum. However, the roof of the caudal part consists of pia and ependyma, a central defect in which constitutes the **median aperture** of the fourth ventricle, or the **foramen of**

Magendie. The latter provides communication between the lumen of the ventricle and the cisterna magna of the subarachnoid space (Fig. 6.5). The rostral part of the roof of the fourth ventricle is partly formed by the superior cerebellar peduncles on either side, the space between them being bridged by the thin superior medullary velum (Fig. 6.2).

The fourth ventricle extends rostrally as far as the pontomesencephalic junction, where it becomes continuous with the **cerebral aqueduct**. The cerebral aqueduct is a narrow channel which passes throughout the length of the midbrain, beneath the inferior and superior colliculi. The simple, tubular configuration of the cerebral aqueduct, in comparison to the rest of the cerebral ventricular system, reflects the relatively undifferentiated nature of the midbrain in comparison to the forebrain. At the rostral margin of the midbrain, the cerebral aqueduct opens into the **third ventricle**. This is a midline, narrow, slit-like cavity, the lateral walls of which are formed by the thalamus and hypothalamus on either side (Fig. 6.2 and see Fig. 12.2). The roof of the third ventricle is formed by pia-ependyma, which spans between two nerve fibre bundles, the **striae medullaris thalami**, which are situated along the dorsomedial border of the thalamus on either side. In the rostral part of the third ventricle lies an aperture, the **interventricular foramen**, or **foramen of Monro**, which is located between the column of the fornix and the anterior pole of the thalamus.

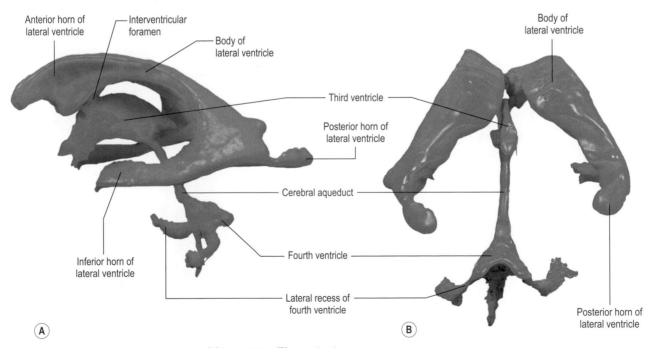

Anterior horn of lateral ventricle
Interventricular foramen
Body of lateral ventricle
Body of lateral ventricle
Third ventricle
Posterior horn of lateral ventricle
Cerebral aqueduct
Inferior horn of lateral ventricle
Fourth ventricle
Lateral recess of fourth ventricle
Posterior horn of lateral ventricle

(A) (B)

Fig. 6.1 Resin cast of the ventricular system. (A) Lateral view; **(B)** posterior view.

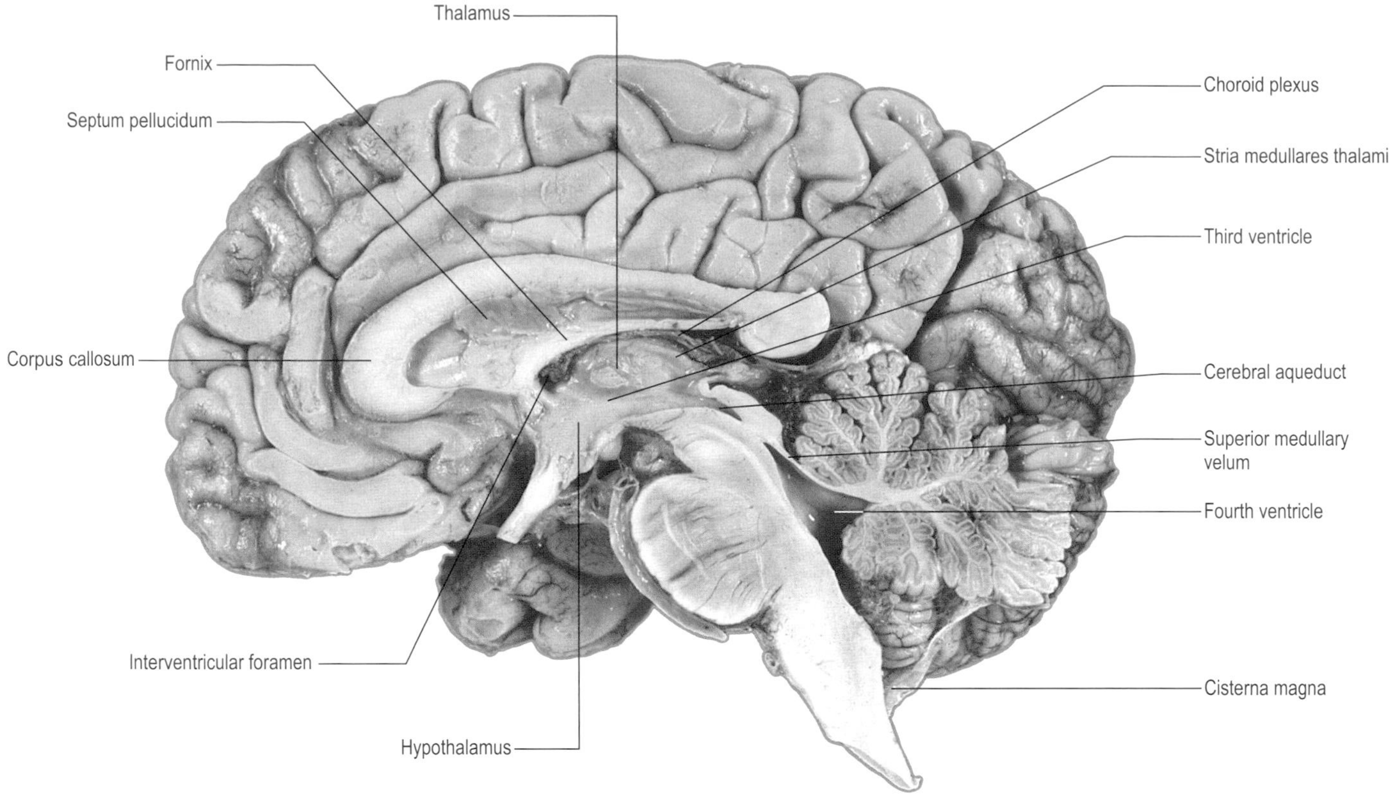

Thalamus

Fornix

Septum pellucidum

Choroid plexus

Stria medullares thalami

Third ventricle

Corpus callosum

Cerebral aqueduct

Superior medullary velum

Fourth ventricle

Interventricular foramen

Cisterna magna

Hypothalamus

Fig. 6.2 Median sagittal section of the brain showing the ventricular system.

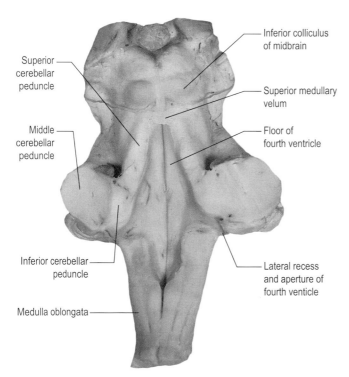

Superior cerebellar peduncle

Inferior colliculus of midbrain

Superior medullary velum

Middle cerebellar peduncle

Floor of fourth ventricle

Inferior cerebellar peduncle

Lateral recess and aperture of fourth venticle

Medulla oblongata

Fig. 6.3 Dorsal aspect of the brainstem showing the floor of the fourth ventricle. The cerebellum has been removed by severing the cerebellar peduncles.

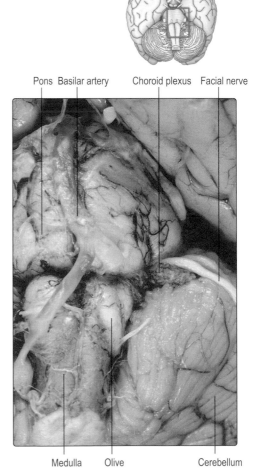

Pons Basilar artery   Choroid plexus Facial nerve

Medulla   Olive   Cerebellum

Fig. 6.4 Cerebellopontine angle. The point of continuity between the lateral recess of the fourth ventricle and the subarachnoid space is indicated by a small tuft of choroid plexus, which protrudes through the lateral aperture.

The interventricular foramen provides communication, on either side, with the extensive **lateral ventricle** located within the cerebral hemisphere (Fig. 6.6 and see Fig. 16.15). The lateral ventricle is approximately C-shaped. It consists of an anterior (frontal) horn, a body, posterior (occipital) horn and an inferior (temporal) horn. The anterior horn of the lateral ventricle is that part lying anterior to the interventricular foramen. The lateral wall of the anterior horn is formed by the head of the caudate nucleus and its roof is the corpus callosum (see Figs 13.3–13.7). The medial wall is formed by the **septum pellucidum** (Fig. 6.2). This thin sheet spans between the corpus callosum and fornix in the midline and separates the anterior horns of the two lateral ventricles. The body of the lateral ventricle extends behind the interventricular foramen, having as its floor the thalamus and the tail of the caudate nucleus. More posteriorly, a small posterior horn extends towards the occipital pole but the principal course of the ventricle sweeps downwards and forwards to form the extensive inferior horn, which lies in the temporal lobe. In the floor of the inferior horn lies the hippocampus, while in its roof runs the much attenuated tail of the caudate nucleus (see Figs 13.9–13.12 and 16.15).

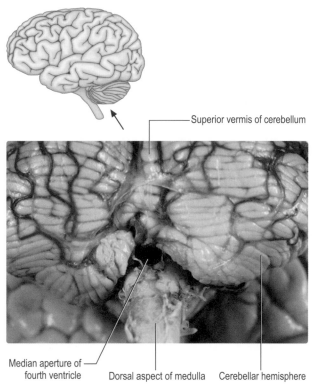

Superior vermis of cerebellum

Median aperture of fourth ventricle

Dorsal aspect of medulla

Cerebellar hemisphere

Fig. 6.5 Posterior view of the brain. The cerebellum and brainstem have been slightly separated to show the median aperture of the fourth ventricle.

Topographical anatomy of ventricular system

- The ventricular system consists of the lateral ventricles, third ventricle, cerebral aqueduct and fourth ventricle.

- The lateral ventricle is located within each cerebral hemisphere and is approximately C-shaped. It communicates, via the interventricular foramen, with the third ventricle.

- The third ventricle is a midline, slit-like cavity. Its lateral walls consist of the thalamus and hypothalamus. Caudally, the third ventricle becomes continuous with the cerebral aqueduct.

- The cerebral aqueduct extends throughout the midbrain, linking the third and fourth ventricles.

- The fourth ventricle is located between the brainstem (pons and medulla) and the cerebellum. A median aperture and two lateral apertures communicate with the subarachnoid space surrounding the brain.

Cerebrospinal fluid

The ventricular system, together with the cranial and spinal subarachnoid spaces, contains cerebrospinal fluid (CSF; Fig. 6.7). This is produced by the **choroid plexus**, which is located in the lateral, third and fourth ventricles (Figs 6.2, 6.6 and see Fig. 16.15). The choroid plexus is formed by invagination of the vascular pia mater into the ventricular lumen, where it becomes highly convoluted, producing a sponge-like appearance. The

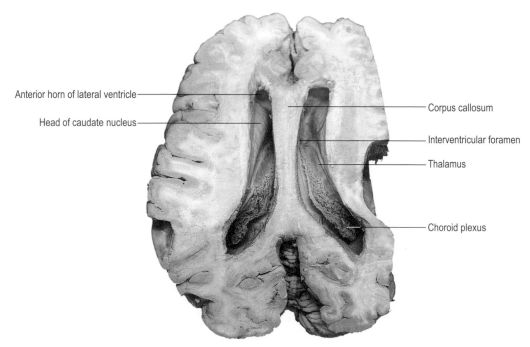

Anterior horn of lateral ventricle

Head of caudate nucleus

Corpus callosum

Interventricular foramen

Thalamus

Choroid plexus

Fig. 6.6 Lateral ventricle. Superior aspect of a dissection of the cerebral hemispheres in which much of the corpus callosum has been removed to reveal the lumen of the lateral ventricles.

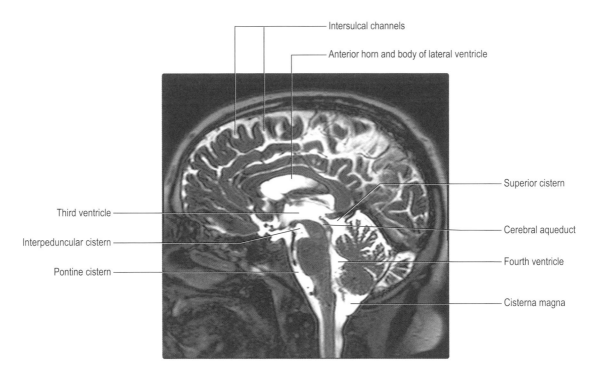

Intersulcal channels

Anterior horn and body of lateral ventricle

Superior cistern

Third ventricle

Interpeduncular cistern

Pontine cistern

Cerebral aqueduct

Fourth ventricle

Cisterna magna

Fig. 6.7 Sagittal T$_2$-weighted MR image of the brain demonstrating CSF within the ventricular system and subarachnoid space. *(Courtesy of Professor A Jackson, Wolfson Molecular Imaging Centre, University of Manchester, Manchester, UK.)*

choroid plexus enters the third and fourth ventricles through their roofs and the lateral ventricle through the choroid fissure, along the line of the fimbria/fornix (see Figs 16.14, 16.15).

CSF is produced partly by an active secretory process and partly by passive diffusion. It is a colourless fluid containing little protein and few cells. The volume of CSF in the combined ventricular and subarachnoid spaces is approximately 150 mL. CSF is produced continuously, at a rate sufficient to fill these spaces several times each day. This means that an efficient mechanism is required for the circulation of CSF and its reabsorption (Figs 6.8–6.10).

Most CSF is produced by the choroid plexus of the lateral ventricle. From here it flows through the interventricular foramen into the third ventricle and thence, by way of the cerebral aqueduct, into the fourth ventricle. CSF leaves the ventricular system through the three apertures of the fourth ventricle and, thus, enters the subarachnoid space. Most CSF passes through the median aperture to enter the cisterna magna, located between the medulla and cerebellum. A lesser amount flows through the lateral apertures to enter the subarachnoid space in the region of the cerebellopontine angles. The majority of CSF then flows superiorly, round the cerebral hemispheres, to the sites of reabsorption. Within the subarachnoid space, CSF serves partially to cushion the brain from sudden movements of the head.

CSF is reabsorbed into the venous system by passing into the dural venous sinuses, principally the superior sagittal sinus. Along the sinuses are located numerous **arachnoid villi**, which consist of invaginations of arachnoid mater through the dural wall and into the lumen of the sinus (Fig. 6.9). Reabsorption occurs at these sites because the hydrostatic pressure in the subarachnoid space is higher than that in the lumen of the sinus and also because of the greater colloid osmotic pressure of venous blood compared with CSF. With age, the arachnoid villi become hypertrophic to form **arachnoid granulations** (Fig. 6.10).

Hydrocephalus

Obstruction of the flow of CSF within the ventricular system (e.g. by tumours) or the subarachnoid space (e.g. by adhesions following head injury or meningitis) leads to a rise in fluid pressure causing swelling of the ventricles (**hydrocephalus**). The clinical effects are similar to those of a brain tumour and consist of headaches, unsteadiness and mental impairment. Swelling of the optic discs (**papilloedema**) is seen on ophthalmoscopy. Decompression of the dilated ventricles is achieved by inserting a shunt connecting the ventricles to the jugular vein or the abdominal peritoneum.

Cerebrospinal fluid

- Each ventricle contains choroid plexus, which secretes CSF.

- CSF flows in the direction: lateral ventricles → third ventricle → cerebral aqueduct → fourth ventricle → subarachnoid space.

- The combined ventricular system and subarachnoid space contains about 150 mL CSF, this volume being produced several times each day.

- CSF is reabsorbed into the venous system through arachnoid villi, which project principally into the superior sagittal sinus.

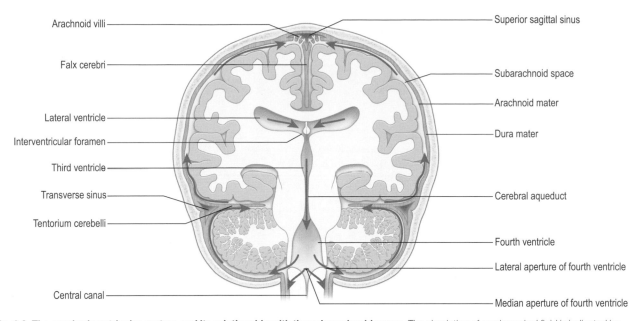

Arachnoid villi

Falx cerebri

Lateral ventricle

Interventricular foramen

Third ventricle

Transverse sinus

Tentorium cerebelli

Central canal

Superior sagittal sinus

Subarachnoid space

Arachnoid mater

Dura mater

Cerebral aqueduct

Fourth ventricle

Lateral aperture of fourth ventricle

Median aperture of fourth ventricle

Fig. 6.8 The cerebral ventricular system and its relationship with the subarachnoid space. The circulation of cerebrospinal fluid is indicated by arrows.

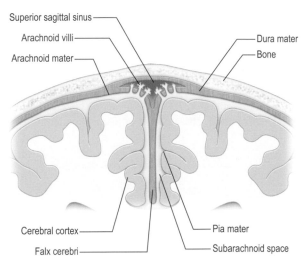

Superior sagittal sinus

Arachnoid villi

Arachnoid mater

Dura mater

Bone

Cerebral cortex

Falx cerebri

Pia mater

Subarachnoid space

Fig. 6.9 Transverse section through the superior sagittal sinus showing arachnoid villi.

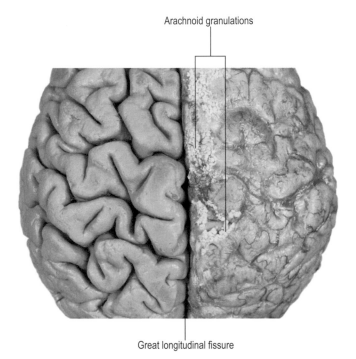

Arachnoid granulations

Great longitudinal fissure

Fig. 6.10 Superior aspect of the cerebral hemispheres showing arachnoid granulations on the right side. On the left side, the arachnoid mater has been removed.

7 | Vasculature of the central nervous system

Vasculature of the spinal cord

Arterial supply of the spinal cord

Three longitudinal arterial vessels run the length of the spinal cord (Fig. 7.1). These are the single **anterior spinal artery** and the paired **posterior spinal arteries**. The anterior spinal artery arises in a Y-shaped configuration from the two vertebral arteries at the level of the medulla oblongata (Fig. 7.2) and descends along the ventral surface of the cord in the midline. The posterior spinal arteries arise from either the vertebral arteries or the posterior inferior cerebellar arteries and run caudally on the posterolateral surface of the cord.

The anterior and posterior spinal arteries alone are insufficient to supply the cord below cervical levels and, therefore, they receive serial reinforcement by anastomosis with **radicular arteries** derived from segmental vessels, including the ascending cervical, intercostal and lumbar arteries. Radicular arteries pass through the intervertebral foramina and divide into anterior and posterior

branches, which run with the dorsal and ventral spinal nerve roots, respectively. One particularly large radicular artery (the **great radicular artery**, or **artery of Adamkiewicz**) may arise from a lateral intercostal or lumbar artery at any level between T8 and L3.

 Disorders of the blood supply of the spinal cord

The blood supply of the spinal cord is most vulnerable in the thoracic region and in the anterior portion of the cord. **Occlusion of the anterior spinal artery**, usually secondary to dissection of the descending thoracic aorta, leads to an acute thoracic cord syndrome with paraplegia and incontinence. The spinothalamic modalities of pain and temperature are preferentially lost, whereas the proprioceptive functions of the dorsal columns are relatively preserved.

Venous drainage of the spinal cord

The venous drainage of the cord follows a basically similar pattern to the arterial supply (Fig. 7.1). Six longitudinal interconnecting venous channels exist. These consist primarily of **anterior** and

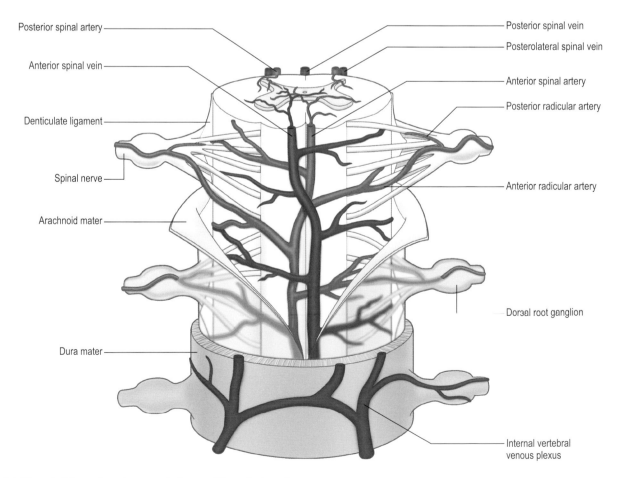

Fig. 7.1 The arterial supply and venous drainage of the spinal cord.

Posterior spinal artery
Anterior spinal vein
Denticulate ligament
Spinal nerve
Arachnoid mater
Dura mater

Posterior spinal vein
Posterolateral spinal vein
Anterior spinal artery
Posterior radicular artery
Anterior radicular artery
Dorsal root ganglion
Internal vertebral venous plexus

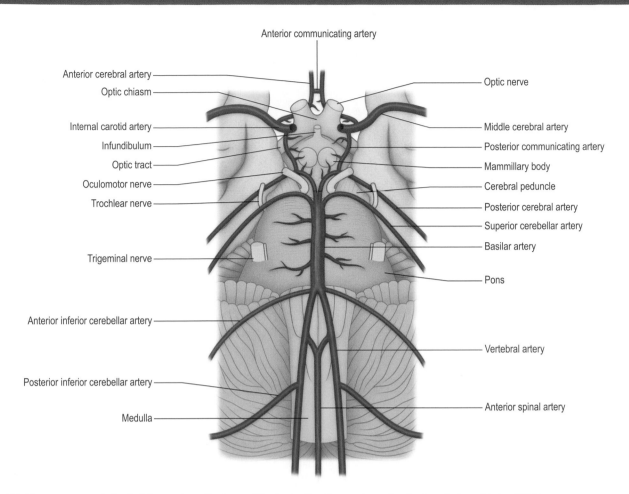

Fig. 7.2 The arrangement of arterial vessels on the base of the brain. The diagram shows the circulus arteriosus (circle of Willis).

posterior spinal veins, which run in the midline. More irregular, sometimes incomplete, bilaterally paired **anterolateral** and **posterolateral veins** are situated near the lines of attachment of the ventral and dorsal nerve roots, respectively. All of these vessels drain via **anterior** and **posterior radicular veins** into the **internal vertebral venous plexus** (epidural venous plexus), which is situated between the dura mater and the vertebral periosteum. The internal venous plexus communicates with an **external vertebral venous plexus** and thence with the ascending lumbar veins, the azygos and hemiazygos veins.

Vasculature of the spinal cord

- The spinal cord is supplied by the anterior and posterior spinal arteries, supplemented by radicular arteries.
- Venous drainage is by anterior and posterior spinal veins, which drain, via radicular veins, into the internal vertebral venous plexus.

Vasculature of the brain

Arterial supply of the brain

The brain is supplied with blood by two pairs of vessels, the **internal carotid arteries** and the **vertebral arteries** (Figs 7.2, 7.3 and see Figs 7.4, 7.6, 7.7). The internal carotid artery arises from the common carotid artery and enters the middle fossa of the cranial cavity through the carotid canal. Its course then follows a series of characteristic bends, known as the **carotid syphon** (Fig. 7.4), after which it passes forwards through the cavernous sinus and then upwards on the medial aspect of the anterior clinoid process, reaching the surface of the brain lateral to the optic chiasm. Along its course, the internal carotid artery gives rise to a number of pre-terminal branches.

- **Hypophyseal arteries** arise from the intra-cavernous section of the internal carotid to supply the neurohypophysis. They also form the pituitary portal system of vessels by which releasing factors are carried from the hypothalamus to the adenohypophysis (Chapter 16).
- The **ophthalmic artery** passes into the orbit through the optic foramen. It supplies the structures of the orbit, the frontal and ethmoidal sinuses, the frontal part of the scalp and dorsum of the nose.
- The **anterior choroidal artery** supplies the optic tract, the choroid plexus of the lateral ventricle, the hippocampus and some of the deep structures of the hemisphere, including the internal capsule and globus pallidus.
- The **posterior communicating artery** passes backwards to join the posterior cerebral artery, thus forming part of the circle of Willis (see below).

Lateral to the optic chiasm, the internal carotid artery divides into its two terminal branches, the **anterior** and **middle cerebral arteries**. The anterior cerebral artery courses medially, above the optic nerve, and then passes into the great longitudinal fissure, between the frontal lobes of the cerebral hemispheres. As it does so, it is joined to the corresponding vessel of the opposite side by the short **anterior communicating artery**. Within the great longitudinal fissure, the anterior cerebral artery follows the dorsal curvature of the corpus callosum (see Fig. 13.23), branches ramifying over the medial surface of the frontal and parietal lobes, which it supplies (Fig. 7.5). The territory supplied by the anterior cerebral artery, therefore, includes the motor and sensory cortices for the lower limb. Fine terminal branches also extend out of the

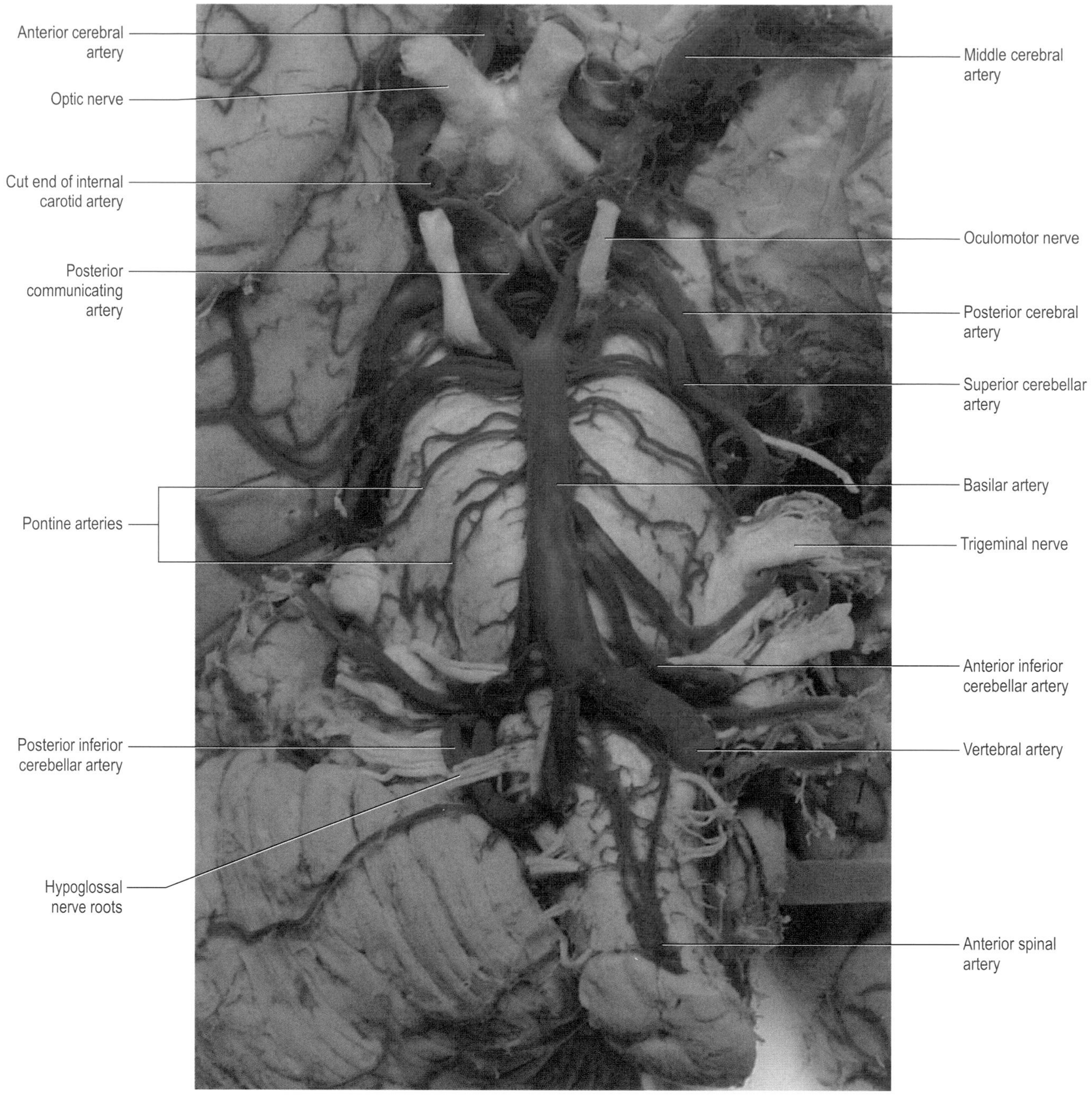

Anterior cerebral artery

Optic nerve

Cut end of internal carotid artery

Posterior communicating artery

Pontine arteries

Posterior inferior cerebellar artery

Hypoglossal nerve roots

Middle cerebral artery

Oculomotor nerve

Posterior cerebral artery

Superior cerebellar artery

Basilar artery

Trigeminal nerve

Anterior inferior cerebellar artery

Vertebral artery

Anterior spinal artery

Fig. 7.3 Arteries on the base of the brain. The arterial system has been injected with a red resin.

great longitudinal fissure to supply a narrow lateral band of frontal and parietal cortices.

The middle cerebral artery is the largest of the three cerebral arteries and its cortical territory is the most extensive (Fig. 7.5). It passes laterally from its origin to enter the lateral fissure within which it subdivides, its branches supplying virtually the whole of the lateral surface of the frontal, parietal and temporal lobes. This territory includes the primary motor and sensory cortices for the whole of the body, excluding the lower limb. It also serves the auditory cortex and the insula within the depths of the lateral fissure.

Since the structures supplied by branches of the internal carotid artery are normally perfused almost entirely from this source, they are often referred to as being supplied by the 'internal carotid system'.

The **vertebral artery** arises from the subclavian artery, ascends through the foramina transversaria of the cervical vertebrae and enters the cranial cavity through the foramen magnum, alongside

the ventrolateral aspect of the medulla (Figs 7.2, 7.3, 7.6, 7.7). Along its course, the vertebral artery gives rise to a number of branches, including the anterior and posterior spinal arteries, which supply the medulla and spinal cord. Its largest branch is the **posterior inferior cerebellar artery**, which supplies the inferior aspect of the cerebellum. As they pass rostrally, the two vertebral arteries converge, uniting at the junction of the medulla and pons to form the midline **basilar artery**.

The basilar artery runs the length of the pons, which it supplies by means of many small pontine branches. It also gives rise to the **anterior inferior cerebellar artery**, which supplies the anterior and inferior portion of the cerebellum, and the **labyrinthine artery**, which passes into the internal acoustic meatus to supply the inner ear. At the junction of the pons and midbrain, the basilar artery divides into two pairs of vessels, the **superior cerebellar arteries** and the **posterior cerebral arteries**. The superior cerebellar artery supplies the superior aspect of the cerebellum. The posterior cerebral artery curves around the

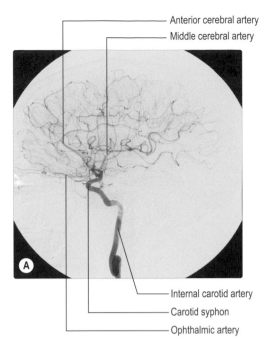

Anterior cerebral artery
Middle cerebral artery

Internal carotid artery
Carotid syphon
Ophthalmic artery

(A)

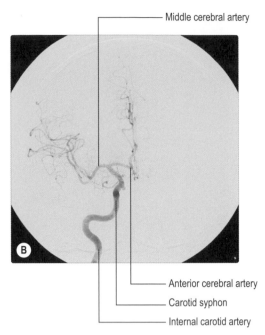

Middle cerebral artery

Anterior cerebral artery
Carotid syphon
Internal carotid artery

(B)

Fig. 7.4 Carotid angiograms. Radio-opaque material has been introduced into the internal carotid artery in order to display its intra-cranial course and the distribution of its branches. **(A)** Left carotid, lateral view; **(B)** right carotid, frontal view. *(Courtesy of Professor PD Griffiths, Academic Unit of Radiology, University of Sheffield, Sheffield, UK).*

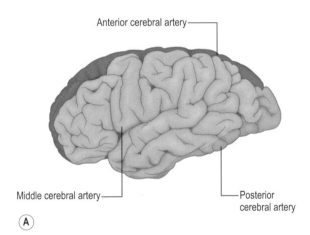

Anterior cerebral artery

Middle cerebral artery
Posterior cerebral artery

(A)

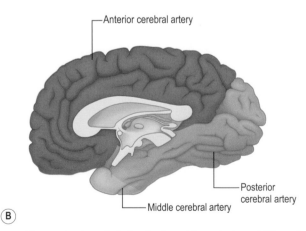

Anterior cerebral artery

Posterior cerebral artery
Middle cerebral artery

(B)

Fig. 7.5 The cerebral cortical distribution of the anterior, middle and posterior cerebral arteries. (A) Lateral aspect; **(B)** medial aspect.

midbrain to supply the visual cortex of the occipital lobe and the inferomedial aspect of the temporal lobe (Fig. 7.5).

The brain regions (brainstem, cerebellum and occipital lobe) served by the vertebral and basilar arteries and their branches are described as being supplied by the 'vertebrobasilar system'.

The internal carotid and vertebrobasilar systems are joined by two thin vessels, the **posterior communicating arteries**, which pass rostrocaudally between the ends of the internal carotid arteries and the posterior cerebral arteries.

This completes an anastomosis of vessels on the base of the brain, known as the **circulus arteriosus** or **circle of Willis** (Figs 7.2, 7.3), which encircles the optic chiasm and the floor of the hypothalamus and midbrain. The anastomotic arrangement of vessels provides the possibility that obstruction or narrowing of the proximal parts of the cerebral arteries, which would be expected to lead to insufficiency in the perfusion of their territories, might be compensated for by circulation of blood through the communicating arteries. The actual significance of this arrangement is dependent on the size of the communicating arteries, which is highly variable between individuals. From the arteries that constitute the circle of Willis, numerous small vessels penetrate the surface of the brain. These are known as **perforating arteries** (also central or ganglionic arteries) and consist of two main groups:

1. **Anterior perforating arteries**, arising from the anterior cerebral artery, anterior communicating artery and the region of origin of the middle cerebral artery. They enter the brain in the region between the optic chiasm and the termination of the olfactory tract, known as the **anterior perforated substance** (see Fig. 16.17). These vessels supply large parts of the basal ganglia, the optic chiasm, the internal capsule and the hypothalamus.

2. **Posterior perforating arteries**, arising from the posterior cerebral and posterior communicating arteries. They enter the brain in the region between the two crura cerebri of the midbrain, known as the **posterior perforated substance** (see Fig. 16.17), to supply the ventral portion of the midbrain and parts of the subthalamus and hypothalamus.

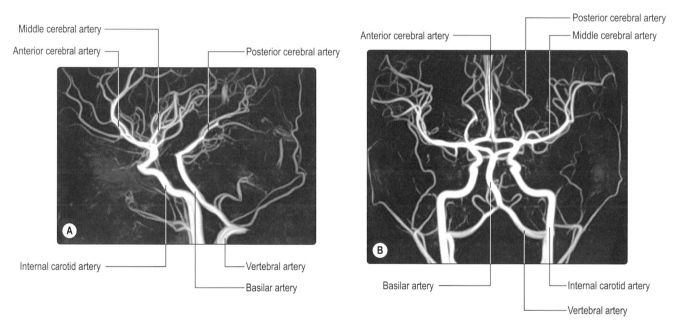

Fig. 7.6 Vertebral angiograms. Radio-opaque material has been introduced into the vertebral artery in order to display its intra-cranial course and the distribution of its branches. (A) Lateral view; (B) frontal view. *(Courtesy of Professor PD Griffiths, Academic Unit of Radiology, University of Sheffield, Sheffield, UK).*

Fig. 7.7 'Time-of-flight' MR arteriograms. The scans were performed on a 3.0T MR scanner. This method does not require the injection of contrast media into the patient; instead it relies on complex MR sequences to produce signal from structures with flow, while suppressing signal from stationary tissues. (A) Lateral view; (B) frontal view. *(Courtesy of Professor PD Griffiths, Academic Unit of Radiology, University of Sheffield, Sheffield, UK).*

Disorders of the blood supply of the brain

One of the most common causes of neurological disability is **stroke**, resulting from blockage or rupture of vessels in the cerebral circulation. The sudden occlusion of a cerebral artery leads to death of brain tissue (**infarction**). Rupture of a blood vessel causes bleeding into the brain (**cerebral haemorrhage**). These events lead to the rapid development of a focal neurological syndrome. Strokes related to the carotid artery and its cerebral branches are associated with focal epilepsy, a contralateral sensory/motor deficit and a psychological deficit (e.g. aphasia). Strokes involving the vertebrobasilar circulation lead to a focal brainstem syndrome. Recovery of function can occur, but it may take up to 2 years and can be incomplete.

An **aneurysm** is an abnormal, balloon-like swelling of an artery. A surgical emergency arises when an aneurysm ruptures and blood projects around the brain in the subarachnoid space (**subarachnoid haemorrhage**) and into the brain (**intracerebral haemorrhage**). A sudden severe headache and neck stiffness are followed by coma and neurological deficits. Neurosurgery or intra-arterial 'coiling' are required to seal the aneurysm to prevent further bleeding and allow recovery.

An **angioma**, or **arteriovenous malformation**, is a congenital collection of swollen blood vessels that can rupture, causing cerebral haemorrhage, or that can 'steal' blood from adjacent brain regions, leading to epilepsy and a focal cerebral syndrome.

Arterial supply of the brain

- The brain is supplied by paired internal carotid and vertebral arteries.

- The internal carotid artery terminates lateral to the optic chiasm, giving rise to the anterior and middle cerebral arteries.

- The anterior cerebral artery passes into the great longitudinal fissure and supplies the medial aspect of the cerebral hemisphere.

- The middle cerebral artery passes into the lateral fissure and supplies the lateral aspect of the cerebral hemisphere.

- The vertebral arteries ascend on the ventrolateral aspect of the medulla, uniting to form the midline basilar artery, which extends the length of the pons. Along their course the vertebral and basilar arteries give rise to branches that supply the cerebellum and brainstem.

- The principal terminal branch of the basilar artery is the posterior cerebral artery, which supplies the occipital lobe of the cerebral hemisphere.

- The anterior communicating artery links together the two anterior cerebral arteries. Posterior communicating arteries pass between the internal carotid artery and the posterior cerebral artery, on each side. This anastomosis of vessels constitutes the circle of Willis.

- Small perforating arteries arise from the circle of Willis to supply the hypothalamic area, the basal ganglia and the internal capsule.

Venous drainage of the brain

Three sorts of vessels contribute to the venous drainage of the brain viz: deep veins, superficial veins and the dural venous sinuses (Figs 7.8–7.10). None of these vessels contains valves.

Deep cerebral veins drain the internal structures of the forebrain (Fig. 7.8). Of particular note are the **thalamostriate vein** and the **choroidal vein**, which drain the basal ganglia, thalamus, internal capsule, choroid plexus and hippocampus. Within each cerebral hemisphere, these vessels merge to form the **internal cerebral vein**. The two internal cerebral veins then unite in the midline to form the **great cerebral vein** (of Galen), which lies beneath the splenium of the corpus callosum. This short vessel is continuous posteriorly with the straight sinus (see below), which lies in the midline of the tentorium cerebelli, along its course of attachment to the posterior part of the falx cerebri.

Superficial veins lie within the subarachnoid space (Fig. 7.9). **Superior cerebral veins** primarily drain the lateral surface of the cerebral hemispheres and empty into the superior sagittal sinus. The **superficial middle cerebral vein** runs along the line of the lateral fissure and empties into the cavernous sinus (see below). In addition, two major anastomotic channels exist, the superior (great) anastomotic vein and the inferior anastomotic vein, which drain into the superior sagittal sinus and the transverse sinus, respectively.

The deep and superficial cerebral veins drain into the **dural venous sinuses** (Figs 7.9, 7.10; see also Chapter 5), which are channels formed between the two layers of dura mater. Major venous sinuses are located in the attached borders of the falx cerebri and the tentorium cerebelli, and on the floor of the cranial cavity.

Along the line where the falx cerebri attaches to the interior of the cranium lies the **superior sagittal sinus**. This receives blood primarily from the superior cerebral veins, which ramify over the lateral surface of the cerebral hemispheres. The free border of the falx encloses the smaller **inferior sagittal sinus**, into which flow veins on the medial aspect of the hemisphere. Within the tentorium cerebelli, along the line of its attachment to the falx, lies the large **straight sinus**. Into this, run both the great cerebral

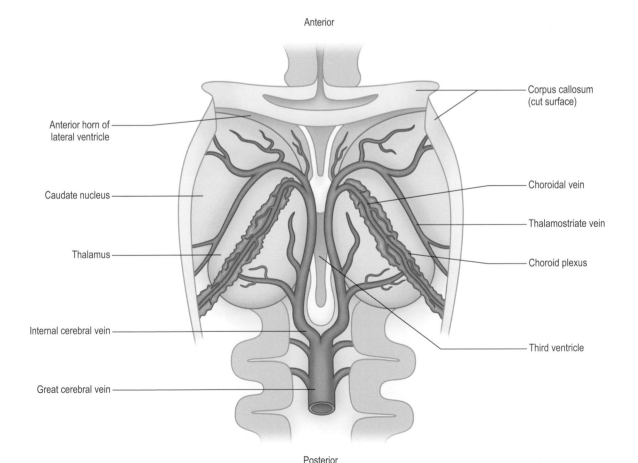

Anterior

Corpus callosum (cut surface)

Anterior horn of lateral ventricle

Caudate nucleus

Thalamus

Internal cerebral vein

Great cerebral vein

Choroidal vein

Thalamostriate vein

Choroid plexus

Third ventricle

Posterior

Fig. 7.8 The deep cerebral veins. The brain is viewed from above and the corpus callosum has been removed to reveal the third and lateral ventricles.

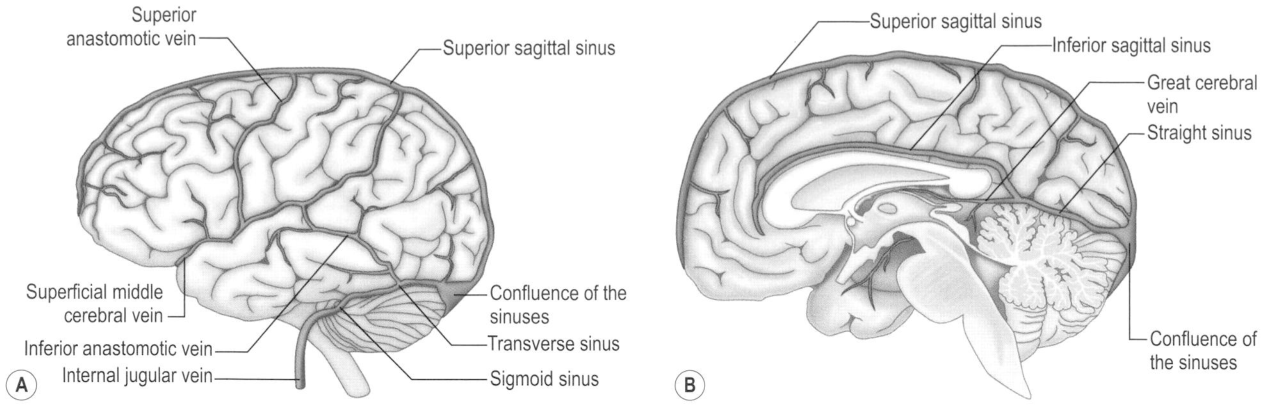

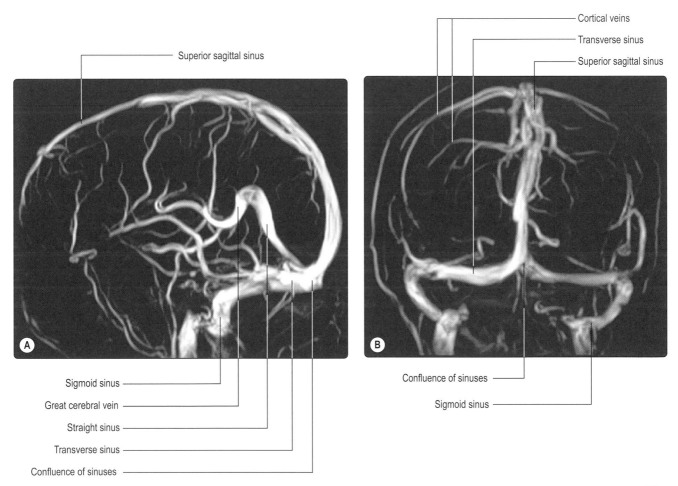

Fig. 7.9 Venous drainage of the brain. (A) Lateral view; **(B)** sagittal view.

In Fig. 7.9 (A), labels: Superior anastomotic vein, Superior sagittal sinus, Superficial middle cerebral vein, Inferior anastomotic vein, Internal jugular vein, Confluence of the sinuses, Transverse sinus, Sigmoid sinus.

In Fig. 7.9 (B), labels: Superior sagittal sinus, Inferior sagittal sinus, Great cerebral vein, Straight sinus, Confluence of the sinuses.

Fig. 7.10 (A) labels: Superior sagittal sinus, Sigmoid sinus, Great cerebral vein, Straight sinus, Transverse sinus, Confluence of sinuses.

Fig. 7.10 (B) labels: Cortical veins, Transverse sinus, Superior sagittal sinus, Confluence of sinuses, Sigmoid sinus.

Fig. 7.10 Phase contrast MR venograms. The scans were performed on a 3.0T MR scanner. (A) Lateral view; (B) frontal view. *(Courtesy of Professor PD Griffiths, Academic Unit of Radiology, University of Sheffield, Sheffield, UK).*

vein, which drains the deep structures of the forebrain, and the inferior sagittal sinus.

The superior sagittal sinus and the straight sinus converge at the **confluence of the sinuses**, which lies adjacent to the internal occipital protuberance (see Fig. 5.1). From here, blood flows laterally on either side in the **transverse sinus**, which lies along the line of attachment of the tentorium to the occipital bone. The transverse sinus is continuous with the **sigmoid sinus**, which, in turn, joins the **internal jugular vein** at the level of the jugular foramen.

The **cavernous sinus** (Fig. 7.11) lies lateral to the body of the sphenoid bone. It receives blood from the middle cerebral vein and drains into the internal jugular vein (via the inferior petrosal sinus) and into the transverse sinus (via the superior petrosal sinus). The two cavernous sinuses are connected by intercavernous sinuses that lie anterior and posterior to the hypophysis, forming a venous circle around it (the circular sinus). The dural venous sinuses are also connected to extracranial veins via **emissary veins**, which pass through the bones of the skull.

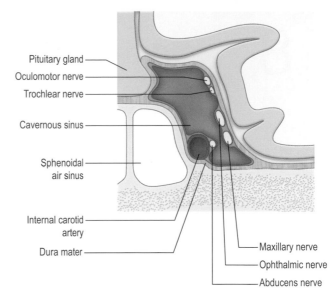

Fig. 7.11 Transverse section through the cavernous sinus.

Labels: Pituitary gland, Oculomotor nerve, Trochlear nerve, Cavernous sinus, Sphenoidal air sinus, Internal carotid artery, Dura mater, Maxillary nerve, Ophthalmic nerve, Abducens nerve

---

Diseases of the venous sinuses

Thrombosis of the sagittal sinuses is a rare complication of childbirth, blood clotting disorders and ear infection. Obstruction of the venous drainage of the brain leads to cerebral swelling (**oedema**) and the syndrome of **raised intracranial pressure**. Cerebral damage caused by venous infarction manifests as epileptic seizures and focal paralysis of the limbs.

In **cavernous sinus thrombosis**, there is acute pain and swelling of the orbit and contents, with ophthalmoplegia, ptosis and numbness of the face.

Venous drainage of the brain

- Venous drainage of the brain involves deep veins, superficial veins and dural venous sinuses.

- Deep cerebral veins drain into the great cerebral vein, which is continuous with the straight sinus.

- Superficial veins empty principally into the superior sagittal sinus and the cavernous sinus.

- The superior sagittal sinus and straight sinuses meet at the confluence of the sinuses.

- From the confluence of the sinuses, venous blood flows, via the transverse sinus and sigmoid sinus, into the internal jugular vein.

The spinal cord and its associated spinal nerves are of immense functional importance. These structures act to:

- Receive afferent fibres from sensory receptors of the trunk and limbs
- Control movements of the trunk and limbs
- Provide autonomic innervation for most of the viscera

The internal organisation of the cord permits many functions to operate in an automatic or reflex fashion. In addition, extensive connections with the brain, through ascending and descending nerve fibre tracts, both convey afferent information to higher centres and mediate their controlling influence over spinal mechanisms.

External features of the spinal cord

Topographical anatomy

The spinal cord occupies the vertebral (or spinal) canal within the vertebral column, which provides support and protection (Figs 8.1, 8.2). Rostrally, the cord is continuous with the medulla oblongata of the brainstem.

The spinal cord is essentially a segmental structure; from rostral to caudal, it consists of 8 cervical (C), 12 thoracic (T), 5 lumbar (L) and 5 sacral (S) segments and 1 coccygeal segment (Fig. 8.3). The cord is approximately cylindrical in shape but its diameter

varies considerably at different levels. It bears two enlargements, cervical and lumbar. The **cervical enlargement** consists of cord segments C4–T1 and provides innervation for the upper limb via the **brachial plexus** (see Fig. 3.11). The **lumbar enlargement** is made up of segments L1–S3 and is associated with innervation of the lower limb via the **lumbosacral plexus** (see Fig. 3.13). Caudal to the lumbar enlargement, the cord tapers abruptly to form a conical termination, the **conus medullaris**. From the tip of the conus, a strand of connective tissue, the **filum terminale** (Fig. 8.4), extends caudally and is attached to the dorsal surface of the first coccygeal vertebra.

Until the third month of fetal life, the spinal cord occupies the entire length of the vertebral canal. Thereafter, the rate of elongation of the vertebral column exceeds that of the spinal cord; as a result, at birth the cord terminates at the level of the third lumbar vertebra and in adult life, it terminates at about the level of the intervertebral disc between L1 and L2 (Figs 8.3, 8.4).

The approximate location of spinal cord segments relative to the bony vertebrae may be identified in the living adult subject by reference to the posterior spinous processes of the vertebrae. As a rule of thumb, cervical cord segments lie approximately one spine higher than their corresponding vertebrae (e.g. C7 cord segment lies adjacent to C6 vertebra), thoracic segments lie approximately two spines higher, and lumbar segments three to four spines higher than their corresponding vertebrae (Fig. 8.3).

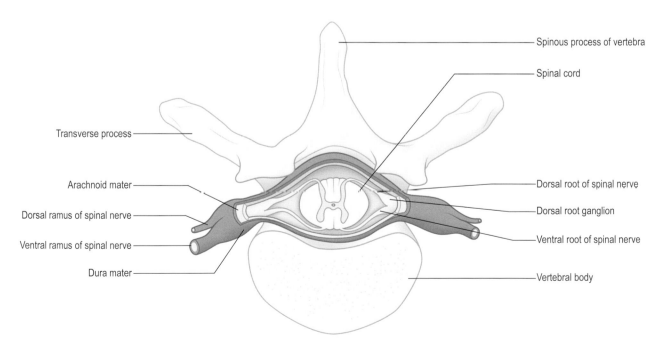

Fig. 8.1 Transverse section through the thoracic region. The diagram shows the relationship between the spinal cord, spinal nerves and vertebral column.

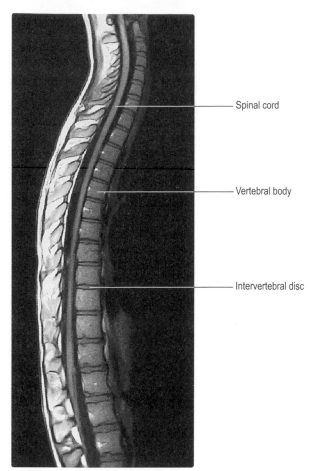

Fig. 8.2 MR image of the vertebral column and spinal cord in the living subject. *(Courtesy of Professor A Jackson, Wolfson Molecular Imaging Centre, University of Manchester, Manchester, UK.)*

Spinal cord

Vertebral body

Intervertebral disc

Topographical anatomy

- The spinal cord provides sensory, motor and autonomic innervation for the trunk and limbs.

- The cord possesses two enlargements: cervical (C4–T1),

  associated with innervation of the upper limbs, and lumbar (L1–S3), innervating the lower limbs.

- The cord terminates at vertebral level L1–L2 in the adult.

Spinal nerves

The spinal cord bears 31 bilaterally paired spinal nerves, each pair being associated with its corresponding cord segment. The spinal nerves originate as two linear series of nerve fascicles, or rootlets, attached to the dorsolateral and ventrolateral aspects of the cord (Fig. 8.5). Groups of six to eight contiguous fascicles that are attached to each cord segment coalesce to form **dorsal** and **ventral nerve roots**. The dorsal and ventral roots of each cord segment then pass to their corresponding **intervertebral foramen** (Fig. 8.6), in or near which they join to form the spinal nerve proper. While the spinal nerves are mixed nerves, containing both afferent and efferent neurones, the dorsal and ventral roots are functionally distinct. The dorsal roots contain **primary afferent neurones**, running from peripheral sensory receptors to the spinal cord and brainstem. The nerve cell bodies of these neurones are located in **dorsal root ganglia** (Fig. 8.1; see also Fig. 1.10), which appear as small enlargements on the dorsal roots near their convergence with the ventral roots at the entrance to the intervertebral foramina. The ventral roots of the spinal nerves carry **efferent neurones**, the cell bodies of which are located in

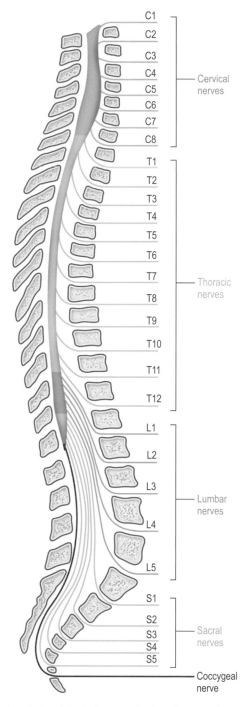

Fig. 8.3 The relationships between spinal cord segments, spinal nerves and vertebral column.

the spinal grey matter. These are comprised of motor neurones, which innervate skeletal muscle, and preganglionic neurones of the autonomic nervous system.

The C1–C7 spinal nerves exit from the vertebral canal above the first seven cervical vertebrae; C8 spinal nerve exits below the seventh cervical vertebra and the remainder leave below their corresponding vertebrae (Fig. 8.3). Because of the different lengths of the spinal cord and the vertebral canal, only in the cervical region do the spinal cord segments lie adjacent to their corresponding vertebral bodies. Below this level, successive spinal nerve roots follow an increasingly oblique and long downwards course to reach their respective intervertebral foramina. This is most marked for the lumbar and sacral roots, which descend below the termination of the cord in a leash-like arrangement, the **cauda equina** (Figs 8.3, 8.4).

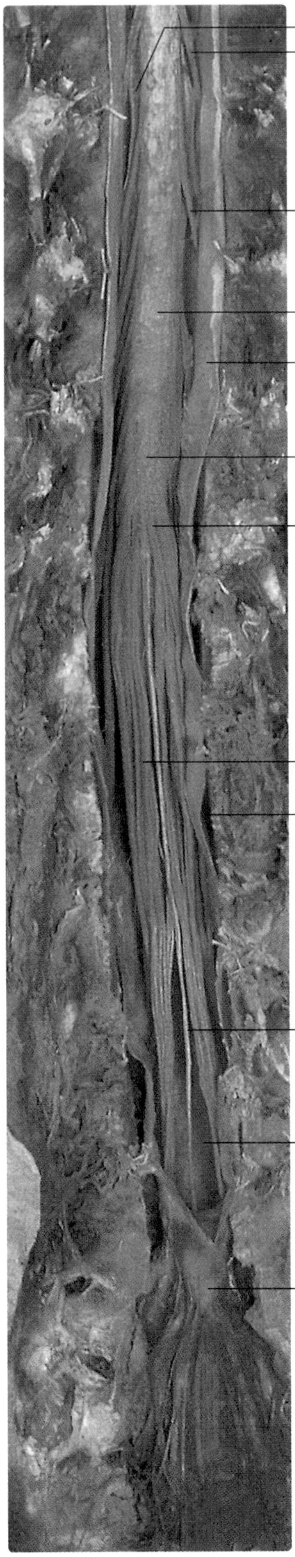
Denticulate ligament
Dorsal roots of spinal nerves
Lumbar enlargement
Dura mater
Conus medullaris
Termination of the spinal cord at L1
Cauda equina
Epidural space
Filum terminale
Subarachnoid space
Termination of the subarachnoid space at S2

Fig. 8.4 Dorsal aspect of the spinal cord caudal to T9–T10. The dura/arachnoid mater have been cut longitudinally and reflected to reveal the spinal cord and nerve roots, including the cauda equina, within the subarachnoid space.

Immediately after leaving the intervertebral foramina, spinal nerves divide to produce a thin **dorsal (posterior) ramus** and a much larger **ventral (anterior) ramus** (Fig. 8.1). The dorsal ramus supplies the muscles and skin of the back region. The ventral ramus supplies the muscles and skin of the front of the body and also the limbs.

Spinal nerve injury

The spinal nerve roots are vulnerable to compression by degenerative changes in the joints of the spinal column (**spondylosis**) and by **prolapse of the intervertebral discs**. Prolapsed intervertebral discs in the cervical spine cause pain in the neck, radiating to the arm and hand, accompanied by tingling sensations (paraesthesiae), weakness and wasting of the muscles corresponding to the radicular distribution, and numbness of the skin corresponding to the dermatomal distribution, together with loss of the tendon reflexes subserved by that particular root (Fig. 8.7). Similarly, lumbar prolapsed intervertebral discs lead to back pain and radiation of pain into the legs, known as **sciatica**. A large lumbosacral prolapsed disc may compress the cauda equina and cause paralysis of the legs and bladder and incontinence, demanding urgent neurosurgery.

The peripheral distribution of spinal nerves, including their pattern of cutaneous innervation (dermatomes) and innervation of muscle groups (myotomes), is described in Chapter 3.

Spinal meninges

The spinal cord, like the brain, is invested by three concentric meningeal coverings: the pia mater, arachnoid mater and dura mater (see Figs 1.17, 8.4, 8.5).

The innermost covering, the pia mater, is a delicate, vascular membrane that is closely applied to the surface of the cord and nerve roots. Along a line midway between the dorsal and ventral roots of the spinal nerves is attached a flat, membranous continuation of the pia, called the **denticulate ligament**. The ligament has a free lateral border for much of its length but, intermittently, lateral projections tether the spinal cord to the arachnoid, and through it to the dura (Figs 8.4, 8.5).

The arachnoid mater lies between the pia and dura. It is a translucent membrane that invests the cord like a loose-fitting bag. Between the pia and arachnoid lies the subarachnoid space. This contains CSF, which is produced in the cerebral ventricular system (Chapter 6).

The outer covering of the cord, the dura mater, is a tough, fibrous membrane. It envelops the cord loosely, as does the arachnoid with which it is in contact, though separated by a theoretical plane, the **subdural space**. The dura is separated from the bony wall of the vertebral canal by the **epidural space**.

Although the spinal cord terminates at vertebral level L1–L2, the arachnoid and dural sheaths and, therefore, the subarachnoid space continue caudally to S2. As the spinal nerve roots pass towards their intervertebral foramina they evaginate the arachnoid and dura, forming meningeal root sleeves that extend as far as the fusion of dorsal and ventral roots. Thereafter, the arachnoid and dura become continuous with the epineurium ensheathing the spinal nerve.

Lumber puncture and epidural anaesthesia

The lowest part of the spinal canal does not contain spinal cord; consequently, hollow needles can be safely inserted into the subarachnoid space in order to remove CSF for diagnostic purposes (**lumbar puncture**) or to inject radio-opaque substances for the radiological delineation of the spinal canal and its contents (**myelography**). Similarly, anaesthetics may be introduced into the epidural space in surgical procedures (**epidural block**).

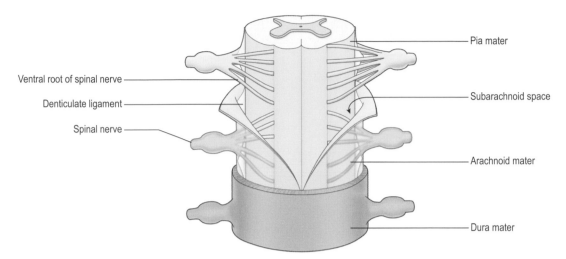

Fig. 8.5 **Ventral aspect of the spinal cord, showing relationships of the spinal nerve roots and the meninges.**

Pia mater

Ventral root of spinal nerve

Denticulate ligament

Spinal nerve

Subarachnoid space

Arachnoid mater

Dura mater

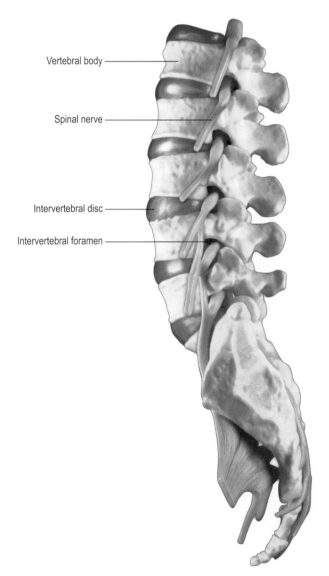

Vertebral body

Spinal nerve

Intervertebral disc

Intervertebral foramen

Fig. 8.6 **Lateral aspect of the spinal column in the lumbar region, illustrating the intervertebral foramina and the emerging spinal nerves.**

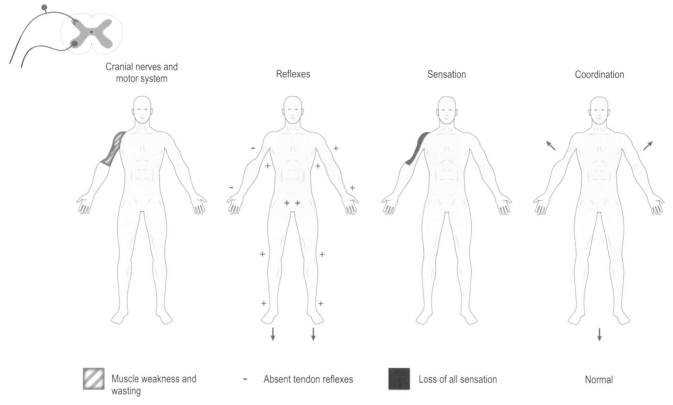

Cranial nerves and motor system   Reflexes   Sensation   Coordination

Muscle weakness and wasting   − Absent tendon reflexes   Loss of all sensation   Normal

Fig. 8.7 Spinal nerve root lesion at the level of C5. Refer also to Fig. 1.48.

Spinal nerves and meninges

- The 31 pairs of spinal nerves attach to the spinal cord as dorsal and ventral roots, carrying afferent and efferent nerve fibres, respectively.

- The cell bodies of afferent neurones are located in dorsal root ganglia. The cell bodies of efferent neurones reside in the spinal grey matter.

- Spinal nerves exit the vertebral canal via intervertebral foramina.

- Below the termination of the cord, spinal nerve roots descend as the cauda equina.

- The cord and nerve roots are susceptible to traumatic injury, e.g. prolapsed intervertebral discs, cervical spondylosis, spinal dislocation.

- The cord is invested by three meninges (pia, arachnoid and dura mater).

- The subarachnoid space contains CSF.

- CSF may be removed by lumbar puncture at L2–L3 or L3–L4.

- Epidural anaesthesia of lumbar and sacral spinal nerves is possible at the same level.

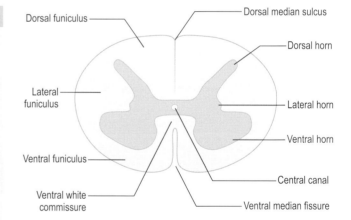

Fig. 8.8 Transverse section through the spinal cord showing the general disposition of grey and white matter.

Internal structure of the spinal cord

The spinal cord is incompletely divided into two symmetrical halves by a **dorsal median sulcus** and a **ventral median fissure** (Fig. 8.8). In the centre of the cord is the small **central canal**, which is continuous rostrally with the cerebral ventricular system. Surrounding the central canal is the spinal **grey matter**, consisting of nerve cell bodies, their dendrites and synaptic contacts. The outer part of the cord consists of **white matter**, which contains ascending and descending nerve fibres. Some of these serve to join neighbouring and distant cord segments for the integration of their functions, while others run between the cord and the brain. Many of the fibres that share a common origin, course and termination are grouped together in fascicles, forming the long **tracts** of the spinal cord.

Different cord levels vary in the relative amounts and configuration of grey and white matter (Fig. 8.9). Higher levels contain greater amounts of white matter. This is because ascending tracts gain fibres at each successive level, whereas the opposite is true of descending tracts.

Grey matter of the spinal cord

The grey matter is approximately H-shaped, or butterfly-shaped, with four protrusions, the **dorsal (posterior)** and **ventral (anterior) horns**, extending dorso- and ventrolaterally towards the attachment zones of the dorsal and ventral root fascicles, respectively. The size and shape of the dorsal and ventral horns varies according to the level (Fig. 8.9). Many afferent nerve fibres entering via the dorsal roots terminate in the dorsal horn, while the ventral horn contains the cell bodies of motor neurones that exit through the ventral nerve roots and innervate skeletal muscle. Both dorsal and ventral horns are, therefore, particularly well-developed at cervical and lumbar levels, in association with innervation of the upper and lower limbs. Thoracic and upper lumbar segments additionally possess a small **lateral** or intermediolateral horn, located between the dorsal and ventral horns, that contains the cell bodies of **preganglionic sympathetic neurones** (Figs 8.8, 8.9B).

The grey matter of the spinal cord may be divided, on the basis of its cytoarchitecture, into ten zones, known as **Rexed's laminae**, which are numbered sequentially from dorsal to ventral (Fig. 8.10). Some of these laminae are equated with cell groupings of particular functional types.

Dorsal horn

Afferent fibres entering through the dorsal roots divide into ascending and descending branches. They mostly terminate near their point of entry but may travel for varying distances in either direction, running in the **dorsolateral fasciculus** or **Lissauer's tract**, which is located superficial to the tip of the dorsal horn (see Fig. 8.15). Dorsal root afferents may, therefore, establish synaptic contacts over several segments of spinal grey matter. Dorsal root fibres terminate extensively within the grey matter but most densely in the dorsal horn. Cutaneous afferents tend to terminate in superficial (dorsal) laminae, while proprioceptive and muscle afferents project mostly to deeper laminae.

The tip of the dorsal horn, approximating to Rexed's lamina II, is also known as the **substantia gelatinosa**. This region receives collaterals of the smallest diameter myelinated (group A delta) and unmyelinated (group C) afferents that are associated with nociception. These neurones are excitatory and use glutamic acid and the peptide substance P as neurotransmitters. In the substantia gelatinosa, complex interactions occur with other types of afferent terminal, interneurones, and with descending pathways from the brain, which control the transmission of pain information to ascending spinothalamic and spinoreticular tract neurones. The cell bodies of these ascending tract neurones are distributed throughout the dorsal horn but are most concentrated in the region of lamina III, also known as the **nucleus proprius** (Fig. 8.11). The modulation of ascending nociceptive information by synaptic interactions in the dorsal horn is often referred to as the 'gate

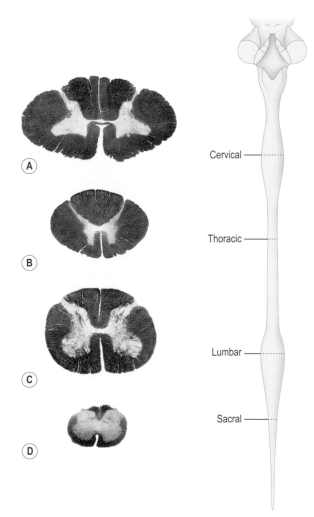

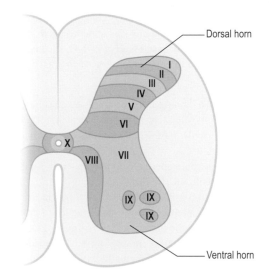

Fig. 8.10 **Lamination of spinal grey matter (Rexed's laminae).**

Fig. 8.9 **Transverse sections through the spinal cord at (A) cervical, (B) thoracic, (C) lumbar and (D) sacral levels.** The histological method employed (Weigert–Pal) stains white matter (myelinated nerve fibres), leaving grey matter (nerve cell bodies) relatively unstained.

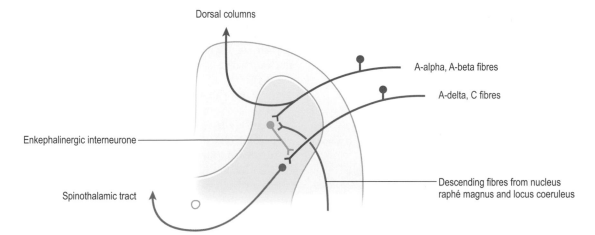

Fig. 8.11 **Simplified neuronal connections within the dorsal horn that modulate the transmission of nociceptive input.**

control' of pain. For example, input from large diameter afferents (groups A-alpha and A-beta), carrying tactile information, inhibits transmission of nociceptive impulses to ascending tract neurones, which is thought to explain why rubbing a sore spot can relieve pain. The basic mechanism underlying this phenomenon is that the large diameter afferents excite dorsal horn interneurones that use the endogenous opioid peptide enkephalin as a neurotransmitter. These interneurones in turn establish presynaptic contacts with the terminals of nociceptive primary afferent neurones. By the process of presynaptic inhibition, they decrease the release of transmitter from these afferent terminals and, thus, decrease the excitation of ascending tract neurones. Certain descending pathways from the brain can also profoundly influence the transmission of nociceptive information at this level. Thus descending serotonergic fibres originating from the nucleus raphé magnus of the medulla (see Figs 9.6, 9.15) and noradrenergic fibres from the locus coeruleus of the upper pons (see Figs 9.10, 9.16) can excite the enkephalinergic dorsal horn interneurones, thereby inhibiting the onward transmission of nociceptive input. The action of endogenous enkephalin is via opiate receptors located on the terminals of nociceptive primary afferents. The analgesic properties of opiate agonists, such as morphine, are partly a result of their action at this site.

Deeper in the dorsal horn, lamina VII contains a number of important cell groups. At cord levels C8–L3 lie the cells of **Clarke's column** (thoracic nucleus, nucleus dorsalis), which are the origin of ascending fibres of the dorsal spinocerebellar tract. The cells of Clarke's column receive afferent input from muscle spindles, Golgi tendon organs, tactile and pressure receptors. At thoracic and upper lumbar levels, the lateral part of lamina VII also contains preganglionic sympathetic neurones that constitute the lateral horn, while at sacral levels (S2–S4), it contains preganglionic parasympathetic neurones.

Ventral horn

In the ventral horn, lamina IX corresponds to groups of motor neurones that innervate skeletal muscle. These are of two types:
1. **Alpha motor neurones**, which innervate extrafusal muscle fibres
2. **Gamma motor neurones**, which innervate intrafusal muscle fibres (within muscle spindles)

The ventral horn is particularly well-developed in the cervical and lumbar enlargements, owing to the presence of motor neurones innervating the upper and lower limbs, respectively. Generally speaking, neurones innervating axial musculature (neck and trunk) tend to be located medially, while those innervating limb muscles are positioned more laterally. In the ventral horn of cord segments C3–C5 is located the **phrenic nucleus**, a group of motor neurones that innervate the diaphragm via the phrenic nerve and are, thus, essential for breathing. Cells in the ventral horn receive direct input from certain dorsal root afferents (e.g. from muscle spindles for mediation of the stretch reflex). Importantly, they also receive input from pathways descending from higher centres concerned with motor control.

Grey matter of the spinal cord

- Internally, the spinal cord consists of a central core of grey matter (cell bodies and synaptic connections) and an outer mantle of white matter (nerve fibres).

- Within the grey matter, the dorsal horn is the main site of termination of primary afferent fibres. It includes the substantia gelatinosa, which is important in the transmission of nociceptive impulses to the brain.

- The lateral horn contains preganglionic sympathetic neurones.

- The ventral horn contains alpha and gamma motor neurones, also known as lower motor neurones.

 Motor neuronopathies

The lower motor neurones of the spinal cord may be selectively affected by two diseases:

Poliomyelitis is an acute viral infection of neurones, leading to rapid paralysis and wasting of the limb and respiratory muscles. The disability is often asymmetrical and frequently affects the legs. Recovery occurs but may be incomplete.

Motor neurone disease is a chronic degenerative disorder that affects both lower motor neurones and the descending tracts to the spinal cord (upper motor neurones). Degeneration of ventral horn cells causes weakness, wasting, hypotonia and fasciculation of the limb muscles (**progressive muscular atrophy**). Degeneration of descending pathways leads to weakness and spasticity of the limb muscles (**primary lateral sclerosis**). With progression, both upper and lower motor neurones degenerate (**amyotrophic lateral sclerosis**).

Spinal reflexes

A reflex is an involuntary, stereotyped pattern of response brought about by a sensory stimulus. Although the qualitative nature of an established reflex response is constant, it may vary considerably in a quantitative sense (e.g. in delay, duration and extent), as a result of intersegmental and supraspinal influences.

Anatomically, the pathways mediating reflex actions consist of afferent neurones conveying impulses from sensory receptors to the CNS (spinal cord or brainstem) and efferent neurones running from the CNS to the effector organ (muscle or gland). In all but the simplest reflexes, interneurones within the CNS are interposed between the afferent and efferent components. The internal organisation of the spinal cord and brainstem thus subserves a number of more or less complex reflex functions, some of which are both relatively well-understood and clinically important.

Stretch reflex

If a muscle with intact innervation is stretched, it responds by contracting, and this is known as the **stretch** or **myotatic reflex**. Anatomically, this is the simplest of reflexes. It is mediated by just two neurones – one afferent and one efferent – which are linked to form a **monosynaptic reflex arc** (Fig. 8.12). The reflex arc consists of afferent neurones that convey impulses from muscle stretch receptors to the CNS and motor neurones that convey impulses back to the muscle.

The stretch receptors within muscles consist of sensory nerve endings that attach to the central, non-contractile, region of specialised muscle cells called **intrafusal muscle fibres** (see also Chapter 3). Intrafusal muscle fibres are oriented parallel to the long axis of the muscle and occur in encapsulated groups called **muscle spindles**. Stretch applied to the muscle in which they lie stimulates the sensory endings. Their afferent fibres carry impulses to the CNS, where they make monosynaptic excitatory contact with the alpha motor neurones that innervate the **extrafusal muscle fibres** comprising the bulk of the same muscle, causing them to contract.

There are two types of intrafusal muscle fibre: **nuclear bag** and **nuclear chain** fibres. These bear two types of sensory ending (see Fig. 3.4):
1. **Primary** or **annulospiral endings**. These are mostly associated with nuclear bag muscle fibres and give rise to group Ia afferent nerve fibres.
2. **Secondary** or **flower-spray endings**. These are mostly associated with nuclear chain muscle fibres and give rise to group II afferents.

Primary endings are exquisitely sensitive to the velocity of stretch and they desensitise rapidly once the new muscle length is achieved. For this reason, they are sometimes called 'dynamic endings'. Secondary endings essentially only signal changes in muscle length, but not the rate of change, and they desensitise slowly. They are sometimes referred to as 'static endings'.

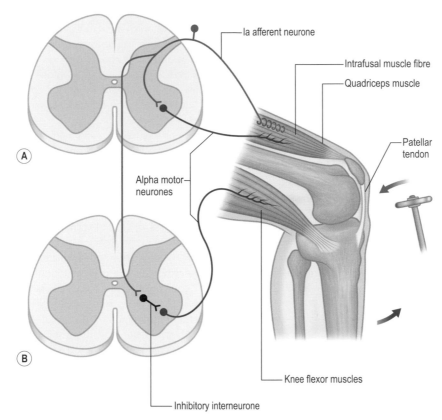

Fig. 8.12 The stretch reflex and reciprocal innervation. (A) The quadriceps stretch reflex is illustrated, whereby striking the patellar tendon elicits extension of the knee. **(B)** Reciprocal innervation. While stretching of the quadriceps muscle causes its reflex contraction, the motor neurones of antagonistic muscles (knee flexors) are inhibited by interneuronal connection within the spinal cord.

Stretch reflexes are crucially important for the control of skeletal muscle tone. The term muscle tone refers to the degree of contraction of a muscle or, in other words, the proportion of motor units that are active at any one time. Muscle tone is reflected in the compliance of the muscle on palpation and its resistance to passive stretch/movement. Thus a muscle with high tone feels firm, or rigid, and resists passive stretch, while a muscle with low tone is soft, or flaccid, and offers little resistance to passive stretch. Since stretch reflexes operate to maintain muscles at a constant length in opposition to imposed stretch, they are important in the control of body posture. By their action, activity is maintained in neck, trunk and lower limb extensor muscles (anti-gravity muscles) that support an upright body posture against the force of gravity and are stretched when these body parts become flexed.

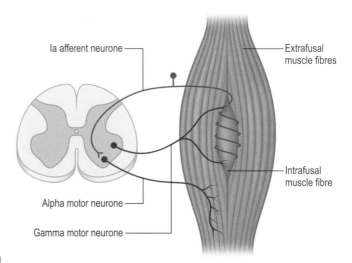

Fig. 8.13 Gamma reflex loop.

Tendon reflexes

Tendon reflexes (deep tendon reflexes or tendon jerks) are monosynaptic stretch reflexes, elicited during clinical examination, by percussion of the tendon of a muscle. This causes rapid, brief stimulation of dynamic stretch receptors. Each tendon reflex is subserved by specific spinal cord segments:

Reflex	Cord segments
Biceps reflex (biceps jerk)	C5/C6
Brachioradialis reflex (supinator jerk)	C5/C6
Triceps reflex (triceps jerk)	C6/**C7**
Quadriceps reflex (knee jerk)	L3/L4
Achilles tendon reflex (ankle jerk)	**S1**/S2

In addition to alpha motor neurones, which innervate extrafusal muscle fibres, the ventral horn of the spinal cord (and motor cranial nerve nuclei) contain an additional population of efferent neurones – **gamma motor neurones** – which innervate the polar,

contractile elements of intrafusal muscle fibres (Fig. 8.13). The function of gamma motor neurones is to control the sensitivity of the stretch receptors. Thus, when gamma motor neurones are activated, the resultant contraction of the intrafusal muscle fibre applies tension to the sensory endings. This lowers the threshold of the stretch receptors to externally applied stretch and, thus, increases the sensitivity of the stretch reflex. This mechanism is referred to as the **gamma reflex loop** (Fig. 8.13).

There are two types of gamma motor neurone. So-called 'dynamic' gamma motor neurones innervate nuclear bag fibres, while 'static' gamma motor neurones innervate nuclear chain fibres.

Like alpha motor neurones, gamma motor neurones are under the influence of descending pathways from the brain and the two types of motor neurone can be separately controlled. Abnormal activity of these descending pathways, which occurs in many pathological conditions, therefore induces changes in the sensitivity of stretch reflexes. This is evidenced by abnormalities in tendon reflexes and in muscle tone. When upper motor neurones are damaged, for example in stroke, this results in overactivity of dynamic gamma motor neurones. As a consequence, tendon reflexes are hypersensitive (hyperreflexia) and muscle tone is increased during initial muscle stretch (spasticity). In disorders of the basal ganglia, such as Parkinson's disease (Chapter 14), there is overactivity of static gamma motor neurones. This results in hypertonia of muscles throughout the extent of passive movement (rigidity), while the tendon reflexes remain normal.

The tendons of skeletal muscles contain mechanoreceptors called **Golgi tendon organs**. These give rise to class Ib afferent fibres that enter the spinal grey matter and, via an interneurone, inhibit alpha motor neurones running to the muscle of origin. This arrangement is thought to fulfil a protective function and it underlies the abrupt relaxation that occurs, following initial contraction, on rapid passive stretch of a spastic muscle (the **clasp-knife reaction**).

When a stretch reflex is elicited (e.g. the quadriceps reflex, by tapping the patellar tendon), primary afferent fibres from the muscle spindle excite not only the alpha motor neurones of the stretched muscle but also interneurones that inhibit the alpha motor neurones of antagonistic muscles (e.g. the knee flexors, Fig. 8.12). This illustrates the general principle of **reciprocal innervation** of agonist and antagonist muscle groups.

Flexor reflex

Noxious cutaneous stimulation of the limbs causes flexion withdrawal from the offending stimulus. This is mediated by a **polysynaptic reflex**, in which one or more interneurones are interposed between afferent and efferent neurones. Primary afferent fibres activate interneurones within the spinal grey matter, which in turn excite alpha motor neurones innervating the limb flexor muscles (Fig. 8.14). Flexion of a limb about several joints requires the coordinated action of more than one spinal segment and this is achieved by collateralisation of primary afferents and interneurones.

All forms of cutaneous stimulation have the potential to elicit the flexor reflex, but this is normally prevented by descending pathways from the brain, unless the stimulus is painful. In certain pathological conditions, the descending inhibitory influence is lost and even innocuous cutaneous stimulation can cause limb withdrawal. The extensor plantar response (Babinski reflex) is characterised by extension (dorsiflexion) of the great toe and splaying of the other toes in response to stimulation of the sole of the foot. Physiologically, it is a flexor reflex and is present in infants before myelination of the corticospinal tract has taken place. Thereafter, the reflex is absent, being suppressed by descending corticospinal influences (stimulation of the sole of the foot then causing a flexor plantar response, with curling of the toes). When the descending influence is lost (e.g. following a stroke in the internal capsule) the extensor plantar reflex re-emerges. A positive Babinski reflex is regarded as pathognomonic of damage to the corticospinal tract.

Activation of the flexor reflex in a weight-bearing limb (e.g. by standing on a pin) simultaneously causes reflex extension of the contralateral limb to take the weight of the body. This is called the **crossed extensor reflex** (Fig. 8.14). It is mediated by axon collaterals that cross the midline of the cord and excite the alpha motor neurones of contralateral limb extensor muscles.

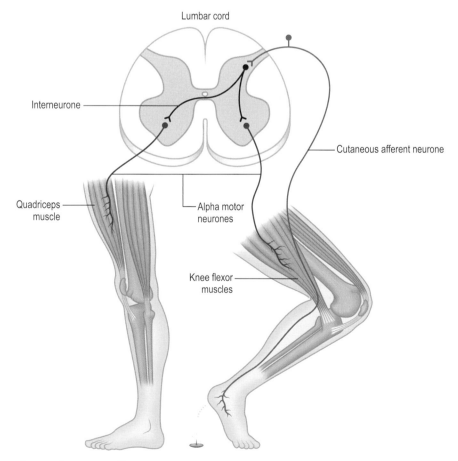

Fig. 8.14 Flexor reflex and crossed extensor reflex.

Spinal reflexes

- The internal organisation of the cord subserves a number of important reflex functions.

- The monosynaptic stretch reflex mediates muscle contraction in response to stretch of muscle spindles.

- The sensitivity of the stretch reflex is regulated by gamma motor neurones, which provide

motor innervation to the spindle fibres.

- The stretch reflex is responsible for maintenance of muscle tone and posture and is clinically tested as the deep tendon reflexes.

- The polysynaptic flexor reflex mediates limb withdrawal from noxious stimuli.

White matter of the spinal cord

The grey matter of the spinal cord is completely surrounded by white matter, which consists of ascending and descending nerve fibres. The white matter of each side can be roughly divided into dorsal, lateral and ventral columns or **funiculi** (sing., funiculus), separated by the dorsal and ventral horns (Fig. 8.8). Nerve fibres sharing common origins, terminations and functions are organised into **tracts** or **fasciculi** (sing., fasciculus: Latin for small bundle). Some fibres interconnect adjacent or distant cord segments and mediate intersegmental coordination, while other fibres are longer and serve to join the spinal cord with the brain. The **intersegmental** (or **propriospinal**) fibres occupy a narrow band immediately peripheral to the grey matter. This is known as the **fasciculus proprius** (Fig. 8.15). Nerve fibres running between the spinal cord and the brain constitute the **ascending** and **descending tracts** of the spinal cord (8.15–8.17 and 8.19–8.24).

Ascending spinal tracts

Ascending tracts carry impulses from pain, thermal, tactile, muscle and joint receptors to the brain. Some of this information eventually reaches a conscious level (the cerebral cortex), while some is destined for subconscious centres (e.g. the cerebellum).

Pathways that carry information to a conscious level share certain common characteristics.

There is a sequence of three neurones between the peripheral receptor and the cerebral cortex.

- The first neurone (**first-order neurone** or **primary afferent neurone**) enters the spinal cord through the dorsal root of a spinal nerve and its cell body lies in a dorsal root ganglion. The central process may collateralise extensively and make synaptic connections that mediate spinal reflexes and intersegmental coordination. The main fibre remains on the ipsilateral side of the cord and terminates in synaptic contact with the second neurone, which is located either in the spinal grey matter or in the medulla oblongata of the brainstem, depending on the modality being served.

- The second neurone (**second-order neurone**) has its cell body in the cord or medulla oblongata. Its axon crosses over (decussates) to the opposite side of the CNS and ascends to the thalamus, where it terminates upon the third neurone.

- The third neurone (**third-order neurone**) has its cell body in the thalamus. Its axon passes to the somatosensory cortex in the parietal lobe of the ipsilateral cerebral hemisphere.

Two main tract systems in the spinal cord fit into this pattern: the dorsal (posterior) columns and the spinothalamic tracts.

Dorsal columns

The **dorsal columns** are located between the dorsal median sulcus and the dorsal horn. The dorsal columns are comprised of two tracts, incompletely separated by a thin septum: the **fasciculus gracilis**, situated medially and the **fasciculus cuneatus**, situated laterally. The tracts carry impulses concerned with proprioception (movement and joint position sense) and discriminative (fine) touch.

The dorsal columns contain the axons of primary afferent neurones that have entered the cord through the dorsal roots of spinal nerves (Fig. 8.16). The fasciculus gracilis consists of fibres that join the cord at sacral, lumbar and lower thoracic levels and, thus, includes those from the lower limb. Fibres of the fasciculus cuneatus enter via the upper thoracic and cervical dorsal roots and, thus, include those from the upper limb. Since the dorsal

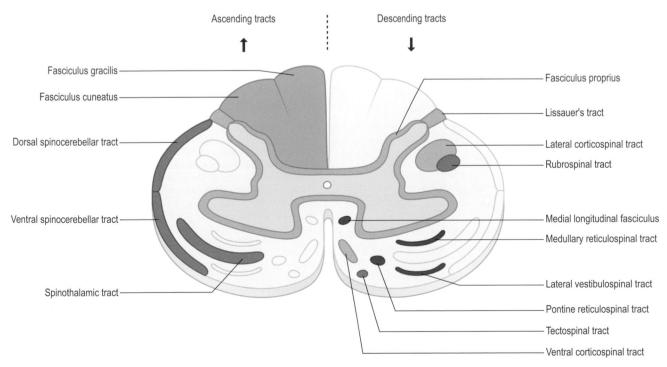

Ascending tracts ↑   Descending tracts ↓

Fasciculus gracilis
Fasciculus cuneatus
Dorsal spinocerebellar tract
Ventral spinocerebellar tract
Spinothalamic tract

Fasciculus proprius
Lissauer's tract
Lateral corticospinal tract
Rubrospinal tract
Medial longitudinal fasciculus
Medullary reticulospinal tract
Lateral vestibulospinal tract
Pontine reticulospinal tract
Tectospinal tract
Ventral corticospinal tract

Fig. 8.15 Ascending and descending tracts of the spinal cord. All ascending and descending tracts are present bilaterally. In this figure, ascending tracts are emphasised on the left side and descending tracts are emphasised on the right side. In addition, the location of Lissauer's tract and the fasciculus proprius (which contain both ascending and descending fibres) are shown.

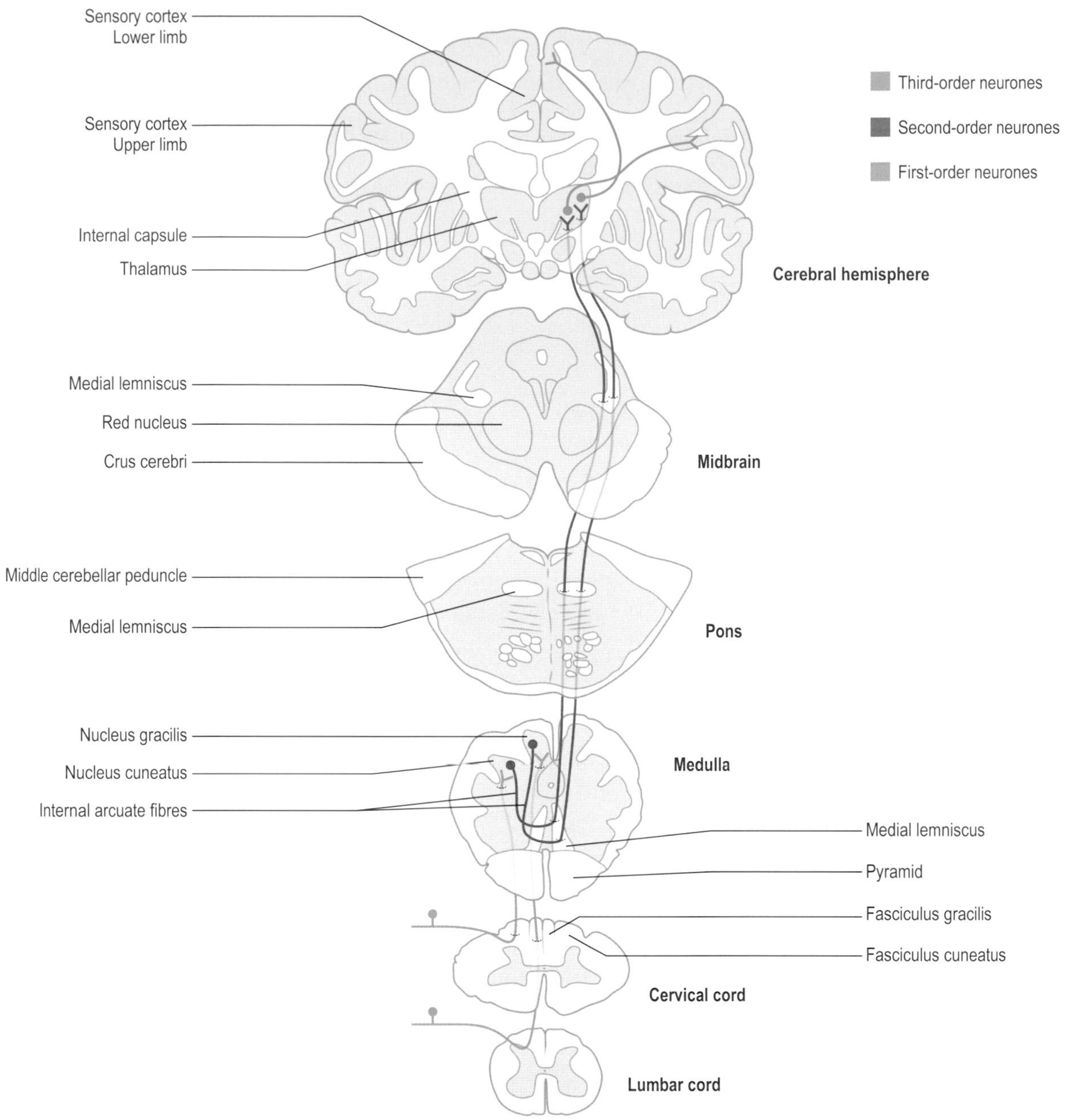

Third-order neurones

Second-order neurones

First-order neurones

Sensory cortex
Lower limb

Sensory cortex
Upper limb

Internal capsule

Thalamus

Cerebral hemisphere

Medial lemniscus

Red nucleus

Crus cerebri

Midbrain

Middle cerebellar peduncle

Medial lemniscus

Pons

Nucleus gracilis

Nucleus cuneatus

Internal arcuate fibres

Medulla

Medial lemniscus

Pyramid

Fasciculus gracilis

Fasciculus cuneatus

Cervical cord

Lumbar cord

Fig. 8.16 Dorsal columns. The central pathways carrying conscious proprioception and discriminative touch are illustrated.

columns contain primary afferent neurones, they carry information relating to the ipsilateral side of the body. Fibres ascend without interruption to the medulla oblongata, where they terminate upon second-order neurones, the cell bodies of which are located in the **nucleus gracilis** and **nucleus cuneatus** (see also Fig. 9.6).

The axons of the second-order neurones decussate in the medulla as **internal arcuate fibres** and, thereafter, ascend through the brainstem as the **medial lemniscus**. The medial lemniscus terminates in the **ventral posterior (VP) nucleus** of the thalamus upon third-order thalamocortical neurones. These in turn project to the somatosensory cortex, located in the postcentral gyrus of the parietal lobe.

Spinothalamic tract

The **spinothalamic tract** (sometimes referred to as the anterolateral system) lies lateral and ventral to the ventral horn of the spinal grey matter. It carries information related to pain and thermal sensations and also non-discriminative (course) touch and pressure. Some authorities identify distinct lateral and ventral spinothalamic tracts conveying pain and temperature or touch and

Lesions of the dorsal columns

Tabes dorsalis is a late manifestation of syphilitic infection of the CNS. It chiefly affects the lumbosacral dorsal spinal roots and the dorsal columns of the spinal cord. The loss of proprioception leads to a high steppage and unsteady gait (**sensory ataxia**), which is exacerbated when the eyes are closed (**Romberg's sign**).

Subacute combined degeneration of the spinal cord is a systemic disease resulting from a deficiency of vitamin B_{12} (cyanocobalamin), which also causes pernicious anaemia. The degeneration of the dorsal columns produces sensory ataxia. The lateral columns of the spinal cord are also involved (combined), causing weakness and spasticity of the limbs. The disorder, although uncommon, is an important one since proper treatment with vitamin B_{12} can lead to complete recovery.

In **multiple sclerosis**, an immune disease, specific damage to the fasciculus cuneatus of the cervical spinal cord leads to loss of proprioception in the hands and fingers, causing profound loss of dexterity and inability to identify the shape and nature of objects by touch alone (**astereognosis**).

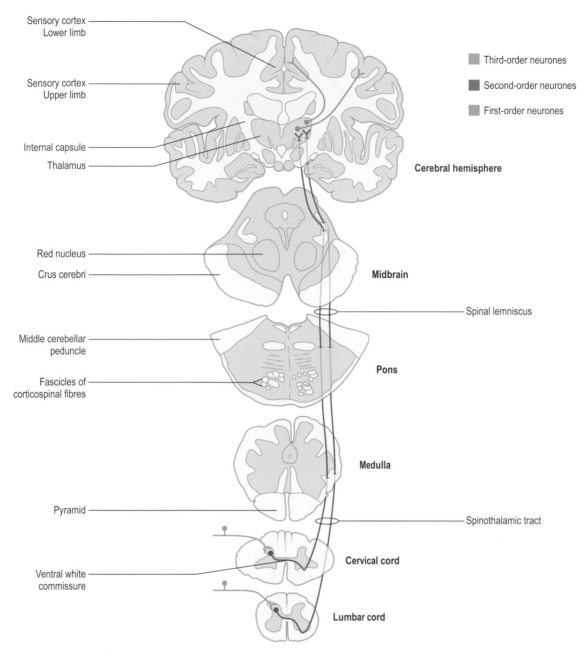

Sensory cortex
Lower limb

Sensory cortex
Upper limb

Internal capsule

Thalamus

Red nucleus

Crus cerebri

Middle cerebellar
peduncle

Fascicles of
corticospinal fibres

Pyramid

Ventral white
commissure

Cerebral hemisphere

Midbrain

Spinal lemniscus

Pons

Medulla

Spinothalamic tract

Cervical cord

Lumbar cord

Third-order neurones

Second-order neurones

First-order neurones

Fig. 8.17 Spinothalamic tract. The central pathways for pain, temperature, touch and pressure are illustrated.

pressure, respectively, but there appears to be little evidence for this in man and fibres carrying these modalities are probably intermingled, at least to some extent.

The spinothalamic tract contains second-order neurones, the cell bodies of which lie widely distributed in the contralateral dorsal horn and receive input from primary afferent fibres that terminate in this region (Fig. 8.17). After leaving the parent cell bodies, spinothalamic axons decussate to the opposite side of the cord by passing through the **ventral white commissure**, which lies ventral to the central canal of the cord, and, thus, enter the contralateral spinothalamic tract. Axons carrying pain and temperature decussate promptly within one segment of their origin, while those carrying touch and pressure may ascend for several segments before crossing.

In the brainstem, the spinothalamic fibres run in close proximity to the medial lemniscus and are known as the **spinal lemniscus**. The majority of fibres terminate in the ventral posterior nucleus of the thalamus, contacting third-order thalamocortical neurones that project to the somatosensory cortex.

The spinothalamic tract is sometimes referred to as the 'neospinothalamic system'. It is highly organised somatotopically; consequently, the location of sensory stimuli, particularly those to the body surface, can be identified with very high accuracy. It is thought to be the route via which sharp, pricking pain (sometimes called 'fast' pain) is conducted.

Spinothalamic tract lesions

The spinothalamic tract can be selectively damaged in **syringomyelia**, in which the central canal becomes enlarged to form a cavity compressing adjacent nerve fibres. The second-order neurones subserving pain and temperature are damaged as they decussate in the ventral white commissure, close to the central canal, causing a selective loss of pain and temperature awareness in the upper limbs. This is termed a **dissociated sensory loss**, since light touch and proprioceptive sensation are retained. The patient injures and burns the hands painlessly, and the joints of the limbs become disorganised without discomfort (**Charcot's joints**).

Selective surgical destruction of the spinothalamic tract (**cordotomy** or **tractotomy**) is sometimes performed for the neurosurgical relief of intractable pain from a variety of causes.

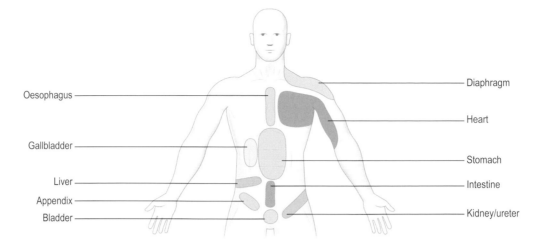

Oesophagus

Gallbladder

Liver

Appendix

Bladder

Diaphragm

Heart

Stomach

Intestine

Kidney/ureter

Fig. 8.18 Principal body regions associated with referred pain from the viscera.

The **spinoreticulothalamic system** represents an additional, phylogenetically older, route by which nociceptive sensory impulses ascend to higher centres. Some second-order neurones arising from the dorsal horn ascend in the ventrolateral region of the cord and then terminate in the brainstem reticular formation, particularly within the medulla. Reticulothalamic fibres then ascend to the intralaminar thalamic nuclei, which in turn activate the cerebral cortex. The spinoreticulothalamic system is poorly organised somatotopically and is thought to be the route via which dull, aching pain (sometimes called 'slow' pain) is transmitted to a conscious level. Activation of spinothalamic and spinoreticular fibres, which may ultimately be perceived as unpleasant or painful, can be modulated by descending pathways from the brain (see Fig. 8.11).

While painful stimuli originating from somatic structures, and particularly from the body surface, can be localised with high precision due to the detailed somatotopic organisation of the ascending pathways and the somatosensory cortex, pain that originates from deep, visceral structures is generally poorly localised. In addition, noxious stimuli originating from visceral structures are sometimes perceived as pain in other parts of the body – a phenomenon known as **'referred pain'** (Fig. 8.18). A classic example is pain from heart disease being felt in the left chest, shoulder and arm. The mechanism underlying referred pain is not entirely understood but it is thought to be due to the convergence of somatic and visceral afferents from corresponding regions onto the same neurones in the dorsal horn of the spinal cord. Such convergence results in misinterpretation as to the source of the noxious stimulus.

Ascending pathways that carry afferent information to a subconscious level are represented principally by the **spinocerebellar tracts**.

Spinocerebellar tracts

Ascending spinocerebellar fibres carry information derived from muscle spindles, mechanoreceptors such as Golgi tendon organs, and tactile receptors, to the cerebellum for the control of posture and the coordination of movement. Four pathways appear to be involved in this process, two carrying information from the lower limb and two from the upper limb. The spinocerebellar system consists of a sequence of only two neurones, the tracts containing second-order neurones whose cell bodies of origin mostly lie in the base of the dorsal horn; they receive input from primary afferent fibres terminating in this region. Some tract axons ascend ipsilateral to their origin while others ascend contralaterally (Fig. 8.19). The dorsal and ventral spinocerebellar tracts are located at the dorsolateral and ventrolateral surfaces of the cord, respectively (see Fig. 8.15) and relay

information from the lower limb. Fibres of the dorsal spinocerebellar tract originate from a prominent group of cells in lamina VII of cord segments T1–L2, known as the thoracic nucleus or **Clarke's column**. The axons ascend ipsilaterally to enter the cerebellum through the **inferior cerebellar peduncle**. Fibres of the ventral spinocerebellar tract originate from cells at lumbosacral cord levels. The fibres decussate, ascend on the contralateral side of the cord and enter the cerebellum via the **superior cerebellar peduncle**. Some axons then re-cross within the cerebellar white matter.

The upper limb equivalent of the dorsal spinocerebellar tract is represented by **cuneocerebellar fibres**. In this pathway, some primary proprioceptive afferents, originating mostly in the cervical enlargement and ascending ipsilaterally in the fasciculus cuneatus (one of the dorsal columns), terminate in the medulla just lateral to the principal cuneate nucleus in a group of cells known as the lateral (external, accessory) cuneate nucleus. From here, axons enter the cerebellum via the inferior cerebellar peduncle. The upper limb equivalent of the ventral spinocerebellar tract is the **rostral spinocerebellar tract**. Axons arise from cells in the cervical enlargement and ascend ipsilaterally in the lateral funiculus, entering the cerebellum mostly through the inferior peduncle.

Spinocerebellar tract neurones terminate in the cerebellar cortex as mossy fibres, predominantly within the vermis and paravermal area.

White matter of the spinal cord: principal ascending tracts

- Ascending tracts carry afferent information to conscious and subconscious levels. Pathways to a conscious level follow a basic plan of three neurones in a sequence from peripheral receptor to cerebral cortex.

- Dorsal columns (fasciculus gracilis and cuneatus) carry proprioception and discriminative touch. They convey first-order neurones ipsilaterally to the nuclei gracilis and cuneatus of the medulla. Second-order neurones decussate and pass to the thalamus. Third-order neurones project to the somatosensory cortex. Lesions (e.g. tabes dorsalis, vitamin B_{12} deficiency) lead to ataxia and loss of discriminative touch ipsilaterally.

- Spinothalamic tract carries pain, temperature, touch and pressure. The tract contains second-order neurones with cell bodies in the dorsal horn. Axons decussate and pass to the thalamus. Third-order neurones project to the somatosensory cortex. Lesions (e.g. syringomyolia) lead to impairment of pain, temperature, touch and pressure sensitivity on the contralateral side.

- Spinocerebellar tracts contain second-order neurones carrying muscle, joint and tactile information involved in motor control. Lesions lead to ataxia (e.g. Friedreich's ataxia).

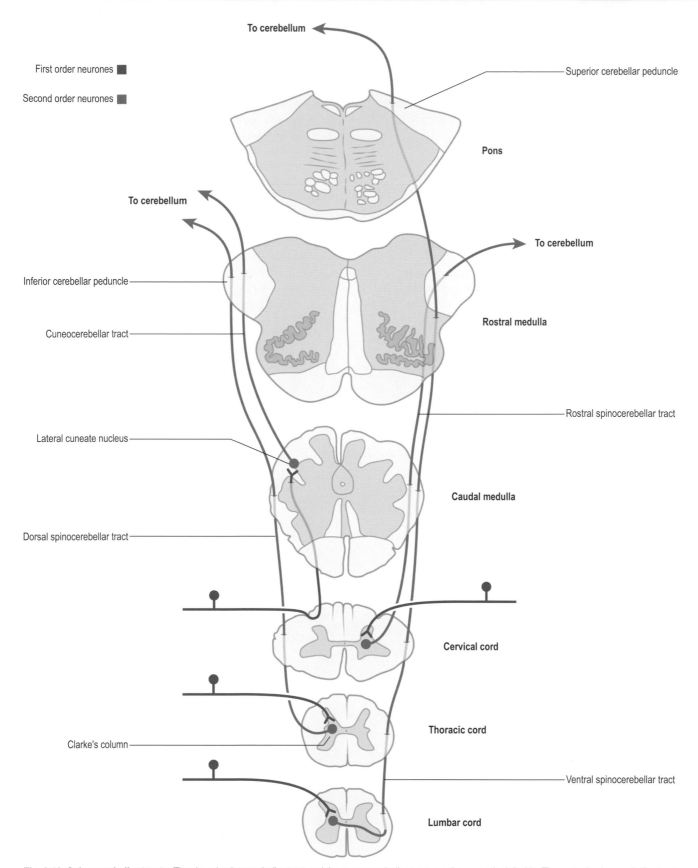

First order neurones ■

Second order neurones ■

To cerebellum

Superior cerebellar peduncle

Pons

To cerebellum

To cerebellum

Inferior cerebellar peduncle

Rostral medulla

Cuneocerebellar tract

Rostral spinocerebellar tract

Lateral cuneate nucleus

Caudal medulla

Dorsal spinocerebellar tract

Cervical cord

Clarke's column

Thoracic cord

Ventral spinocerebellar tract

Lumbar cord

Fig. 8.19 Spinocerebellar tracts. The dorsal spinocerebellar tract and the cuneocerebellar tract are shown on the left side. The ventral spinocerebellar tract and the rostral spinocerebellar tract are shown on the right side.

Descending spinal tracts

Descending tracts of the spinal cord (see Fig. 8.15) originate from the cerebral cortex and brainstem. They are concerned with the control of movement, muscle tone, spinal reflexes, spinal autonomic functions and the modulation of sensory transmission to higher centres.

Corticospinal tracts

The **corticospinal tracts** (Figs. 8.20, 8.21) are particularly concerned with the control of voluntary, discrete, skilled movements, especially those of the distal parts of the limbs. Such movements are sometimes referred to as 'fractionated' movements. Corticospinal tract neurones arise from cell bodies in the cerebral cortex. The cells of origin are widely distributed in the motor and sensory cortices, including the **precentral gyrus** or **primary motor cortex** of the frontal lobe, where the large **Betz cells** give rise to the largest-diameter corticospinal axons. Corticospinal axons leave the cerebral hemispheres by passing through the massive subcortical fibre systems of the **corona radiata** and **internal capsule** to enter the **crus cerebri** of the midbrain (Fig. 8.21).

They then pass through the ventral portion of the pons to reach the medulla oblongata, where they form two prominent columns on its ventral surface. These are called the **pyramids** and, for this reason, the term **pyramidal tract** is used as an alternative name for the corticospinal tract. In the caudal medulla, the fibres within the pyramids undergo subtotal decussation. About 75% to 90% of fibres decussate and enter the contralateral **lateral corticospinal tract**, which is located in the lateral part of the spinal white matter, deep to the dorsal spinocerebellar tract; 10% to 25% of pyramidal fibres remain ipsilateral and enter the **ventral**

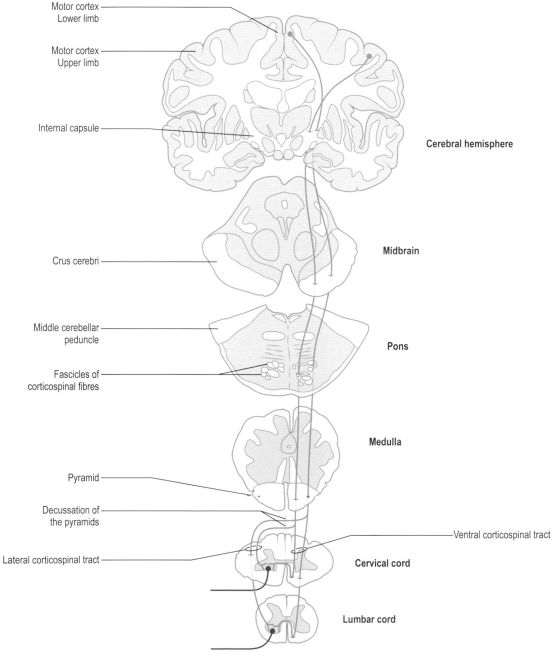

Fig. 8.20 Corticospinal tracts.

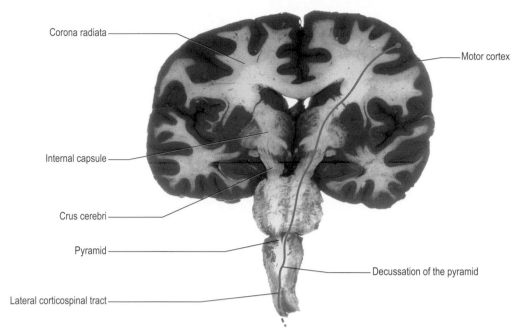

Corona radiata

Motor cortex

Internal capsule

Crus cerebri

Pyramid

Decussation of the pyramid

Lateral corticospinal tract

Fig. 8.21 The course of the corticospinal tract superimposed upon a coronal section of the brain.

corticospinal tract located lateral to the ventral median fissure. They also decussate near to their termination; as a result, the fibres of the pyramidal tract effectively innervate the contralateral side of the spinal cord and control movement of the contralateral side of the body.

 Hereditary spastic paraparesis

Hereditary spastic paraparesis is an inherited degenerative disorder (autosomal dominant) in which progressive weakness affects the legs, leading to marked stiffness of gait. Degeneration of the lateral funiculi, including the lateral corticospinal tract, chiefly affects the thoracic spinal cord, causing a spastic paraparesis with hyperreflexia and extensor plantar responses, but with sparing of sensation and bladder function.

Approximately 55% of corticospinal neurones terminate at cervical levels, 20% at thoracic and 25% at lumbosacral levels. Fibres terminate extensively in the spinal grey matter. Many of those fibres that originate from the motor cortex terminate in the ventral horn, some making monosynaptic contact with motor neurones.

Rubrospinal tract

The **rubrospinal tract** originates from the **red nucleus** of the midbrain tegmentum (Fig. 8.22). It exerts control over the tone of limb flexor muscles, being excitatory to the motor neurones of these muscles. Axons leaving the cells of the red nucleus course ventromedially and cross in the **ventral tegmental decussation**, after which they descend to the spinal cord where they lie ventrolateral to, and partly intermingled with, the lateral corticospinal tract.

The red nucleus receives afferent fibres from the motor cortex and from the cerebellum. The rubrospinal tract, therefore, represents a non-pyramidal route by which the motor cortex and cerebellum can influence spinal motor activity.

Tectospinal tract

Tectospinal tract fibres arise from the **superior colliculus** of the midbrain (Fig. 8.23). Axons pass ventromedially around the periaqueductal grey matter and cross in the **dorsal tegmental**

decussation. In the spinal cord, descending tectospinal fibres lie near the ventral median fissure and they terminate predominantly in cervical segments. The superior colliculus receives visual input and the tectospinal tract is thought to mediate reflex movements in response to visual stimuli.

Vestibulospinal tracts

Vestibulospinal tract fibres arise from the **vestibular nuclei** situated in the pons and medulla, in and near the floor of the fourth ventricle (Fig. 8.24). The vestibular nuclei receive input from the labyrinthine system by way of the vestibular nerve and also from the cerebellum.

Axons from cells of the **lateral vestibular nucleus (Deiters' nucleus)** descend ipsilaterally as the **lateral vestibulospinal tract**, which is located in the ventral funiculus. Lateral vestibulospinal tract fibres mediate powerful excitatory effects upon extensor motor neurones. They serve to control extensor muscle tone in the anti-gravity maintenance of posture.

The **medial vestibular nucleus** contributes descending fibres to the ipsilateral **medial longitudinal fasciculus**, also known as the **medial vestibulospinal tract**, which is located adjacent to the ventral median fissure and descends as far as cervical levels. The medial longitudinal fasciculus contains fibres that link the vestibular nuclei with the nuclei innervating the extraocular muscles (oculomotor, trochlear and abducens nuclei) and is, thus, important in coordinating head and eye movements (Chapter 9, p 93; Chapter 10, pp 103–104).

Reticulospinal tracts

The reticular formation of the pons and medulla gives rise to reticulospinal fibres. Axons arising from the pontine reticular formation descend ipsilaterally as the **medial (or pontine) reticulospinal tract**. Axons from the medulla descend bilaterally in the **lateral (or medullary) reticulospinal tracts**. Both tracts are located in the ventral funiculus.

Reticulospinal fibres influence voluntary movement, reflex activity and muscle tone by controlling the activity of both alpha and gamma motor neurones. They also mediate pressor and depressor effects upon the circulatory system and are involved in the control of breathing.

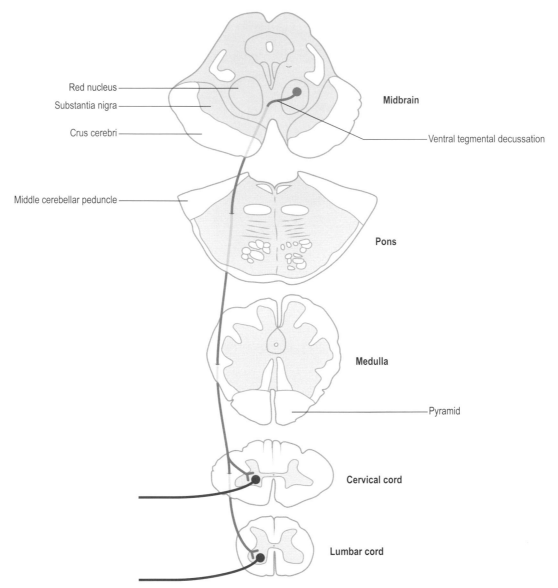

Red nucleus

Substantia nigra

Crus cerebri

Midbrain

Ventral tegmental decussation

Middle cerebellar peduncle

Pons

Medulla

Pyramid

Cervical cord

Lumbar cord

Fig. 8.22 Rubrospinal tract.

White matter of the spinal cord: principal descending tracts

- Corticospinal tract controls discrete, skilled movements, particularly of the distal extremities. It originates from motor and sensory cortices. Fibres descend through the internal capsule, crus cerebri and ventral pons to reach the medullary pyramid. Most fibres (75%–90%) decussate to form the lateral corticospinal tract, the remainder forming the ipsilateral ventral corticospinal tract.

- Rubrospinal tract controls limb flexor muscles and originates from the red nucleus of the midbrain. Fibres cross in the ventral tegmental decussation.

- Tectospinal tract is involved in reflex responses to visual input. It originates from the contralateral superior colliculus and fibres cross in the dorsal tegmental decussation.

- Vestibulospinal tracts descend from the vestibular nuclei. The lateral vestibulospinal tract originates from the ipsilateral lateral vestibular nucleus and mediates excitation of limb extensor muscles.

- Reticulospinal tracts descend from the pons and medulla. They are involved in the control of reflex activities, muscle tone and vital functions.

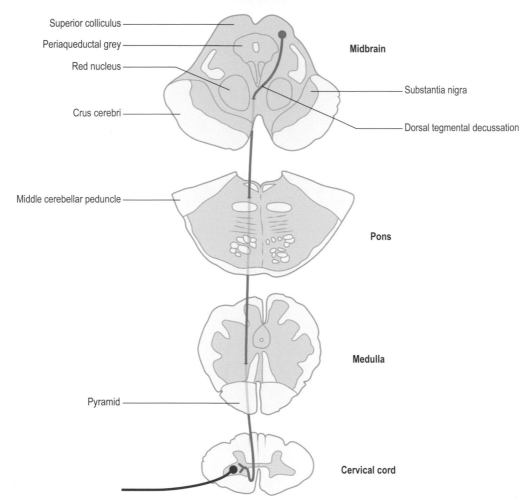

Superior colliculus

Periaqueductal grey

Red nucleus

Crus cerebri

Midbrain

Substantia nigra

Dorsal tegmental decussation

Middle cerebellar peduncle

Pons

Medulla

Pyramid

Cervical cord

Fig. 8.23 Tectospinal tract.

 Lesions of the spinal cord

Focal lesions of the spinal cord and the nerve roots produce clinical manifestations in 2 ways:

1. The lesion destroys function at the segmental level.
2. The lesion interrupts descending motor and ascending sensory tracts.

Damage to different parts of the spinal cord, therefore, is accompanied by distinctive clinical syndromes (Fig. 8.25).

Acute lesions of the spinal cord follow occlusion of the anterior spinal artery and trauma, causing fractures of the spine. Chronic compression of the spinal cord and emerging nerve roots is caused by infection and tumours of the spine, meninges and nerve roots and by prolapsed intervertebral discs. Subacute and chronic lesions of the spinal cord are commonly due to the immune disorder of multiple sclerosis.

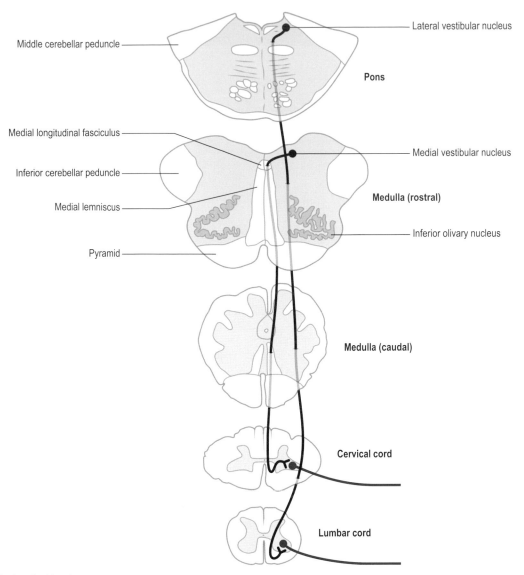

Fig. 8.24 Vestibulospinal tracts.

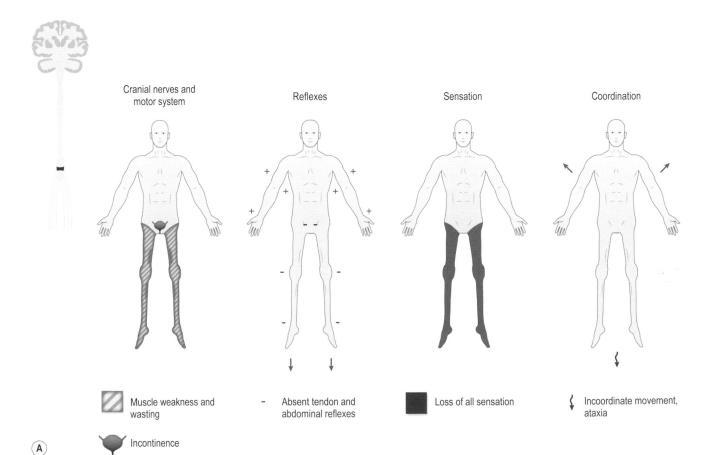

| Cranial nerves and motor system | Reflexes | Sensation | Coordination |

<table>
<tr><td>▨ Muscle weakness and wasting</td><td>– Absent tendon and abdominal reflexes</td><td>■ Loss of all sensation</td><td>〈 Incoordinate movement, ataxia</td></tr>
<tr><td>● Incontinence</td><td></td><td></td><td></td></tr>
</table>

(A)

Fig. 8.25 (A) Lumbosacral spinal cord lesion. A lumbosacral cord lesion causes weakness, wasting and fasciculation of muscles, areflexia of the lower limbs (lower motor neurone lesion), incontinence, sensory loss below the level of the lesion and 'sensory' ataxia. Refer also to Fig. 1.48.

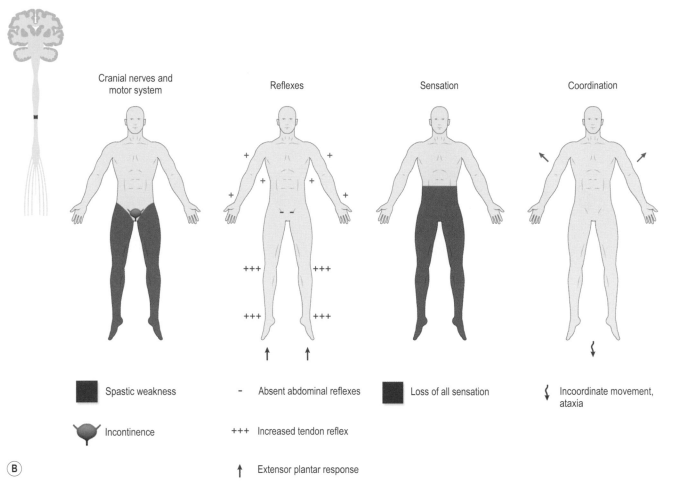

Cranial nerves and motor system	Reflexes	Sensation	Coordination

■ Spastic weakness — Absent abdominal reflexes ■ Loss of all sensation ⟨ Incoordinate movement, ataxia

Incontinence +++ Increased tendon reflex

(B)

↑ Extensor plantar response

Fig. 8.25, cont'd (B) Thoracic spinal cord lesion. A thoracic cord lesion causes a spastic paraparesis, hyperreflexia and extensor plantar responses (upper motor neurone lesion), incontinence, sensory loss below the level of the lesion and 'sensory' ataxia. Refer also to Fig. 1.48.

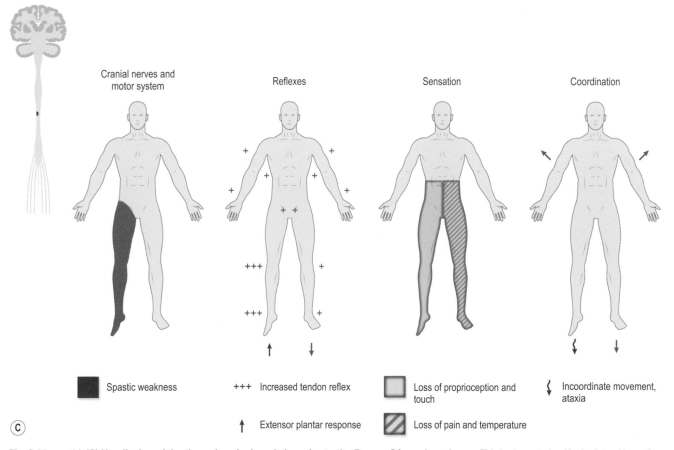

Cranial nerves and motor system	Reflexes	Sensation	Coordination

■ Spastic weakness +++ Increased tendon reflex ▢ Loss of proprioception and touch ⟨ Incoordinate movement, ataxia

(C) ↑ Extensor plantar response ▨ Loss of pain and temperature

Fig. 8.25, cont'd (C) Hemilesion of the thoracic spinal cord gives rise to the Brown–Séquard syndrome. This is characterised by ipsilateral loss of proprioception and upper motor neurone signs (hemiplegia/monoplegia) plus contralateral loss of pain and temperature sensation. Refer also to Fig. 1.48.

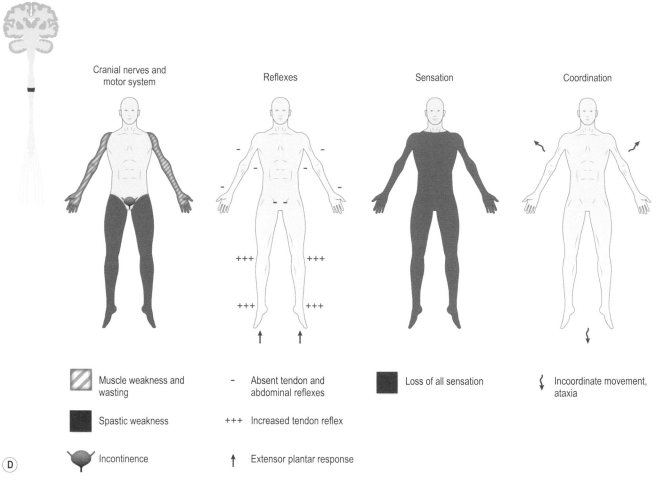

Cranial nerves and motor system	Reflexes	Sensation	Coordination

▨ Muscle weakness and wasting	− Absent tendon and abdominal reflexes	■ Loss of all sensation	∿ Incoordinate movement, ataxia
■ Spastic weakness	+++ Increased tendon reflex		
Incontinence	↑ Extensor plantar response		

(D)

Fig. 8.25, cont'd (D) Lower cervical spinal cord lesion. A lower cervical cord lesion causes weakness, wasting and fasciculation of muscles, and areflexia of the upper limbs (lower motor neurone lesion). In addition, there is spastic paraparesis, hyperreflexia and extensor plantar responses (upper motor neurone lesion) in the lower limbs, incontinence, sensory loss below the level of the lesion and 'sensory' ataxia. Refer also to Fig. 1.48.

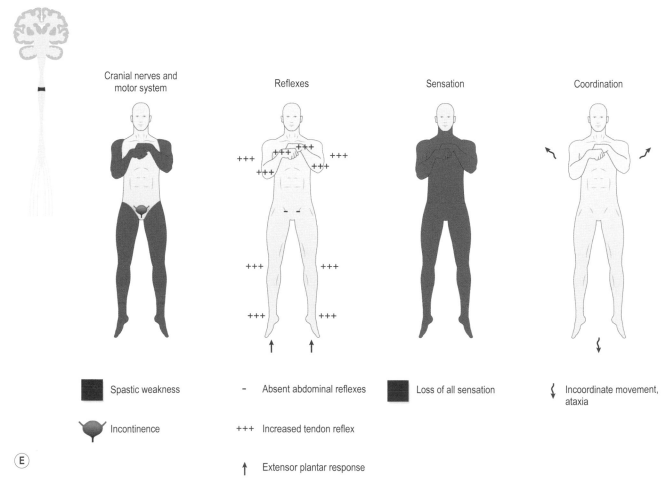

Cranial nerves and motor system	Reflexes	Sensation	Coordination

■ Spastic weakness	− Absent abdominal reflexes	■ Loss of all sensation	∿ Incoordinate movement, ataxia
Incontinence	+++ Increased tendon reflex		
	↑ Extensor plantar response		

(E)

Fig. 8.25, cont'd (E) Upper cervical spinal cord lesion. A high cervical cord lesion causes spastic tetraplegia with hyperreflexia, extensor plantar responses (upper motor neurone lesion), incontinence, sensory loss below the level of the lesion and 'sensory' ataxia. Refer also to Fig. 1.48.

The brainstem consists of the medulla oblongata, pons and midbrain. The archaic term 'bulb' is applied to the brainstem in compound anatomical names given to nerve fibres originating from, or terminating in, the brainstem (e.g. 'corticobulbar' refers to axons that arise in the cerebral cortex and terminate in the brainstem). It is also used clinically to denote the medulla in such terms as 'bulbar palsy' and 'pseudobulbar palsy', which describe syndromes associated with medullary dysfunction.

The brainstem lies upon the basal portion of the occipital bone (clivus), its dorsal aspect being largely covered by the cerebellum with which it has rich interconnections. Caudally, the medulla is continuous with the spinal cord just below the foramen magnum. Rostrally, the midbrain is continuous with the diencephalon of the forebrain.

The brainstem contains numerous ascending and descending fibre tracts. Some of these pass throughout its whole length, having their origin in the spinal cord or cerebral hemisphere, respectively; others have their origin or termination within the nuclei of the brainstem itself. Some of these brainstem nuclei receive afferent fibres from, or send efferent fibres into, cranial nerves, 10 pairs of which (III–XII) attach to the surface of the brainstem; these are known as the **cranial nerve nuclei** (see Fig. 10.2). In addition, the brainstem contains a complex and heterogeneous matrix of neurones known as the **reticular formation**, within which a number of individually identified nuclei exist. The reticular formation has several important functions, including control over the level of consciousness, the perception of pain and regulation of the cardiovascular and respiratory systems. It also has extensive connections with the cranial nerve nuclei, with the cerebellum, and with brainstem and spinal motor mechanisms, through which it influences movement, posture and muscle tone. The brainstem contains the cells of origin of important monoaminergic (dopaminergic, noradrenergic, serotonergic) neurones that have widespread projections throughout the CNS and are important in sensory, motor, autonomic and cognitive functions.

External features of the brainstem

Dorsal surface of the brainstem

The dorsal surface of the brainstem can be viewed if the overlying cerebellum is removed by cutting the three pairs of nerve fibre bundles, or **peduncles**, by which it is attached on each side (Figs 9.1, 9.2). On the dorsal surface of the medulla, the midline is marked by a dorsal median sulcus, continuous with that of the spinal cord. In the caudal part of the medulla, the **dorsal columns** (**fasciculus gracilis** and **fasciculus cuneatus**, containing first-order sensory neurones) continue rostrally from the spinal cord to their termination in the **nucleus gracilis** and **nucleus cuneatus**, the locations of which are marked by two small elevations, the gracile and cuneate tubercles.

The caudal two-thirds of the medulla contains the rostral continuation of the central canal of the spinal cord and is, therefore, sometimes referred to as the 'closed' portion of the medulla. Passing rostrally, the central canal moves progressively more dorsal until, in the rostral medulla, it opens out into the lumen of the fourth ventricle. This portion of the medulla is sometimes referred to as the 'open' medulla. The floor of the

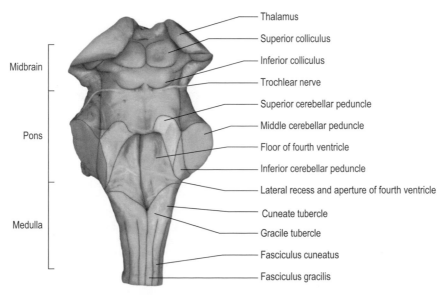

Midbrain

Pons

Medulla

Thalamus
Superior colliculus
Inferior colliculus
Trochlear nerve
Superior cerebellar peduncle
Middle cerebellar peduncle
Floor of fourth ventricle
Inferior cerebellar peduncle
Lateral recess and aperture of fourth ventricle
Cuneate tubercle
Gracile tubercle
Fasciculus cuneatus
Fasciculus gracilis

Fig. 9.1 Dorsal aspect of the brainstem.

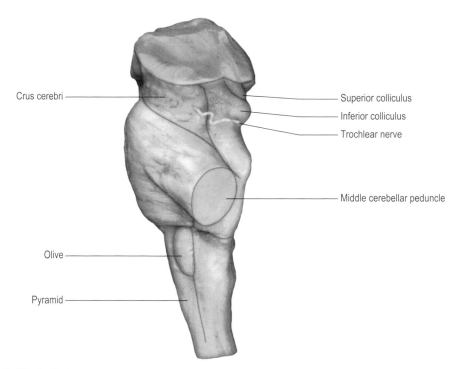

Fig. 9.2 Lateral aspect of the brainstem.

fourth ventricle forms a shallow, rhomboid depression on the dorsal surface of the rostral medulla and the pons. The transition from medulla to pons is not clearly delineated on the dorsal surface of the brainstem but, approximately, the caudal third of the floor of the fourth ventricle constitutes the dorsal aspect of the rostral medulla, while the rostral two-thirds of the ventricular floor is made up of the dorsal aspect of the pons. The fourth ventricle is widest at the level of the pontomedullary junction. Here, a **lateral recess** of the ventricle extends to the lateral margins of the brainstem. At this point, a small lateral aperture (**foramen of Luschka**) provides passage for CSF within the fourth ventricle to reach the subarachnoid space surrounding the brain (see Fig. 6.4). The lateral walls of the rostral part of the fourth ventricle are made up of the **superior** and **inferior cerebellar peduncles**, connecting the brainstem with the cerebellum. In the rostral pons, the walls converge until, at the pontomesencephalic junction, the fourth ventricle becomes continuous with a small channel, the **cerebral aqueduct**, which passes throughout the length of the midbrain.

The dorsal aspect of the midbrain is marked by four paired elevations, the **superior** and **inferior colliculi** (singular: colliculus; Latin for 'little hill'), which are parts of the visual and auditory systems, respectively. The **trochlear nerve** (cranial nerve IV) emerges immediately caudal to the inferior colliculus.

Ventral surface of the brainstem

On the ventral surface of the medulla, prominent longitudinal columns, the pyramids, run on either side of the ventral median fissure (Figs 9.3, 9.4). The pyramid gives its name to the underlying **pyramidal** or **corticospinal tract**, which consists of descending fibres originating from the ipsilateral cerebral cortex. In the caudal medulla, 75–90% of these fibres cross over in the **decussation of the pyramids** (Figs 9.3, 9.4, 9.5), partly obscuring the ventral median fissure as they do so, to form the lateral corticospinal tract of the spinal cord. Lateral to the pyramid lies an elongated elevation, the **olive**, within which lies the **inferior olivary nucleus** (see Fig. 9.7). This has connections primarily with the cerebellum and is involved in the control of movement.

The transition from medulla to pons is clearly delineated on the ventral surface of the brainstem. The ventral part of the pons is dominated by a transverse system of fibres (the **transverse pontine fibres** or **pontocerebellar fibres**) that originate from cells in the ventral pons (**pontine nuclei**) and which, after decussation, pass through the contralateral **middle cerebellar peduncle** to enter the cerebellar hemisphere. The pontine nuclei receive **corticopontine fibres** from the ipsilateral cerebral cortex (including the motor cortex) and constitute an important connection between cerebral and cerebellar cortices involved in the coordination of movement. The massive system of transverse pontine fibres obscures the underlying corticospinal tract.

The ventral surface of the midbrain consists, on either side, of a large column of descending fibres, the **crus cerebri** or **basis pedunculi**. In the midline, the two crura cerebri are separated by a depression called the interpeduncular fossa. The crus cerebri is continuous rostrally with the internal capsule of the cerebral hemisphere (see Fig. 1.30) and consists of corticobulbar and corticospinal fibres that have left the cerebral hemisphere via the internal capsule on their way to the brainstem and spinal cord. The nerve fibres descending through the crus are primarily motor in function.

External features of the brainstem

- The brainstem consists of the modulla oblongata, pons and midbrain.

- On the dorsal aspect of the brainstem can be seen the dorsal columns, the floor of the fourth ventricle and the superior and inferior colliculi.

- The dorsal aspect of the rostral medulla and the pons form the floor of the fourth ventricle; the lateral and median apertures of the fourth ventricle permit the passage of CSF into the

subarachnoid space. The cerebral aqueduct runs through the midbrain, beneath the colliculi.

- On the ventral aspect of the brainstem can be seen the pyramids, transverse pontine fibres and the crura cerebri.

- The inferior, middle and superior cerebellar peduncles connect the cerebellum to the medulla, pons and midbrain, respectively.

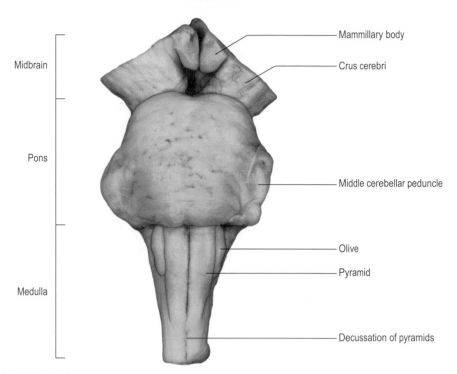

Fig. 9.3 Ventral aspect of the brainstem.

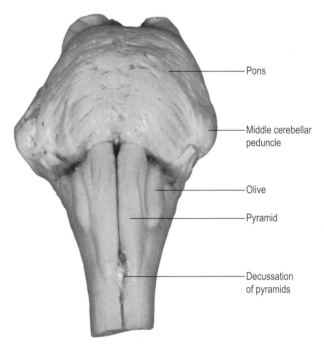

Fig. 9.4 Ventral aspect of the brainstem showing the decussation of the pyramids.

Internal structure of the brainstem

Caudal medulla

At the transition from spinal cord to medulla, the pattern of grey and white matter undergoes considerable rearrangement (Fig. 9.5). The ventral horn becomes much attenuated. The dorsal horn is replaced by the caudal part of the **trigeminal sensory nucleus (nucleus of the spinal tract of the trigeminal nerve)**. The trigeminal sensory nucleus is regarded as the brainstem homologue of the dorsal horn, since it receives primary afferent fibres conveying general sensation from the head, which enter the brainstem in the trigeminal nerve. It is a large nucleus that extends the whole length of the brainstem and into the upper segments of

the spinal cord. This latter, caudal part of the trigeminal nucleus is particularly associated with the modalities of pain and temperature. The trigeminal nerve attaches to the pons and, therefore, fibres that terminate in the parts of the trigeminal nucleus caudal to this level descend in a tract (**the spinal tract of the trigeminal**), which lies immediately superficial to the nucleus.

In the ventral medulla, the majority of fibres of the pyramid undergo decussation and then pass laterally, dorsally and caudally to form the lateral corticospinal tract.

Mid-medulla

On the ventral surface of the mid-medulla the pyramids are prominent, above their decussation. On the dorsal surface, the ascending fibres of the dorsal columns reach their termination in the gracile and cuneate nuclei, which appear beneath their respective tracts (Fig. 9.6). The dorsal columns consist of first-order sensory neurones; the cell bodies of these neurones lie in the dorsal root ganglia of spinal nerves and have central processes that ascend ipsilaterally through the cord and into the medulla. They terminate in the nuclei gracilis and cuneatus, upon the cell bodies of second-order neurones. The axons of the second-order neurones course ventrally and medially as **internal arcuate fibres**, decussating in the midline. Thereafter, they turn rostrally forming a distinct tract, the **medial lemniscus**, which runs through the rostral medulla, the pons and midbrain, to terminate upon third-order neurones in the ventral posterior nucleus of the thalamus (see also Fig. 8.16).

Rostral medulla

Passing into the rostral medulla, a number of new features appear, mostly related to the ventricular system and cerebellar connections. On the ventral surface of the medulla, the descending fibres of the pyramids remain conspicuous. Immediately dorsal to the medial aspect of the pyramid run the ascending fibres of the medial lemniscus, on either side of the midline (Fig. 9.7). In the midline is located the medullary part of the brainstem raphé nuclear complex, represented at this level by the **nucleus raphé magnus**, a major origin of serotonergic neurones. Dorsolateral to the pyramid and lateral to the medial

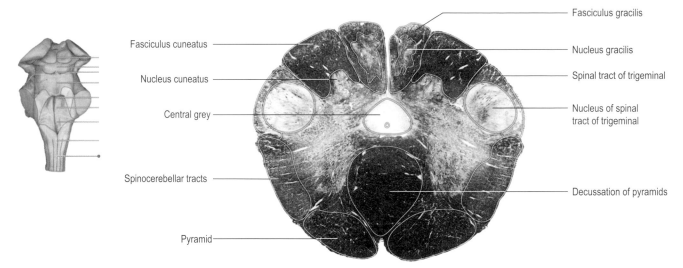

Fasciculus cuneatus

Nucleus cuneatus

Central grey

Spinocerebellar tracts

Pyramid

Fasciculus gracilis

Nucleus gracilis

Spinal tract of trigeminal

Nucleus of spinal tract of trigeminal

Decussation of pyramids

Fig. 9.5 Transverse section through the caudal medulla at the level of the decussation of the pyramids. The sections shown in Figs 9.5–9.13 have been stained by the Weigert–Pal method. Areas rich in nerve fibres stain darkly, whereas areas rich in cell bodies are relatively pale.

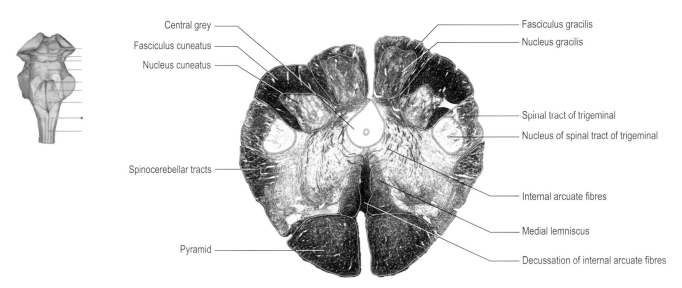

Central grey

Fasciculus cuneatus

Nucleus cuneatus

Spinocerebellar tracts

Pyramid

Fasciculus gracilis

Nucleus gracilis

Spinal tract of trigeminal

Nucleus of spinal tract of trigeminal

Internal arcuate fibres

Medial lemniscus

Decussation of internal arcuate fibres

Fig. 9.6 Transverse section through the mid-medulla at the level of the great sensory decussation.

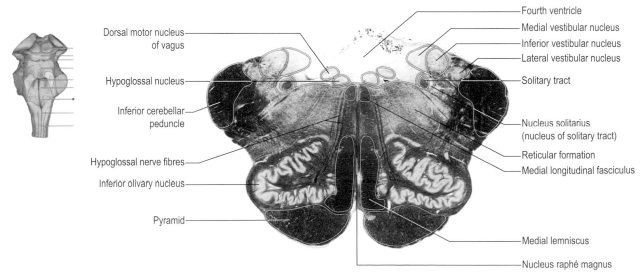

Dorsal motor nucleus of vagus

Hypoglossal nucleus

Inferior cerebellar peduncle

Hypoglossal nerve fibres

Inferior olivary nucleus

Pyramid

Fourth ventricle

Medial vestibular nucleus

Inferior vestibular nucleus

Lateral vestibular nucleus

Solitary tract

Nucleus solitarius (nucleus of solitary tract)

Reticular formation

Medial longitudinal fasciculus

Medial lemniscus

Nucleus raphé magnus

Fig. 9.7 Transverse section through the rostral medulla at the level of the inferior olivary nucleus.

lemniscus is the **inferior olivary nucleus**, lying within the prominence of the olive. The inferior olivary nucleus has roughly the form of a crenated bag with an opening, or hilum, facing medially, through which afferent and efferent fibres pass. The nucleus is concerned with the control of movement and receives afferents from the motor and sensory cortices of the cerebral hemisphere and from the red nucleus of the midbrain. Its main efferent connection is to the cerebellum via the inferior cerebellar peduncle. Within the cerebellum, axons originating from the inferior olivary nucleus, known as climbing fibres, end in excitatory synapses in the dentate nucleus and upon Purkinje cells of the cerebellar cortex.

Dorsal to the inferior olivary nucleus and lateral to the medial lemniscus lie second-order sensory fibres ascending to the ventral posterior thalamus from the trigeminal nucleus (the **trigeminothalamic tract** or **trigeminal lemniscus**) and from the spinal cord (spinothalamic fibres, referred to in the brainstem as the **spinal lemniscus**).

The dorsal surface of the rostral medulla forms part of the floor of the fourth ventricle. Both immediately beneath and deep beneath the floor of the ventricle lie a number of cranial nerve nuclei, some of which can be clearly identified in simply stained sections, others of which cannot. Immediately beneath the ventricular floor, just lateral to the midline, lies the **hypoglossal nucleus**, which contains motor neurones innervating the muscles of the tongue via the hypoglossal nerve. Lateral to the hypoglossal nucleus lies the **dorsal motor nucleus of the vagus**, containing preganglionic parasympathetic neurones that run in the vagus nerve. The most caudal aspect of the ventricular floor is known as the **area postrema**. At this point, the blood-brain barrier, which limits the passage of certain chemicals from the blood to the brain, is absent. This region is the central site of action of substances that cause vomiting (emetics). In the lateral part of the floor of the fourth ventricle are located the **vestibular nuclei**, which receive primary afferent fibres from the vestibular nerve. Ventromedial to the hypoglossal nucleus, close to the midline, is located the **medial longitudinal fasciculus**. This consists of both ascending and descending fibres and can be identified also in the pons and midbrain. Within the brainstem, it links the vestibular nuclei with the nuclei supplying the extraocular muscles (abducens, trochlear and oculomotor nuclei) and subserves conjugate eye movements and the coordination of head and eye movements.

The dorsolateral part of the rostral medulla is dominated by the **inferior cerebellar peduncle**, or **restiform body**. This consists of fibres passing between the medulla and the cerebellum.

Prominent among these are olivocerebellar fibres (from the inferior olivary nucleus), connections between the vestibular nuclei and the cerebellum, and the fibres of the dorsal spinocerebellar tract, conveying proprioceptive information from the lower limb. On the dorsal and lateral aspects of the inferior cerebellar peduncle lie the **dorsal** and **ventral cochlear nuclei**, which receive afferent fibres from the cochlear nerve. Medial to the inferior cerebellar peduncle and ventral to the vestibular nuclei lies the **nucleus solitarius** (or nucleus tractus solitarius, solitary nucleus), surrounding a small, dense fascicle of fibres, the **tractus solitarius** (or solitary tract). The nucleus solitarius receives visceral afferent fibres entering the brainstem in the facial, glossopharyngeal and vagus nerves. Deep beneath the ventricular floor, ventral to the nucleus solitarius and just dorsal to the inferior olivary nucleus, is located the **nucleus ambiguus**. This sends motor fibres into the glossopharyngeal and vagus nerves and cranial roots of the accessory nerve and, thence, to the muscles of the pharynx and larynx.

Pons

The pons may be divided into a ventral, or basal, portion and a dorsal portion, also known as the **tegmentum**. The ventral portion is marked by numerous transversely oriented fascicles of **pontocerebellar fibres** (**transverse pontine fibres**) that originate from scattered cell groups, the **pontine nuclei**, and pass into the contralateral side of the cerebellum through the massive middle cerebellar peduncle (**brachium pontis**) (Figs 9.8, 9.9). Corticospinal fibres (which continue caudally into the medullary pyramid) appear as small, separate bundles running longitudinally between the fascicles of transverse pontine fibres.

The ascending fibres of the medial lemniscus become separated from the pyramid and displaced dorsally, together with the spinal lemniscus and trigeminothalamic tract (trigeminal lemniscus), by intervening transverse pontocerebellar fibres. The medial lemniscus also rotates through 90° so that it lies almost horizontally, marking the boundary between ventral and tegmental portions of the pons. In the caudal to mid-pons (Fig. 9.9), an additional group of transversely running fibres is located close to the ascending lemniscal fibres but dorsal to the pontocerebellar fibres. This is the **trapezoid body**, which consists of acoustic fibres crossing the brainstem from the cochlear nuclei. They ascend into the midbrain as the **lateral lemniscus** (Fig. 9.10) and terminate in the inferior colliculus.

Beneath the floor of the fourth ventricle, in the pontine tegmentum, lie a number of cranial nerve nuclei. These include

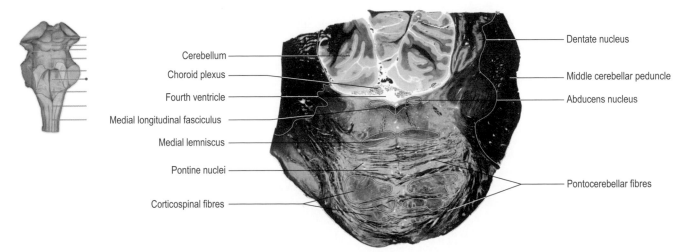

Cerebellum
Choroid plexus
Fourth ventricle
Medial longitudinal fasciculus
Medial lemniscus
Pontine nuclei
Corticospinal fibres

Dentate nucleus
Middle cerebellar peduncle
Abducens nucleus
Pontocerebellar fibres

Fig. 9.8 Transverse section through the caudal pons.

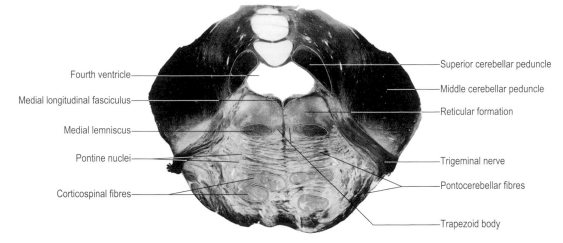

Fourth ventricle
Medial longitudinal fasciculus
Medial lemniscus
Pontine nuclei
Corticospinal fibres

Superior cerebellar peduncle
Middle cerebellar peduncle
Reticular formation
Trigeminal nerve
Pontocerebellar fibres
Trapezoid body

Fig. 9.9 Transverse section through the mid-pons at the level of the trigeminal nerve.

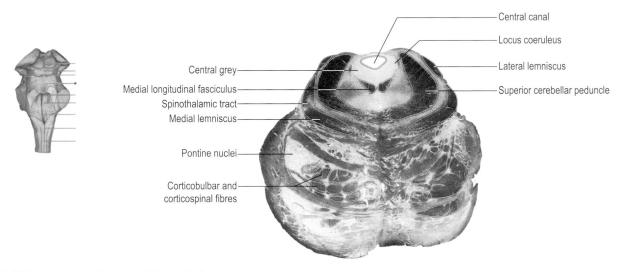

Central grey
Medial longitudinal fasciculus
Spinothalamic tract
Medial lemniscus
Pontine nuclei
Corticobulbar and corticospinal fibres

Central canal
Locus coeruleus
Lateral lemniscus
Superior cerebellar peduncle

Fig. 9.10 Transverse section through the rostral pons.

the **abducens nucleus** (innervating the lateral rectus muscle), the **facial motor nucleus** (innervating the muscles of facial expression) and the **trigeminal motor nucleus** (innervating the muscles of mastication), which each supply motor axons to their respective cranial nerves. Also the trigeminal sensory nucleus, already encountered in the medulla, reaches its maximum extent in the pons, adjacent to the origin of the trigeminal nerve.

In the rostral half of the pons, the superior cerebellar peduncles form the lateral walls of the fourth ventricle, the thin superior medullary velum spanning between them to form its roof. The superior peduncle contains some cerebellar afferent fibres, such as the ventral spinocerebellar tract, which conveys proprioceptive information from the lower limb. It consists mainly, however, of ascending cerebellar efferents concerned with the coordination of movement, which are destined for the red nucleus of the midbrain and the ventral lateral nucleus of the thalamus. The superior cerebellar peduncles converge towards the midline as they pass into the midbrain. In the most rostral part of the pons, close to the pontomesencephalic junction (a region called the isthmus), the fourth ventricle becomes greatly attenuated as it merges into the cerebral aqueduct (Fig. 9.10). Central grey matter begins to encompass the lumen (much like the grey matter surrounding the central canal of the spinal cord) and, at this level, lies a group of pigmented neurones, the **locus coeruleus**, which is a major site of noradrenergic neurones.

Midbrain

The midbrain (Figs 9.11–9.13) is, for descriptive purposes, divided into dorsal and ventral portions at the level of the cerebral aqueduct. The dorsal portion is known as the **tectum**, which consists largely of the **inferior** and **superior colliculi (corpora quadrigemina)**. The ventral portion of the midbrain is known as the **tegmentum**. It is bounded ventrally by the massive fibre system of the **crus cerebri**. The term **cerebral peduncle** is sometimes used as a synonym for crus cerebri but, strictly speaking, the cerebral peduncle refers to the whole of the ventral midbrain, on either side, excluding the tectum.

In the caudal part of the midbrain, the inferior colliculus constitutes part of the **ascending acoustic (auditory) projection**. Ascending auditory fibres run in the **lateral lemniscus**, which terminates in the inferior colliculus. Efferent fibres from the inferior colliculus terminate in the **medial geniculate nucleus** of the thalamus, which in turn projects to the auditory cortex of the temporal lobe.

The superior colliculus of the rostral midbrain is part of the visual system. Its main afferents are corticotectal fibres originating from the visual cortex of the occipital lobe and from the frontal eye field of the frontal lobe. These inputs are concerned with controlling movements of the eyes, such as those occurring when a moving object is followed (smooth pursuit) or when the direction of the gaze is altered (saccadic eye movements). In

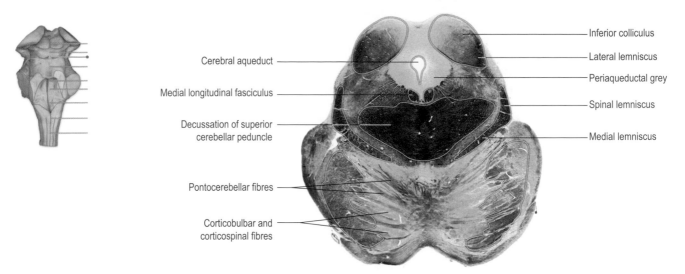

Cerebral aqueduct

Medial longitudinal fasciculus

Decussation of superior
cerebellar peduncle

Pontocerebellar fibres

Corticobulbar and
corticospinal fibres

Inferior colliculus

Lateral lemniscus

Periaqueductal grey

Spinal lemniscus

Medial lemniscus

Fig. 9.11 Transverse section through the brainstem at the level of the pontine–mesencephalic junction.

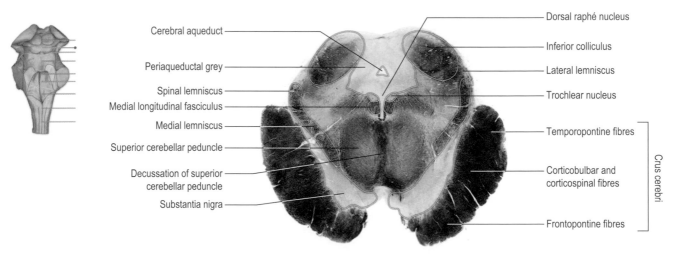

Cerebral aqueduct

Periaqueductal grey

Spinal lemniscus
Medial longitudinal fasciculus
Medial lemniscus

Superior cerebellar peduncle

Decussation of superior
cerebellar peduncle

Substantia nigra

Dorsal raphé nucleus

Inferior colliculus

Lateral lemniscus

Trochlear nucleus

Temporopontine fibres

Corticobulbar and
corticospinal fibres

Frontopontine fibres

Crus cerebri

Fig. 9.12 Transverse section through the caudal midbrain at the level of the inferior colliculus.

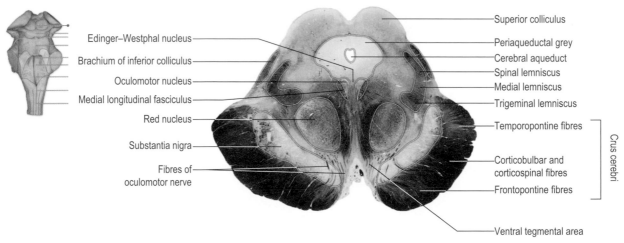

Edinger–Westphal nucleus

Brachium of inferior colliculus

Oculomotor nucleus

Medial longitudinal fasciculus

Red nucleus

Substantia nigra

Fibres of
oculomotor nerve

Superior colliculus

Periaqueductal grey

Cerebral aqueduct

Spinal lemniscus

Medial lemniscus

Trigeminal lemniscus

Temporopontine fibres

Corticobulbar and
corticospinal fibres

Frontopontine fibres

Ventral tegmental area

Crus cerebri

Fig. 9.13 Transverse section through the rostral midbrain at the level of the superior colliculus.

addition, corticotectal fibres from the visual cortex are involved in the **accommodation reflex** (Chapter 10).

A small number of visual fibres running in the optic tract terminate just rostral to the superior colliculus, in the **pretectal nucleus**. This nucleus has connections with nearby midbrain preganglionic parasympathetic neurones **(Edinger–Westphal nucleus)** controlling the smooth muscle of the eye and is part of the circuit mediating the **pupillary light reflex** (Chapter 10).

Ventral to the colliculi, the cerebral aqueduct runs the length of the midbrain. Surrounding the aqueduct is a pear-shaped arrangement of grey matter, the **periaqueductal** (or **central**) **grey**. In the ventral part of the periaqueductal grey, at the levels of the inferior and superior colliculi, respectively, lie the **trochlear** and **oculomotor nuclei**, which innervate the extraocular muscles controlling eye movements. Near the oculomotor nucleus lies the Edinger–Westphal nucleus. Close to these nuclei runs the medial longitudinal fasciculus, which links them to the abducens nucleus in the pons and the vestibular nuclei in the medulla and is important in the control of gaze.

At the level of the inferior colliculus (Figs 9.11, 9.12), the central portion of the tegmentum is dominated by the converging superior cerebellar peduncles (**brachium conjunctivum**). This massive fibre system originates in the cerebellum and courses ventromedially as it runs into the midbrain. Beneath the inferior colliculus, the two superior cerebellar peduncles decussate in the midline. Rostral to the decussation, at the level of the superior colliculus (Fig. 9.13), the central portion of the tegmentum is occupied by the **red nucleus**, in which some of the fibres of the superior cerebellar peduncle terminate. The red nucleus is involved in motor control. Its other major source of afferents is the motor cortex of the frontal lobe. Efferent fibres from the red nucleus cross in the ventral tegmental decussation and descend to the spinal cord in the **rubrospinal tract**. In addition, the red nucleus projects to the inferior olivary nucleus of the medulla, via the **central tegmental tract**.

The most ventral part of the midbrain tegmentum is occupied by the **substantia nigra**. This consists of two subnuclei: the **pars compacta** and the **pars reticulata**. The pars compacta consists of pigmented, melanin-containing neurones that synthesise dopamine as their transmitter. These neurones project to the caudate nucleus and putamen (striatum) of the basal ganglia in the forebrain and constitute the nigrostriatal pathway (Chapter 14). This connection is important for the control of voluntary movement, posture and muscle tone and degeneration of the pars compacta is associated with Parkinson's disease. Dopamine-containing neurones extend dorsomedially from the ventromedial part of the pars compacta into a region known as the ventral tegmental area (VTA; Fig. 9.13). These cells of the VTA are the origin of the ascending mesolimbic dopaminergic pathway and they innervate a number of forebrain structures including the nucleus accumbens, amygdala and septum and the cingulate, orbital and prefrontal cortices (Fig. 9.14). The non-pigmented subdivision of the substantia nigra is called the pars reticulata. It is considered to be a functional homologue of the internal segment of the globus pallidus, which is also part of the basal ganglia, and the two share very similar connections.

Ventral to the substantia nigra lies the massive crus cerebri. This consists entirely of descending cortical efferent fibres that have left the cerebral hemisphere by traversing the internal capsule. Approximately the middle 50% of the crus consists of **corticobulbar** and **corticospinal fibres**. The corticobulbar fibres end predominantly in or near the motor cranial nerve nuclei of the brainstem. The corticospinal (pyramidal) fibres traverse the pons to enter the medullary pyramid and, thence, the corticospinal tracts.

On either side of the corticobulbar and corticospinal fibres, the crus cerebri contains corticopontine fibres that originate from widespread regions of the cerebral cortex and terminate in the pontine nuclei of the ventral pons. From the pontine nuclei connections are established with the cerebellum, via the middle cerebellar peduncle, that are involved in the coordination of movement.

Reticular formation

The reticular formation consists of a complex matrix of neurones that extends throughout the length of the brainstem. This is, in phylogenetic terms, a relatively old part of the brainstem and its neurones fulfil a number of important functions, some of which are necessary for survival. The reticular formation has widespread afferent and efferent connections with other parts of the CNS, which reflect its complex and multimodal functions. Some reticular neurones have long axons that ascend and descend for considerable distances within the brainstem, allowing profuse interactions throughout the neuraxis. Within the reticular formation a number of more-or-less well-defined nuclei can be identified, while some functions are subserved by more dispersed neuronal networks that do not correspond exactly to anatomically identified nuclei. The latter applies to the so-called respiratory and cardiovascular centres. These consist of diffuse neuronal networks located within the lateral medullary and caudal pontine reticular formation that control respiratory movements and cardiovascular function.

Descending **reticulospinal tracts** originate from the medullary and pontine reticular formation (Chapter 8). These predominantly influence muscle tone and posture. Within the reticular formation of the medulla lies a group of particularly large cell bodies, the nucleus reticularis gigantocellularis, which contributes descending fibres to the lateral reticulospinal tract.

Some of the ascending fibres of the reticular formation constitute the so-called **reticular activating system**. These neurones, many of which are cholinergic, receive input, either directly or indirectly, from multiple sensory sources. Through the intermediary of thalamic nuclei (mostly the intralaminar nuclei), they cause activation of the cerebral cortex and heightened arousal.

The **raphé nuclei** are a series of midline nuclei that extend throughout the length of the brainstem (Figs 9.7, 9.12). Many of the neurones are serotonergic, utilising serotonin (5-hydroxytryptamine, 5-HT) as their transmitter. Their axons are widely distributed throughout the CNS, including ascending

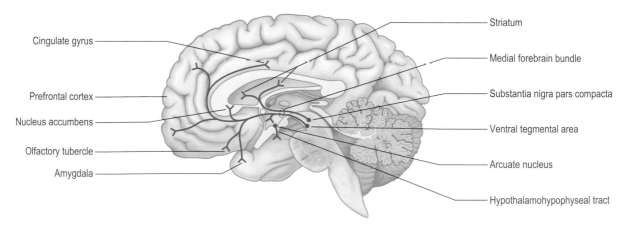

Cingulate gyrus

Prefrontal cortex

Nucleus accumbens

Olfactory tubercle

Amygdala

Striatum

Medial forebrain bundle

Substantia nigra pars compacta

Ventral tegmental area

Arcuate nucleus

Hypothalamohypophyseal tract

Fig. 9.14 Dopaminergic neurones and their principal projections.

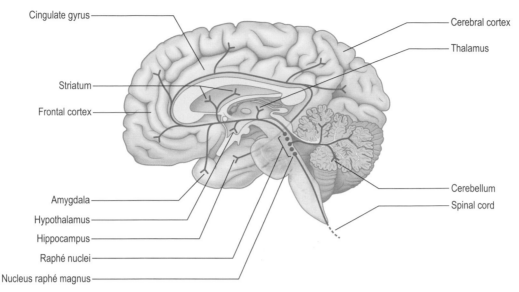

Fig. 9.15 Serotonergic neurones and their principal projections.

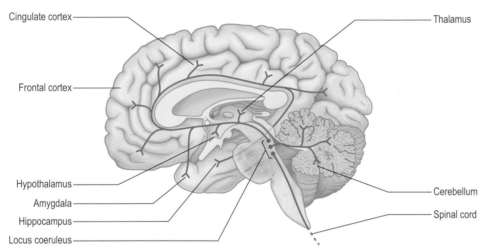

Fig. 9.16 Noradrenergic neurones and their principal projections.

projections to the thalamus, hypothalamus, striatum, amygdala, hippocampus and widespread regions of the cerebral cortex (Fig. 9.15). The functional significance of such diverse connections is not fully understood, but ascending fibres to forebrain structures are involved in mood and cognitive function and in the neural mechanisms of sleep. There are also serotonergic projections to the cerebellum and descending fibres to the spinal cord. The latter originate from the nucleus raphé magnus of the medulla and are involved in the modulation of nociceptive mechanisms in the dorsal horn (see Fig. 8.11). Some of these descending neurones contain enkephalin.

The **locus coeruleus** is a group of pigmented neurones that lies in the rostral pontine tegmentum (Fig. 9.10). It is the principal noradrenergic cell group of the brain, of which there are a number in the brainstem. It projects to the cerebellum and many areas of the forebrain, including the diencephalon, limbic structures and cerebral cortex (Fig. 9.16). The locus coeruleus, like the raphé nuclei, has been implicated in the neural mechanisms regulating sleep, particularly REM (rapid eye movement) sleep. The noradrenergic innervation of the forebrain also appears to be important in higher mental functions such as mood and cognition. Other noradrenergic fibres project throughout the brainstem and spinal cord.

Internal structure of the brainstem

- Cranial nerves III–XII attach to the brainstem, their fibres either originating from, or terminating in, the cranial nerve nuclei.

- The reticular formation controls the level of consciousness, the cardiovascular system and the respiratory system.

- Ascending sensory systems pass through the brainstem en route to the thalamus. First-order proprioceptive fibres in the dorsal columns relay in the dorsal column nuclei. Second-order fibres decussate to form the medial lemniscus. Spinothalamic fibres form the spinal lemniscus. Second-order fibres originating in the trigeminal sensory nucleus constitute the trigeminothalamic tract (trigeminal lemniscus).

- Descending fibre systems end in the brainstem, pass through it and originate within it.

- Corticobulbar fibres terminate in the midbrain, pons and medulla. The corticospinal tract runs through the crus cerebri, the basal part of the pons and the medullary pyramid; 75%-90% of fibres cross in the pyramidal decussation to form the lateral corticospinal tract.

- The reticular formation, red nucleus and vestibular nuclei give rise to descending fibres that pass to the spinal cord.

Brainstem lesions

A unilateral brainstem lesion caused by stroke, tumour or multiple sclerosis causes ipsilateral cranial nerve dysfunction, contralateral spastic hemiparesis, hyperreflexia and an extensor plantar response (upper motor neurone lesion), contralateral hemisensory loss and ipsilateral incoordination (Fig. 9.17). A bilateral lesion destroys the 'vital centres' that control breathing and the circulation, leading to coma and death. This usually follows a massive stroke of the brainstem and is the end result of raised intracranial pressure, due to a space-occupying lesion, which displaces the cerebellar hemispheres down through the foramen magnum to compress the upper brainstem.

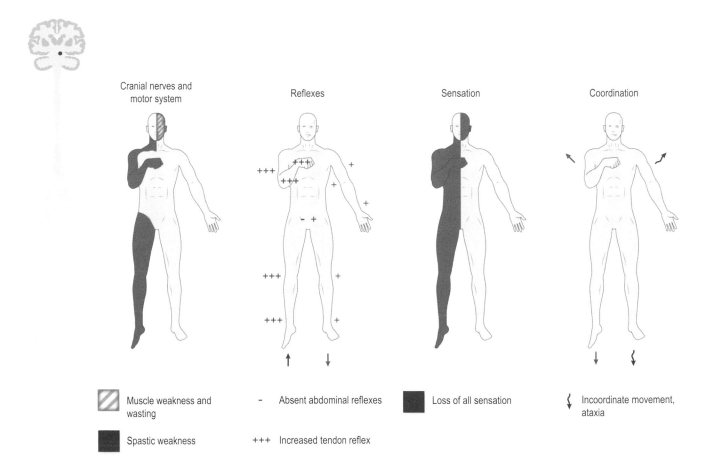

Cranial nerves and motor system

Reflexes

Sensation

Coordination

▨	Muscle weakness and wasting	−	Absent abdominal reflexes
■	Spastic weakness	+++	Increased tendon reflex
		↑	Extensor plantar response

■	Loss of all sensation
⌇	Incoordinate movement, ataxia

Fig. 9.17 Brainstem lesion. Refer also to Fig. 1.48.

Cranial nerves and cranial nerve nuclei

10

There are 12, bilaterally paired, cranial nerves. These carry afferent and efferent nerve fibres between the brain and peripheral structures, principally of the head and neck. The cranial nerves are individually named and numbered (Roman numerals I–XII) according to the rostrocaudal sequence in which they attach to the brain (Fig. 10.1 and Table 10.1):

I	olfactory	VII	facial
II	optic	VIII	vestibulocochlear
III	oculomotor	IX	glossopharyngeal
IV	trochlear	X	vagus
V	trigeminal	XI	accessory
VI	abducens	XII	hypoglossal

The first two cranial nerves attach directly to the forebrain, while the rest attach to the brainstem. The olfactory system is closely associated, both structurally and functionally, with parts of the forebrain collectively referred to as the limbic system; these, including cranial nerve I, are considered together in Chapter 16. The visual system and cranial nerve II are described in Chapter 15. Cranial nerves III–XII are directly connected to various neuronal cell groups, located ipsilaterally within the brainstem and called

the cranial nerve nuclei; these either receive cranial nerve afferents or contain the cell bodies of efferent neurones that have axons leaving the brain in cranial nerves. The locations of these nuclei are illustrated schematically in Fig. 10.2. Some can readily be seen in stained sections of the brainstem (see Figs 9.5–9.13).

Cranial nerve nuclei

Afferent nuclei

Afferent fibres carrying general sensory information (touch, pressure, pain, temperature) from the head enter the brain through the trigeminal nerve at the level of the pons and terminate in the **trigeminal sensory nucleus**. This is a large nucleus that runs the whole length of the brainstem and extends caudally into the cervical spinal cord. Fibres conveying the special senses of motion/positional sense and hearing run in the vestibulocochlear nerve. They terminate in the **vestibular** and **cochlear nuclei**, respectively, which are located in the medulla, in and near to the lateral part of the floor of the fourth ventricle (sometimes referred to as the vestibular area). Visceral afferents,

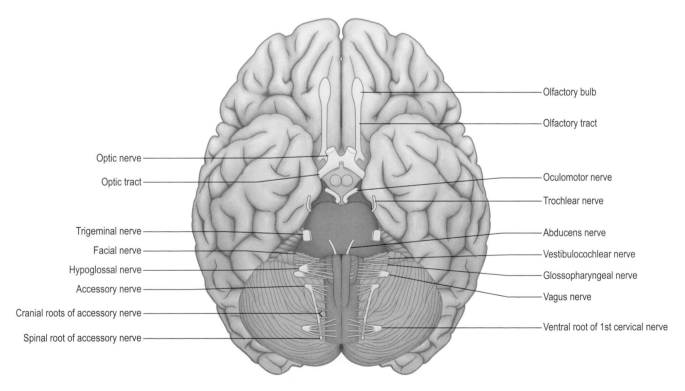

Fig. 10.1 The base of the brain illustrating the locations of the cranial nerves. The points of attachment are shown, except for the trochlear nerve, which arises from the dorsal aspect of the brainstem.

Table 10.1 **Summary of components, connections and functions of the cranial nerves**					
Cranial nerve		Component fibres	Structures innervated	Central connections	Functions
I	Olfactory	Sensory	Olfactory epithelium	Olfactory bulb	Olfaction
II	Optic	Sensory	Retina	Lateral geniculate nucleus; pretectal nucleus	Vision; pupillary light reflex
III	Oculomotor	Motor	Superior, inferior and medial rectus muscles, inferior oblique muscle; levator palpebrae superioris muscle	Oculomotor nucleus	Movement of eyeball; elevation of upper eyelid
		Parasympathetic	Sphincter pupillae and ciliary muscle of the eyeball, via ciliary ganglion	Edinger–Westphal nucleus	Pupillary constriction and accommodation
IV	Trochlear	Motor	Superior oblique muscle	Trochlear nucleus	Movement of eyeball
V	Trigeminal	Sensory	Face, scalp, cornea, nasal and oral cavities, cranial dura mater	Trigeminal sensory nucleus	General sensation
		Motor	Muscles of mastication; tensor tympani	Trigeminal motor nucleus	Opening and closing mouth; tension on tympanic membrane
VI	Abducens	Motor	Lateral rectus muscle	Abducens nucleus	Movement of eyeball
VII	Facial	Sensory	Anterior two-thirds of tongue	Nucleus solitarius	Taste
		Motor	Muscles of facial expression; stapedius muscle	Facial nucleus	Facial movement; tension on bones of middle ear
		Parasympathetic	Salivary and lacrimal glands, via submandibular and pterygopalatine ganglia	Superior salivatory nucleus	Salivation and lacrimation
VIII	Vestibulocochlear	Sensory	Vestibular apparatus; cochlea	Vestibular nuclei; cochlear nuclei	Vestibular sensation (position and movement of head); hearing
IX	Glossopharyngeal	Sensory	Pharynx, posterior third of tongue, Eustachian tube, middle ear	Trigeminal sensory nucleus	General sensation
			Posterior third of tongue; carotid body, carotid sinus	Nucleus solitarius	Taste; chemoreception, baroreception
		Motor	Stylopharyngeus muscle	Nucleus ambiguus	Swallowing
		Parasympathetic	Parotid salivary gland, via otic ganglion	Inferior salivatory nucleus	Salivation
X	Vagus	Sensory	Pharynx, larynx, trachea, oesophagus, external ear	Trigeminal sensory nucleus	General sensation
			Thoracic and abdominal viscera; aortic bodies, aortic arch	Nucleus solitarius	Visceral sensation: chemoreception, baroreception
		Motor	Soft palate, pharynx, larynx, upper oesophagus	Nucleus ambiguus	Speech, swallowing
		Parasympathetic	Thoracic and abdominal viscera	Dorsal motor nucleus of vagus	Innervation of cardiac muscle. Innervation of smooth muscle and glands of cardiovascular system, respiratory and gastrointestinal tracts
XI	Accessory (spinal roots)	Motor	Sternomastoid and trapezius muscles	Spinal cord	Movement of head and shoulder
XII	Hypoglossal	Motor	Intrinsic and extrinsic muscles of tongue	Hypoglossal nucleus	Movement of tongue

The components are colour-coded according to their embryological origin (see also Fig. 1.11 and Fig. 10.2).

including taste fibres, terminate in the **nucleus solitarius** of the medulla.

Efferent nuclei

On the basis of their embryological derivation, the efferent cranial nerve nuclei can be divided into three groups, each lying in a discontinuous longitudinal column.

Nuclei of the somatic efferent cell column

The somatic efferent cell column lies near to the midline and consists of the nuclei that send motor fibres into the III, IV, VI and XII nerves. The **oculomotor nucleus** lies in the ventral apex of the periaqueductal grey of the midbrain at the level of the superior colliculus (see Fig. 9.13). Its efferent fibres run in the oculomotor nerve to innervate the levator palpebrae superioris muscle and all of the extraocular muscles, except the superior oblique and lateral rectus. The **trochlear nucleus** also lies in the midbrain, at the ventral border of the periaqueductal grey, but at the level of the inferior colliculus (see Fig. 9.12). Fibres leave in the trochlear nerve, to innervate the superior oblique muscle of the eye. The **abducens nucleus** is located in the caudal pons beneath the floor of the fourth ventricle (see Fig. 9.8). Its efferents run in the abducens nerve and they innervate the lateral rectus muscle. In the medulla lies the

hypoglossal nucleus (see Fig. 9.7), which innervates the intrinsic and extrinsic muscles of the tongue via the hypoglossal nerve.

Nuclei of the branchiomotor cell column

The branchiomotor cell column innervates striated muscles derived from the embryonic branchial (pharyngeal) arches. In the tegmentum of the mid-pons is located the **trigeminal motor nucleus**, which supplies fibres to the trigeminal nerve and innervates the muscles of mastication, tensor tympani, tensor veli palatini, mylohyoid and the anterior belly of the digastric muscle. In the caudal pontine tegmentum lies the **facial motor nucleus**. This innervates the muscles of facial expression and the stapedius muscle via the facial nerve. Within the medulla lies the **nucleus ambiguus**. This long nucleus sends motor fibres into the glossopharyngeal, vagus and cranial part of the accessory nerve to innervate the muscles of the pharynx and larynx.

Nuclei of the parasympathetic cell column

The parasympathetic cell column consists of preganglionic parasympathetic neurones that send axons into the III, VII, IX and X cranial nerves. The most rostral cell group constitutes the **Edinger–Westphal nucleus**, which lies in the midbrain periaqueductal grey matter adjacent to the oculomotor nucleus (see Fig. 9.13). Its axons leave the brainstem in the oculomotor

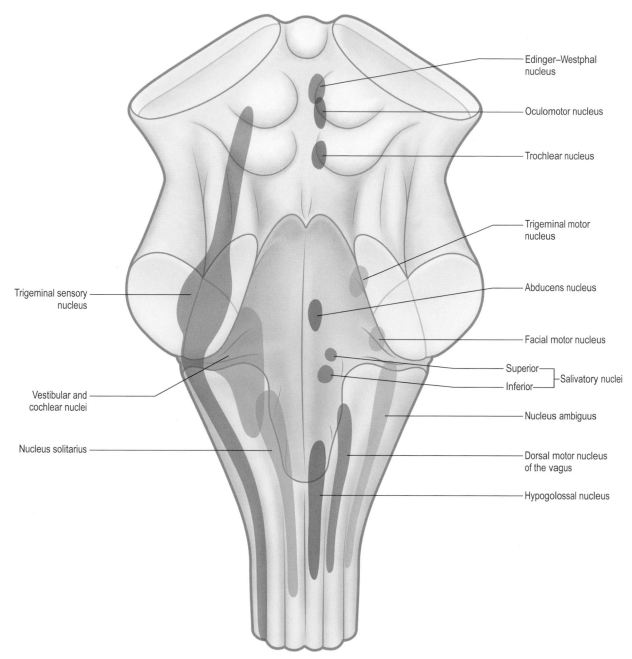

Fig. 10.2 The brainstem viewed from the dorsal aspect. The diagram illustrates the locations of the afferent cranial nerve nuclei (left) and the efferent cranial nerve nuclei (right). On the right, nuclei shaded in the same colour share a common embryological origin (see also Fig. 1.11).

nerve and pass to the ciliary ganglion in the orbit, within which they synapse; from here postganglionic fibres innervate the sphincter pupillae and ciliary muscles within the eye.

In the pontine tegmentum lie two parasympathetic cell groups, the **superior** and **inferior salivatory nuclei**. The superior salivatory nucleus supplies preganglionic fibres to the facial nerve that terminate in the pterygopalatine and submandibular ganglia. Postganglionic fibres from the pterygopalatine ganglion innervate the lacrimal gland and the nasal and oral mucous membranes. Those from the submandibular ganglion innervate the submandibular and sublingual salivary glands. The inferior salivatory nucleus sends preganglionic fibres into the glossopharyngeal nerve. These terminate in the otic ganglion, which in turn sends postganglionic axons to the parotid salivary gland.

The largest preganglionic parasympathetic cell group lies in the medulla and constitutes the **dorsal motor nucleus of the vagus** (see Fig. 9.7). Its rostral portion lies immediately beneath the floor of the fourth ventricle, lateral to the hypoglossal nucleus.

Fibres leave in the vagus nerve and are widely distributed to thoracic and abdominal viscera.

Cranial nerves

III: Oculomotor nerve

The oculomotor nerve carries the majority of somatic motor axons that innervate the extraocular muscles responsible for moving the eye. It also contains preganglionic parasympathetic neurones which, via the intermediary of the ciliary ganglion, control the smooth muscle within the eye.

The motor neurones serving the extraocular muscles have their cell bodies in the **oculomotor nucleus**, which lies at the base of the periaqueductal grey of the midbrain at the level of the superior colliculus (Fig. 10.3). Preganglionic parasympathetic neurones arise from the nearby **Edinger–Westphal nucleus** (Fig. 10.3; see also Fig. 9.13). Fibres from both sources course ventrally through the midbrain tegmentum, many of them traversing the red nucleus, to exit on the medial aspect of the crus

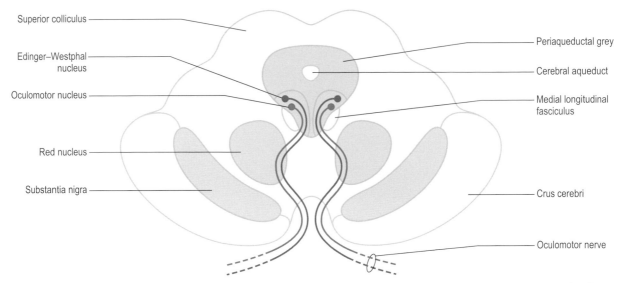

Fig. 10.3 Transverse section through the midbrain at the level of the superior colliculus. The diagram shows the origin and course of oculomotor nerve fibres within the brainstem.

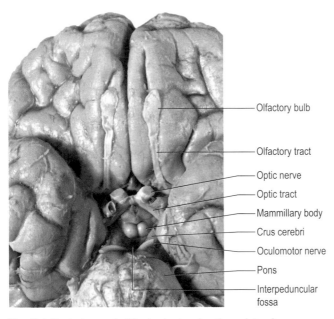

Fig. 10.4 Ventral aspect of the brain showing the points of attachment of cranial nerves I, II and III.

cerebri, within the interpeduncular fossa (Fig. 10.4; see also Fig. 10.9). The oculomotor nerve passes between the posterior cerebral and superior cerebellar arteries (see Fig. 7.2), then runs anteriorly, lying in the wall of the cavernous sinus (see Fig. 7.11), before gaining access to the orbit through the superior orbital fissure. The oculomotor nerve supplies all of the extraocular muscles, with the exception of the superior oblique and lateral rectus and, thus, functions to elevate, depress and adduct the eyeball (Fig. 10.5). It also innervates the striated muscle of the levator palpebrae superioris, serving to elevate the upper eyelid. Preganglionic parasympathetic neurones from the Edinger–Westphal nucleus terminate in the ciliary ganglion, located within the orbit, behind the eyeball. From here, postganglionic neurones run in the **short ciliary nerves** to innervate the sphincter (constrictor) pupillae muscle of the iris and the ciliary muscle contained within the ciliary body (see also Fig. 15.2).

Pupillary light reflex

The amount of light entering the eye is regulated by the size of the pupil. Illumination of the retina causes constriction of the pupil

through contraction of the sphincter pupillae muscle of the iris, thus reducing the amount of light reaching the retina. This is known as the **direct light reflex** (Fig. 10.6). Even if only one retina is illuminated (e.g. during clinical examination) the pupils of both eyes constrict. The constriction of the pupil of the non-illuminated eye is called the **consensual light reflex**. The afferent limb of the light reflex consists of a small contingent of optic tract fibres that pass directly from the eye to the **pretectal area**, just rostral to the superior colliculus, rather than to the lateral geniculate nucleus of the thalamus, where the majority of visual fibres terminate (see also Chapter 15). Neurones of the pretectal area project bilaterally to the Edinger–Westphal nuclei, from which efferent fibres leave in the oculomotor nerve.

Accommodation reflex

Fixation upon a nearby object, by convergence of the optic axes, involves concomitant contraction of the ciliary muscles to increase the convexity of the lens, thus focussing the image. It is also accompanied by pupillary constriction. The phenomenon involves the visual cortex, with corticobulbar fibres activating the parasympathetic neurones of the Edinger–Westphal nuclei bilaterally.

IV: Trochlear nerve

The thin trochlear nerve contains only somatic motor neurones. These arise in the **trochlear nucleus**, which lies in the ventral part of the midbrain periaqueductal grey, at the level of the inferior colliculus (Fig. 10.7). The efferent axons pass dorsally, around the periaqueductal grey, and decussate in the midline. The trochlear nerve emerges from the dorsal aspect of the brainstem (the only cranial nerve to do so) just caudal to the inferior colliculus (Fig. 10.8). The nerve courses round the cerebral peduncle to gain the ventral aspect of the brain (Fig. 10.9), passing between the posterior cerebral and superior cerebellar arteries (see Fig. 7.2), as does the oculomotor nerve. It then runs anteriorly, lying in the lateral wall of the cavernous sinus (see Fig. 7.11) and enters the orbit through the superior orbital fissure. It supplies just one muscle, the **superior oblique**. The action of the superior oblique is complex. Depending on the starting position of the eyeball it can act to depress, abduct or intort the eye. Importantly, with the eye adducted, the superior oblique depresses the visual axis.

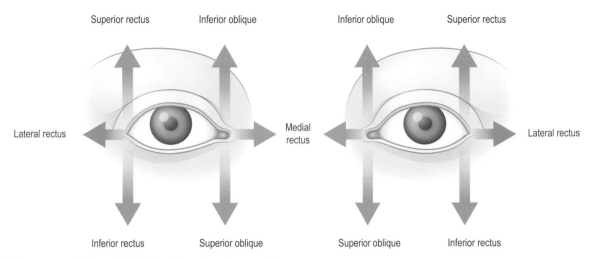

Fig. 10.5 Eye movements brought about by the extraocular muscles.

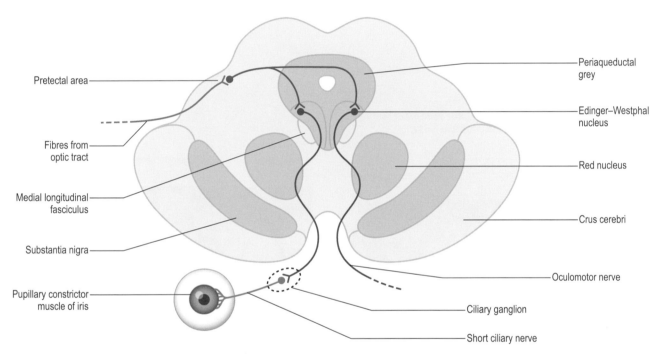

Fig. 10.6 Transverse section through the most rostral part of the midbrain. The diagram shows the pathways involved in the direct and consensual pupillary light reflexes.

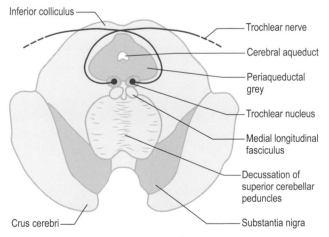

Fig. 10.7 Transverse section through the midbrain at the level of the inferior colliculus. The diagram shows the location of the trochlear nucleus and the course of trochlear nerve fibres.

VI: Abducens nerve

The abducens nerve, like the trochlear, contains only somatic motor neurones. The cell bodies of origin are located in the **abducens nucleus**, which lies beneath the floor of the fourth ventricle in the caudal pons (Fig. 10.10). Efferent axons course ventrally through the pons and emerge from the ventral surface of the brainstem at the junction between the pons and the pyramid of the medulla (Fig. 10.11). The nerve then passes anteriorly, through the cavernous sinus (see Fig. 7.11) and enters the orbit through the superior orbital fissure. The abducens supplies the lateral rectus muscle, which abducts the eye.

V: Trigeminal nerve

The trigeminal nerve has both sensory and motor components. It is the main sensory nerve for the head and, additionally, it innervates the muscles of mastication. It attaches to the brainstem as two adjacent roots (a large sensory and a smaller motor root) on the ventrolateral aspect of the pons, where this merges with the middle cerebellar peduncle (Figs 10.1, 10.9, 10.11).

The sensory fibres within the trigeminal nerve are primary sensory neurones with peripheral processes distributed, via the

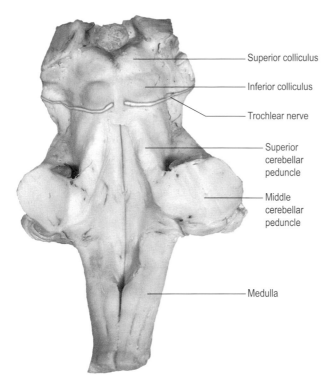

Fig. 10.8 Dorsal aspect of the brainstem, after removal of the cerebellum, showing the origin of the cranial nerve IV.

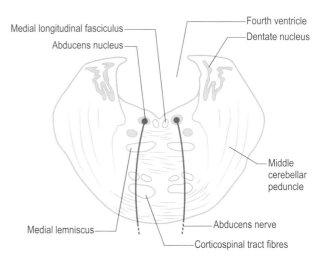

Fig. 10.10 Transverse section through the caudal pons. The diagram shows the location of the abducens nucleus and the course of abducens nerve fibres.

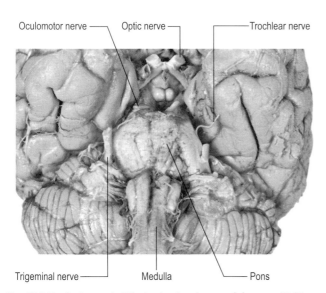

Fig. 10.9 Ventral aspect of the brain showing cranial nerves III, IV and V.

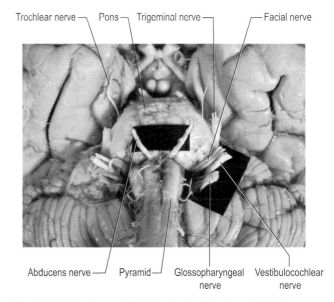

Fig. 10.11 Ventral aspect of the brain showing the points of attachment of cranial nerves VI–IX.

Lesions of cranial nerves III, IV and VI

A third cranial nerve palsy (Fig. 10.12) is caused by a lesion of the oculomotor nucleus within the midbrain or by compression of the peripheral course of cranial nerve III by an aneurysm or tumour. It leads to drooping of the eyelid (**ptosis**), dilation of the pupil that is unresponsive to light and accommodation, and an inability to move the eyeball upwards, downwards or inwards (adduction).

A lesion of the trochlear nerve is manifest by diplopia on looking medially and downwards (e.g. when walking downstairs).

A sixth cranial nerve palsy (Fig. 10.13) is caused by a lesion of the abducens nucleus in the pons or by compression of the peripheral course of the nerve by an aneurysm or tumour. It leads to an inability to move the eye outwards (abduction).

Combined unilateral palsies of cranial nerves III, IV and VI occur from lesions along their peripheral course where the nerves run adjacent to each other, such as within the cavernous sinus, at the entrance to the orbit (superior orbital fissure syndrome) and within the orbit. There they are vulnerable to compression by tumours and aneurysms. The effects of such unilateral lesions are:

• Ptosis.
• Dilation of the pupil that is unresponsive to light or accommodation.
• Paralysis of all eye movements (**ophthalmoplegia**) causing double vision (**diplopia**).

Multiple sclerosis can affect eye movements through demyelination of the medial longitudinal fasciculus in the brainstem, which interferes with conjugate ocular deviation. Typically, on horizontal gaze, the abducting eye moves normally but the adducting eye fails to follow. Adduction is preserved on convergence. **Internuclear ophthalmoplegia** is the term used to describe this disorder (Fig. 10.14). See also Fig. 10.27.

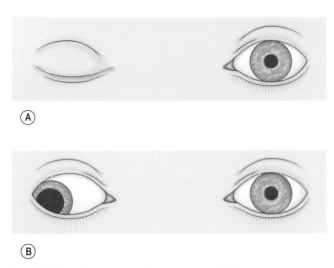

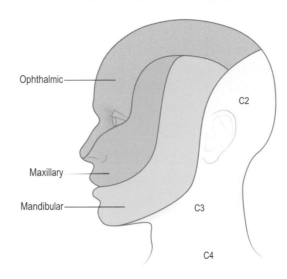

Fig. 10.15 Superficial distribution of sensory fibres in the three divisions of the trigeminal nerve.

Fig. 10.12 Right oculomotor (III) nerve palsy. (A) Shows ptosis on the right. (B) Shows that, with elevation of the eyelid, the eyeball can be seen to be abducted and the pupil dilated.

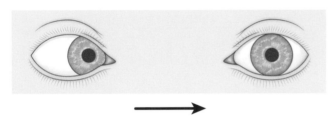

Fig. 10.13 Left abducens (VI) nerve palsy. On looking in the direction of the arrow, the left eye fails to abduct.

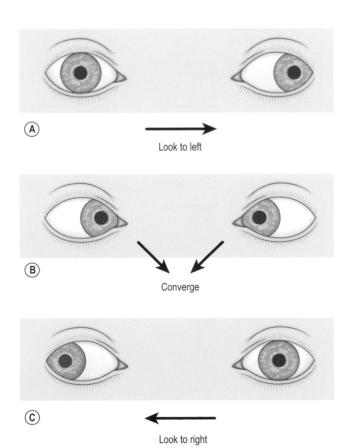

Look to left

Converge

Look to right

Fig. 10.14 Internuclear ophthalmoplegia.

ophthalmic, maxillary and mandibular divisions of the trigeminal, to numerous structures of the head (Fig. 10.15). The sensations of touch, pressure, pain and temperature are relayed from the face and scalp, the cornea, the nasal and oral cavities, including the teeth and gums and the paranasal sinuses. The trigeminal nerve also innervates the intracranial dura mater and intracranial arteries. In addition, proprioceptive fibres are carried from the muscles of mastication and the temporomandibular joint. The cell bodies of afferents in the trigeminal nerve, with the exception of those conveying proprioception, are located in the **trigeminal (or semilunar) ganglion**, located at the convergence of the ophthalmic, maxillary and mandibular nerves. The central processes of these cells terminate in the **trigeminal sensory nucleus** (Fig. 10.16).

The trigeminal sensory nucleus is a large nucleus which extends throughout the length of the brainstem and into the upper cervical spinal cord. It is considered to consist of three subnuclei. The **chief (or principal) sensory nucleus** lies in the pontine tegmentum close to the entry of the trigeminal nerve. The **mesencephalic nucleus** extends rostrally into the midbrain. The **spinal nucleus (or nucleus of the spinal tract of the trigeminal)** extends caudally through the medulla and into the cord, where it becomes continuous with the substantia gelatinosa, of which it is considered to be the brainstem homologue.

There is a segregated distribution of afferent fibre termination in the trigeminal nucleus, depending upon the modality being served. Fibres conveying touch and pressure terminate in the chief nucleus. Those carrying pain and temperature end in the spinal nucleus, reaching their termination by descending in the **spinal tract of the trigeminal**, a fascicle of fibres lying immediately superficial to the nucleus (see Figs 9.5, 9.6). In the upper cervical cord, the spinal tract of the trigeminal becomes continuous with Lissauer's tract, which carries functionally homologous afferents of spinal nerve origin, prior to their termination in the dorsal horn. Proprioceptive afferents derived from the muscles of mastication and the temporomandibular joint have their cell bodies not in the trigeminal ganglion, as might be expected, but in the mesencephalic nucleus of the trigeminal. They are the only primary afferents to have their cell bodies located within the CNS.

Axons arising from second-order neurones in the trigeminal nucleus decussate to form the contralateral **trigeminothalamic tract (trigeminal lemniscus)**. This terminates in the contralateral ventral posterior nucleus of the thalamus, which in turn sends

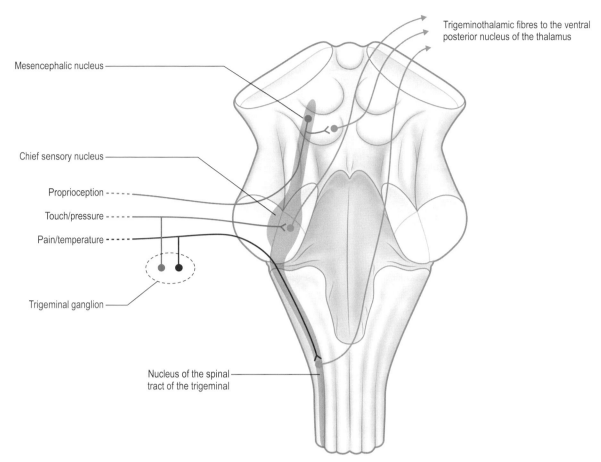

Trigeminothalamic fibres to the ventral posterior nucleus of the thalamus

Mesencephalic nucleus

Chief sensory nucleus

Proprioception

Touch/pressure

Pain/temperature

Trigeminal ganglion

Nucleus of the spinal tract of the trigeminal

Fig. 10.16 The brainstem indicating the location of the trigeminal sensory nucleus and its major connections.

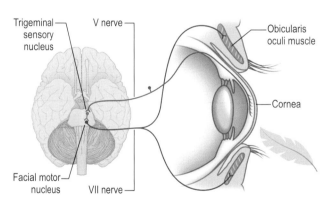

Trigeminal sensory nucleus

V nerve

Obicularis oculi muscle

Cornea

Facial motor nucleus

VII nerve

Fig. 10.17 Corneal reflex. Sensory neurone, blue; motor neurone, red.

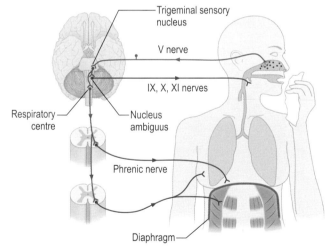

Trigeminal sensory nucleus

V nerve

IX, X, XI nerves

Respiratory centre

Nucleus ambiguus

Phrenic nerve

Diaphragm

Fig. 10.18 Sneeze and cough reflexes. Afferent fibres mediating the sneeze reflex only are illustrated. Sensory neurone, blue; motor neurone, red.

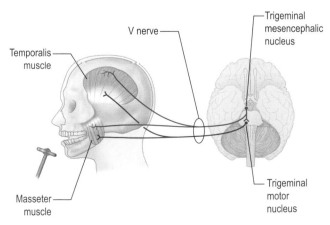

Trigeminal mesencephalic nucleus

V nerve

Temporalis muscle

Masseter muscle

Trigeminal motor nucleus

Fig. 10.19 Jaw jerk. Sensory neurone, blue; motor neurone, red.

fibres to the sensory cortex of the parietal lobe. In addition to this pathway for conscious awareness, the trigeminal nucleus also sends fibres to the cerebellum and establishes a number of reflex connections with certain motor cell groups of the brainstem. Among these is the facial nucleus, through which are mediated facial grimacing and eye closure (**corneal reflex**) in response to noxious stimulation in the territory served by the trigeminal nerve (Fig. 10.17). The **sneeze and cough reflexes** are initiated by afferents running in either the trigeminal nerve (from nasal mucosa) or the vagus nerve (from larynx and trachea) and ending in the trigeminal sensory nucleus. From here, indirect connections are made with diaphragmatic, intercostal and abdominal muscle motor neurones for the forceful expulsion of air, and with the nucleus ambiguus innervating pharyngeal and laryngeal muscles (Fig. 10.18). In the **jaw jerk**, downward percussion of the mandible stimulates proprioceptors in the temporalis and masseter muscles. Afferent fibres run in the trigeminal nerve and establish monosynaptic contact with alpha motor neurones in the trigeminal motor nucleus that serve the same muscles (Fig. 10.19).

The motor axons of the trigeminal nerve arise from cells in the trigeminal motor nucleus, which lies in the pontine tegmentum medial to the chief sensory nucleus (Fig. 10.2). Axons leave the pons in the motor root of the trigeminal and then join the mandibular division of the nerve. They innervate various muscles, the most significant of which are the muscles of mastication (masseter and temporalis, which close the jaw, and the lateral and medial pterygoids, which open the jaw). Trigeminal motor neurones also innervate tensor tympani within the middle ear, tensor veli palatini, mylohyoid and the anterior belly of digastric.

VII: Facial nerve

The facial nerve contains sensory, motor and parasympathetic components (Fig. 10.20). It joins the brainstem at the ventrolateral aspect of the caudal pons (Fig. 10.11), near the pontomedullary junction, in a region known as the **cerebellopontine angle**. The nerve consists of two roots, the more lateral (sometimes called the nervus intermedius) containing sensory and parasympathetic fibres, the more medial root being composed of motor axons.

The sensory fibres of the facial nerve subserve taste sensation from the anterior two-thirds of the tongue, the floor of the mouth and the palate, and also cutaneous sensation from part of the external ear. The cell bodies of primary afferent neurones lie in the **geniculate ganglion** within the facial canal of the petrous temporal bone. The central processes of taste fibres terminate in the rostral part of the **nucleus solitarius** of the medulla. Ascending fibres from the nucleus solitarius project to the ventral posterior nucleus of the thalamus, which in turn sends fibres to the sensory cortex of the parietal lobe. Afferent facial nerve fibres that carry cutaneous sensation terminate in the trigeminal nucleus.

Motor fibres of the facial nerve originate in the **facial motor nucleus** of the caudal pontine tegmentum (Fig. 10.21). The axons initially pass dorsomedially, looping over the abducens nucleus beneath the floor of the fourth ventricle, before leaving the

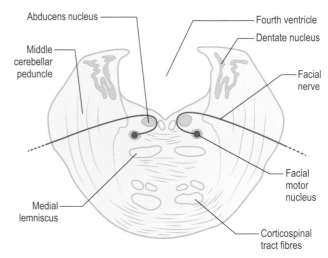

Fig. 10.21 Transverse section through the pons. The diagram shows the origin and course of the motor fibres of the facial nerve.

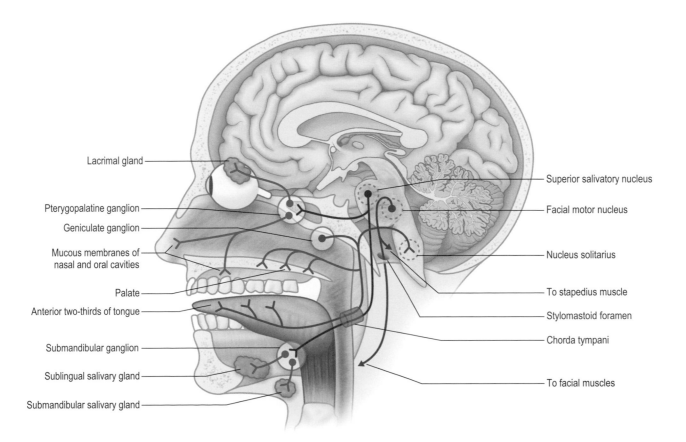

Fig. 10.20 Component fibres of the facial nerve and their peripheral distribution. Blue: sensory; orange: motor; purple: preganglionic parasympathetic; green: postganglionic parasympathetic.

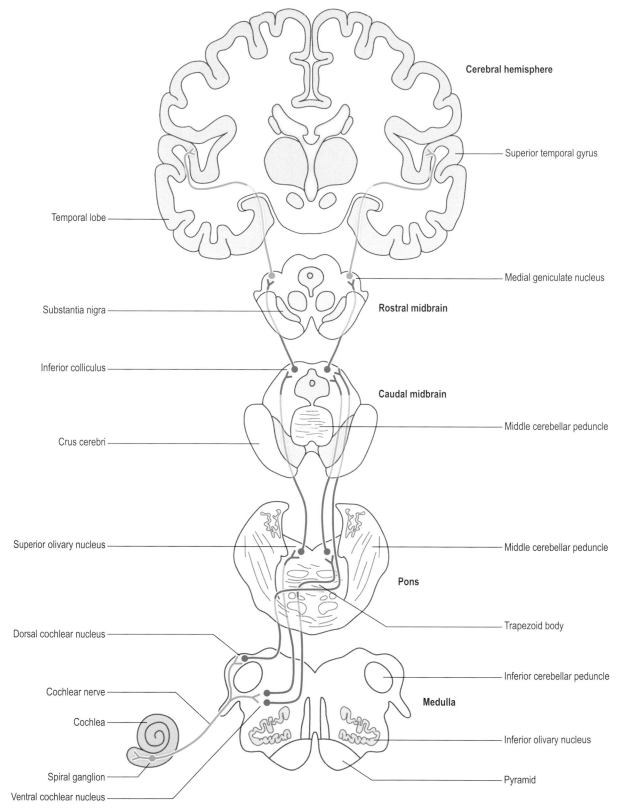

Fig. 10.22 Principal ascending connections of the auditory component of the vestibulocochlear nerve.

brainstem in the motor root of the facial nerve. Motor fibres are distributed to the muscles of facial expression, platysma, stylohyoid, the posterior belly of the digastric muscle and the stapedius muscle of the middle ear.

The facial motor nucleus receives afferents from other brainstem areas for the mediation of certain reflexes and also from the cerebral cortex. Reflex connections are established that mediate protective eye closure in response to visual stimuli or tactile stimulation of the cornea (**corneal reflex**) through fibres from the superior colliculus and the trigeminal sensory nucleus,

respectively. In addition, fibres from the superior olivary nucleus (Fig. 10.22), a part of the central auditory pathway, subserve reflex contraction of the stapedius muscle in response to loud noise.

Corticobulbar fibres from motor cortical areas innervate the facial motor nucleus. Those that control motor neurones supplying the muscles of the upper face (frontalis, orbicularis oculi) are distributed bilaterally. Those that control the motor neurones supplying the muscles of the lower face are entirely crossed. Unilateral upper motor neurone lesions, therefore, give rise to paralysis of the contralateral lower facial muscles.

Preganglionic parasympathetic fibres of the facial nerve originate in the **superior salivatory nucleus** of the pons. Fibres leave the brainstem in the sensory root of the facial nerve (nervus intermedius). From here, they pass to parasympathetic ganglia, namely the submandibular and pterygopalatine ganglia, where they synapse with postganglionic neurones. Postganglionic fibres from the submandibular ganglion innervate the submandibular and sublingual salivary glands. Those from the pterygopalatine ganglion innervate the lacrimal gland and the nasal and oral mucous membranes.

 Bell's palsy

Bell's palsy represents an acute unilateral inflammatory lesion of the facial nerve in its course through the skull. Pain is experienced around the ear and there is paralysis of the facial muscles unilaterally, with failure to close the eye, an absent corneal reflex, hyperacusis on the affected side and loss of taste sensation on the anterior two-thirds of the tongue (see also Fig. 10.27). When the herpes zoster virus is the inflammatory agent, a vesicular rash is apparent in the external auditory canal and the mucous membrane of the oropharynx (**Ramsay Hunt syndrome**).

VIII: Vestibulocochlear nerve

The vestibulocochlear nerve is a sensory nerve that conveys impulses from the inner ear. It has two component parts: the **vestibular nerve**, which carries information related to the position and movement of the head, and the **cochlear nerve**, which carries auditory information. Both divisions contain the axons of first-order sensory neurones, the dendrites of which make contact with hair cells of either the vestibular or auditory apparatus of the inner ear. Both divisions pass together through the internal auditory meatus (which also contains the facial nerve) and attach to the brainstem at the junction of the medulla and pons (Fig. 10.11), in the region known as the cerebellopontine angle.

The vestibular nerve

The vestibular nerve fibres make dendritic contact with **hair cells** of the vestibular portions of the membranous labyrinth; their cell bodies are located in the vestibular ganglion within the internal auditory meatus. The central processes of vestibular fibres mostly end in the **vestibular nuclei** of the rostral medulla. There are four such nuclei (superior, inferior, medial and lateral vestibular nuclei) located close together beneath the lateral part of the floor of the fourth ventricle.

The vestibular nuclei establish contact with a number of other regions for the control of posture, maintenance of equilibrium, coordination of head and eye movements, and the conscious awareness of vestibular stimulation. Fibres from the **lateral vestibular (Deiters') nucleus** descend ipsilaterally in the lateral vestibulospinal tract. The vestibular nuclei also contribute fibres to the **medial longitudinal fasciculus**. This extends throughout the brainstem and into the spinal cord; its descending component is also known as the medial vestibulospinal tract. Vestibulospinal fibres influence the activity of spinal motor neurones concerned with the control of body posture and balance. The ascending part of the medial longitudinal fasciculus establishes connections with the nuclei of the abducens, trochlear and oculomotor nerves for the coordination of head and eye movements. Some efferent fibres from the vestibular nuclei pass through the inferior cerebellar peduncle to the flocculonodular lobe of the cerebellum, which is concerned with the control of equilibrium. Other fibres ascend to the contralateral thalamus (ventral posterior nucleus), which in turn projects to the cerebral cortex. The cortical region responsible for conscious awareness of vestibular sensation is uncertain but is probably adjacent to the 'head' area of the sensory cortex in the parietal lobe or adjacent to the auditory cortex in the temporal lobe.

The cochlear nerve

The cochlear nerve fibres make dendritic contact with hair cells of the **organ of Corti** within the cochlear duct of the inner ear. The cell bodies of these fibres lie within the cochlea and are collectively called the spiral ganglion. The cochlear nerve joins the brainstem at the level of the rostral medulla. Its fibres bifurcate and end in the **dorsal** and **ventral cochlear nuclei**, which lie close to the inferior cerebellar peduncle. From here, the ascending auditory pathway to the thalamus and cerebral cortex (Fig. 10.22) is somewhat more complicated and variable than that for the general senses.

There are several locations between the medulla and thalamus where axons may synapse and not all fibres in the pathway behave in the same manner. From the cochlear nuclei, second-order neurones ascend into the pons, some of them crossing to the other side of the pontine tegmentum as the **trapezoid body**. At this level, some fibres may terminate in the **superior olivary nucleus**. This nucleus is the site of origin of olivocochlear fibres, which leave the brainstem in the vestibulocochlear nerve and end in the organ of Corti. They have an inhibitory function and serve to modulate transmission of auditory information to the cochlear nerve. From the superior olivary nuclei, ascending fibres comprise the **lateral lemniscus**, which runs through the pontine tegmentum to end in the **inferior colliculus** of the midbrain. Some axons within the lateral lemniscus terminate in a small pontine nucleus called the nucleus of the lateral lemniscus. The superior olivary nucleus and the nucleus of the lateral lemniscus are thought to establish reflex connections with motor neurones of the trigeminal and facial motor nuclei, mediating contraction of the tensor tympani and stapedius muscles in response to loud noise. The inferior colliculus sends axons to the **medial geniculate nucleus** of the thalamus. The final step in the ascending auditory pathway consists of axons that originate in the medial geniculate nucleus and pass through the internal capsule to the **primary auditory cortex** of the temporal lobe. This is located predominantly in the **transverse temporal gyri** (Heschl's gyri or convolutions; see Fig. 13.17), which are situated on the upper surface of the **superior temporal gyrus** and, therefore, are largely hidden within the lateral fissure. Throughout the ascending auditory projection, there exists a so-called 'tonotopical' representation of the cochlea, which is analogous to the 'somatotopic' organisation of the pathways for general sensation. Within the brainstem, some ascending fibres decussate while others do not. The representation of the cochlea is, therefore, bilateral at all levels rostral to the cochlear nuclei. For this reason, unilateral lesions of the ascending auditory pathway do not cause monaural deafness but, rather, are manifest as a loss of auditory acuity and an inability to localise the directional origin of sounds.

The region of the temporal lobe surrounding the primary auditory cortex is known as the **auditory association cortex** or **Wernicke's area**. It is here that auditory information is interpreted and given contextual significance. Wernicke's area is important in the processing of language by the brain (Chapter 13).

 Acoustic neuroma

An acoustic neuroma is a benign tumour of the eighth cranial nerve that leads to compression of the nerve and adjacent structures in the **cerebellopontine angle**. Attacks of dizziness accompanied by profound deafness occur (see also Fig. 10.27); with expansion of the tumour, ataxia and paralysis of the cranial nerves (especially V–VII) and the limbs follow. Unilateral and bilateral acoustic neuromas occur in the inherited disease **neurofibromatosis**, in which tumours of the peripheral nerves and skin (neurilemmoma and neurofibroma) can cause cosmetic blemish and deformity.

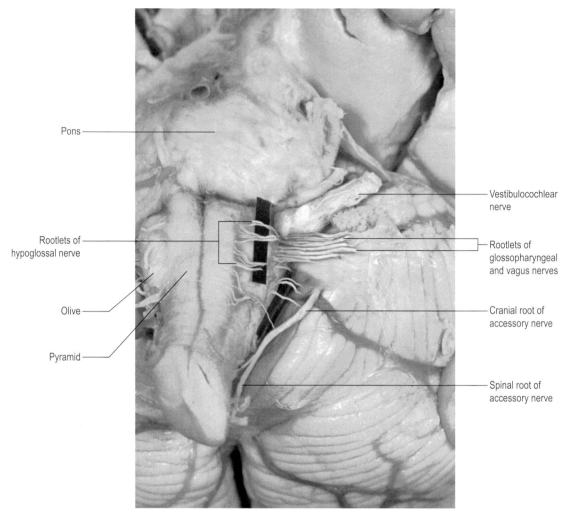

Fig. 10.23 Ventral aspect of the brainstem showing the points of attachment of cranial nerves VIII–XII.

IX: Glossopharyngeal nerve

The glossopharyngeal nerve is principally a sensory nerve, although it also contains preganglionic parasympathetic fibres and a few motor fibres. It attaches to the brainstem as a linear series of small rootlets, lateral to the olive in the rostral medulla (Figs 10.11, 10.23).

The afferent fibres of the glossopharyngeal nerve convey information from:

- Receptors for general sensation in the pharynx, the posterior third of the tongue, Eustachian tube and middle ear
- Taste buds of the pharynx and the posterior third of the tongue
- Chemoreceptors in the carotid body and baroreceptors in the carotid sinus

Within the brainstem, afferent fibres for general sensation end in the trigeminal sensory nucleus. Visceral and taste fibres of the glossopharyngeal nerve terminate in the **nucleus solitarius** of the medulla. Fibres carrying touch information from the pharynx and back of the tongue, and also taste fibres, are important for mediating the **swallowing** and **gag reflexes**, through connections with the nucleus ambiguus and the hypoglossal nucleus (Fig. 10.24).

The motor component of the glossopharyngeal nerve is very small. It arises from cells in the rostral part of the nucleus ambiguus of the medulla and innervates just one muscle, the stylopharyngeus, which is involved in swallowing.

Preganglionic parasympathetic fibres in the glossopharyngeal nerve originate in the **inferior salivatory nucleus** of the rostral medulla. These synapse with postganglionic neurones in the otic ganglion, which in turn innervate the parotid salivary gland.

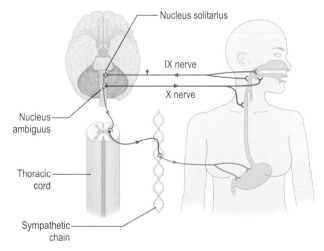

Fig. 10.24 Gag and swallowing reflexes.

X: Vagus nerve

Rootlets of the vagus nerve attach to the lateral aspect of the medulla immediately caudal to the glossopharyngeal nerve (Fig. 10.23). The vagus contains afferent, motor and parasympathetic fibres.

The afferent fibres of the vagus convey information from:

- Receptors for general sensation in the pharynx, larynx, oesophagus, tympanic membrane, external auditory meatus and part of the concha of the external ear

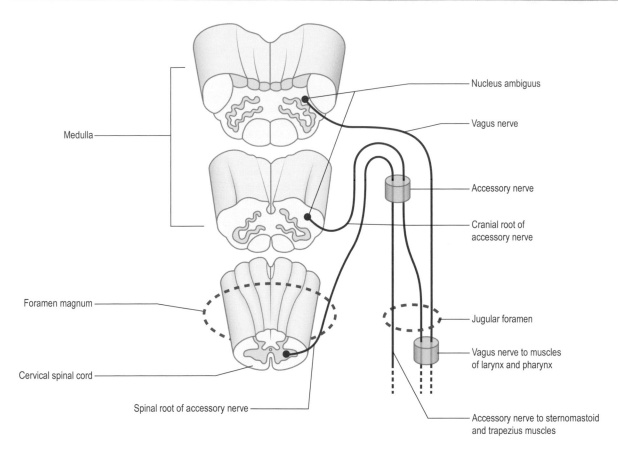

Fig. 10.25 The caudal medulla and rostral spinal cord. The diagram illustrates the origin and course of the motor fibres of the vagus and accessory nerves.

- Chemoreceptors in the aortic bodies and baroreceptors in the aortic arch
- Receptors widely distributed throughout the thoracic and abdominal viscera

Within the brainstem, afferents carrying general sensation end in the trigeminal sensory nucleus, while visceral afferents end in the nucleus solitarius.

The motor fibres of the vagus (Fig. 10.25) arise from the **nucleus ambiguus** of the medulla. They innervate the muscles of the soft palate, pharynx, larynx and upper part of the oesophagus. The nucleus ambiguus is, therefore, crucially important in the control of speech and swallowing. By convention, the most caudal efferents from the nucleus ambiguus are regarded as leaving the brainstem in the cranial roots of the accessory nerve, but these transfer to the vagus nerve proper at the level of the jugular foramen (Fig. 10.25).

The parasympathetic fibres of the vagus nerve originate from the **dorsal motor nucleus of the vagus**, which lies in the medulla immediately beneath the floor of the fourth ventricle (see Fig. 9.7). They are distributed widely throughout the cardiovascular, respiratory and gastrointestinal systems.

XI: Accessory nerve

The accessory nerve is purely motor in function. It consists of two parts: cranial and spinal. The cranial part emerges from the lateral aspect of the medulla as a linear series of rootlets which lie immediately caudal to the rootlets of the vagus nerve (Figs 10.23, 10.25). The cranial root of the accessory nerve carries fibres that have their origin in the caudal part of the nucleus ambiguus of the medulla. At the level of the jugular foramen these fibres join the vagus nerve and are distributed with it to the muscles of the soft palate, pharynx and larynx.

The spinal root of the accessory nerve arises from motor neurones located in the ventral horn of the spinal grey matter at levels C1–C5 (Fig. 10.25). The axons leave the cord not through the ventral roots of spinal nerves but via a series of rootlets that emerge from the lateral aspect of the cord midway between the dorsal and ventral roots. These rootlets course rostrally, coalescing as they do so, and enter the cranial cavity through the foramen magnum. At the side of the medulla, the spinal root of the accessory nerve is joined briefly by the cranial rootlets, but the component fibres separate once again as the nerve leaves the cranial cavity through the jugular foramen. Here the fibres of the cranial root of the accessory, which are derived from the nucleus ambiguus, join the vagus and are distributed with it. The fibres of the spinal root pass to the sternomastoid and trapezius muscles, which serve to move the head and shoulders.

XII: Hypoglossal nerve

The hypoglossal nerve is purely motor in function. It innervates both the extrinsic and intrinsic muscles of the tongue and, therefore, functions both to move the tongue and to change its shape. The axons originate in the hypoglossal nucleus, which lies immediately beneath the floor of the fourth ventricle, near the midline (Fig. 10.26 and see Fig. 9.7). Axons course ventrally through the medulla and emerge from its ventrolateral aspect as a linear series of rootlets located between the pyramid and the olive (Fig. 10.23). The hypoglossal nucleus receives afferents from the nucleus solitarius and the trigeminal sensory nucleus. These are involved in the control of the reflex movements of chewing, sucking and swallowing. It also receives corticobulbar fibres from the contralateral motor cortex, which subserve voluntary movements of the tongue such as occur in speech.

Inferior cerebellar peduncle

Hypoglossal nucleus

Inferior olivary nucleus

Pyramid

Medial lemniscus

Hypoglossal nerve

Fig. 10.26 Transverse section through the medulla. The diagram shows the origin and course of the fibres of the hypoglossal nerve.

Motor neurone disease and lesions of cranial nerves IX–XII

Motor neurone disease is a chronic degenerative disorder seen in those aged over 50 years. The corticobulbar tracts projecting to the nucleus ambiguus and hypoglossal nucleus degenerate, leading to dysphonia (difficulty in phonation), dysphagia (difficulty in swallowing), dysarthria (difficulty in articulation) and weakness and spasticity of the tongue (**pseudobulbar palsy**). There is also degeneration of the nucleus ambiguus and hypoglossal nuclei themselves, leading to dysphonia, dysphagia, dysarthria and weakness, wasting and fasciculation of the tongue (**bulbar palsy**).

The IX, X, XI and XII nerves can be damaged by compression in their peripheral course as they exit the cranium via the foramina of the skull base. Tumours in this area lead to dysphonia and depression of the gag reflex, together with unilateral wasting of the sternomastoid and trapezius muscles (**jugular foramen syndrome**) and unilateral weakness, wasting and fasciculation of the tongue (Fig. 10.27).

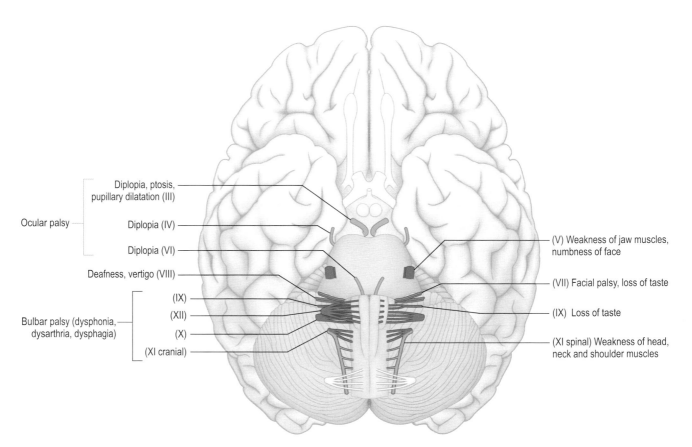

Ocular palsy
- Diplopia, ptosis, pupillary dilatation (III)
- Diplopia (IV)
- Diplopia (VI)

Deafness, vertigo (VIII)

Bulbar palsy (dysphonia, dysarthria, dysphagia)
- (IX)
- (XII)
- (X)
- (XI cranial)

(V) Weakness of jaw muscles, numbness of face

(VII) Facial palsy, loss of taste

(IX) Loss of taste

(XI spinal) Weakness of head, neck and shoulder muscles

Fig. 10.27 Neurological symptoms of cranial nerve lesions.

Cerebellum | 11

The cerebellum is the largest part of the hindbrain. It originates from the dorsal aspect of the brainstem and overlies the fourth ventricle. The cerebellum is connected to the brainstem by three stout pairs of fibre bundles, called the **inferior**, **middle** and **superior cerebellar peduncles** (Figs 11.1, 11.4; see also Figs 9.1–9.3); these join the cerebellum to the medulla, pons and midbrain, respectively. The functions of the cerebellum are entirely motor and it operates at an unconscious level. It controls the maintenance of equilibrium (balance), influences posture and muscle tone and coordinates movement.

External features of the cerebellum

The cerebellum consists of two laterally located **hemispheres**, joined in the midline by the **vermis** (Figs 11.2–11.4). The superior surface of the cerebellum lies beneath the dural tentorium cerebelli and the superior vermis is raised, forming a midline ridge. Conversely, the inferior vermis lies in a deep groove between the hemispheres. The surface of the cerebellum is highly convoluted, the folds, or **folia** (sing., folium), being oriented approximately transversely. Between the folia lie fissures of varying depths. Some of these fissures are landmarks that are used to divide the cerebellum anatomically into three lobes (Figs 11.2–11.5). On the superior surface, the deep **primary fissure** separates the relatively small **anterior lobe** from the much larger **posterior lobe**. On the underside, the conspicuous **posterolateral fissure** demarcates the location of small regions of the hemisphere (the **flocculus**) and vermis (the **nodule**), which together form the **flocculonodular lobe**.

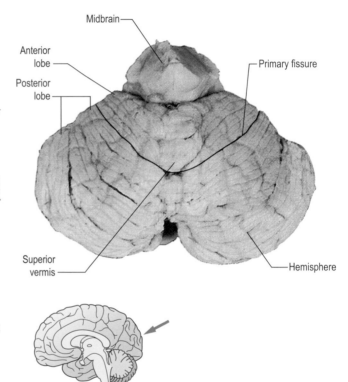

Fig. 11.2 Superior surface of the cerebellum. The cerebellum and brainstem have been detached from the forebrain by cutting through the rostral midbrain.

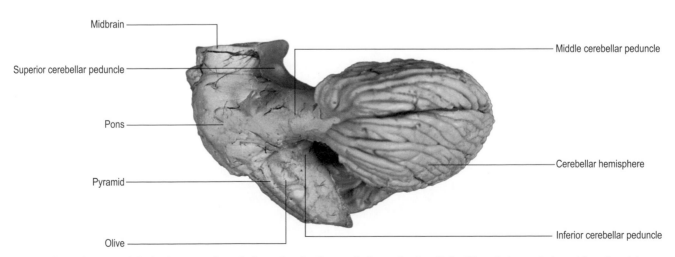

Fig. 11.1 Lateral aspect of the brainstem and cerebellum, showing the cerebellar peduncles. Parts of the anterior, posterior and flocculonodular lobes (q.v.) have been removed to display the peduncles more clearly.

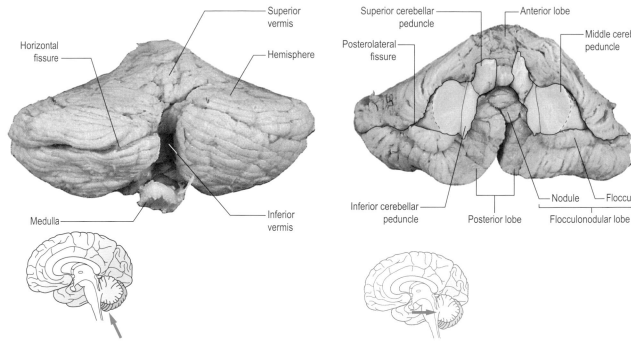

Fig. 11.3 Posterior aspect of the cerebellum.

Fig. 11.4 Anteroinferior aspect of the cerebellum.

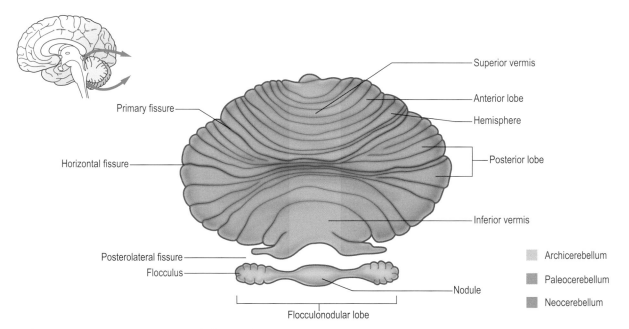

Fig. 11.5 Schematic representation of the cerebellum in which the peduncles have been cut and the surface flattened out. The relationships between the anatomical and functional divisions of the cerebellum are shown.

External features of the cerebellum

- The cerebellum controls the maintenance of equilibrium, posture and muscle tone and it coordinates movement. It operates at an unconscious level.

- The cerebellum is connected to the medulla, pons and midbrain by the inferior, middle and superior cerebellar peduncles, respectively.

- The cerebellum consists of a midline vermis and two laterally located hemispheres.

- Anatomically, the cerebellum is divided into anterior, posterior and flocculonodular lobes.

Internal structure of the cerebellum

The cerebellum basically consists of an outer layer of grey matter, the **cerebellar cortex**, and an inner core of white matter. The white matter is made up largely of afferent and efferent fibres that run to and from the cortex, towards which it extends characteristic, irregular, branch-like projections. This formation is referred to poetically in older literature as the *'arbor vitae'* or *'tree of life'* (Figs 11.6, 11.7). Buried deep within the white matter are four bilaterally paired **cerebellar nuclei** (Figs 11.6–11.8), which constitute the output of the cerebellum to other levels of the neuraxis. They have important connections with the cerebellar cortex and with certain nuclei of the brainstem and thalamus.

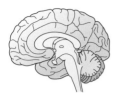

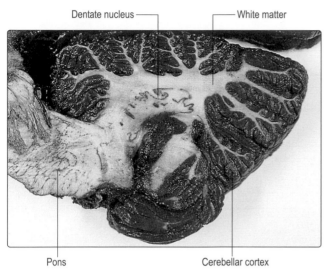

Fig. 11.6 **Parasagittal section through the cerebellum.** Mulligan's stain.

Cerebellar cortex

The cerebellar cortex is highly convoluted, forming numerous transversely oriented folia. Within the cortex lie the cell bodies, dendrites and synaptic connections of the vast majority of cerebellar neurones. The cellular organisation of the cortex is the same in all regions (Figs 11.9, 11.10). It is divided histologically into three layers:

An outer, fibre-rich, **molecular layer**
An intermediate, **Purkinje cell layer**
An inner **granular layer**, which is dominated by the **granule cell**

Afferent projections to the cerebellum arise principally from the spinal cord (spinocerebellar fibres), inferior olivary nucleus (olivocerebellar fibres), vestibular nuclei (vestibulocerebellar fibres) and pons (pontocerebellar fibres). Afferent axons mostly terminate in the cerebellar cortex, where they are excitatory to cortical neurones. Fibres enter the cerebellum through one of the cerebellar peduncles and proceed to the cortex as either **mossy fibres** or **climbing fibres**, depending upon their origin (Fig. 11.10). All afferents originating elsewhere than the inferior olivary nucleus end as mossy fibres. Mossy fibres branch to supply several folia and end in the granular layer, in synaptic contact with granule cells. The axons of granule cells pass towards the surface of the cortex and enter the molecular layer. Here they bifurcate to produce two **parallel fibres** that are oriented along the long axis of the folium.

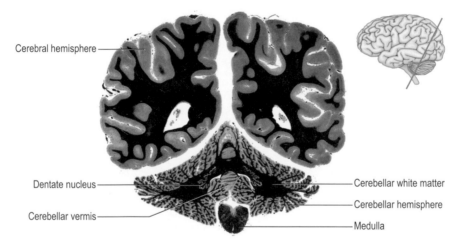

Fig. 11.7 **Coronal section of the brain at the level of the dentate nucleus; myelin stain.** *(Section courtesy of the National Museum of Health and Medicine, Armed Forces Institute of Pathology, Washington, DC, USA.)*

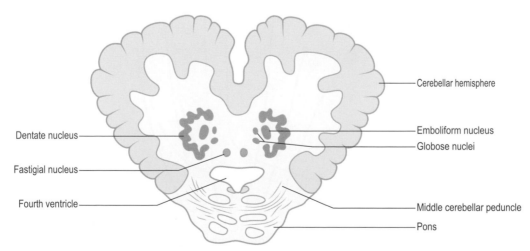

Fig. 11.8 **Horizontal section through the cerebellum and brainstem at the level of the fourth ventricle, showing the cerebellar nuclei.**

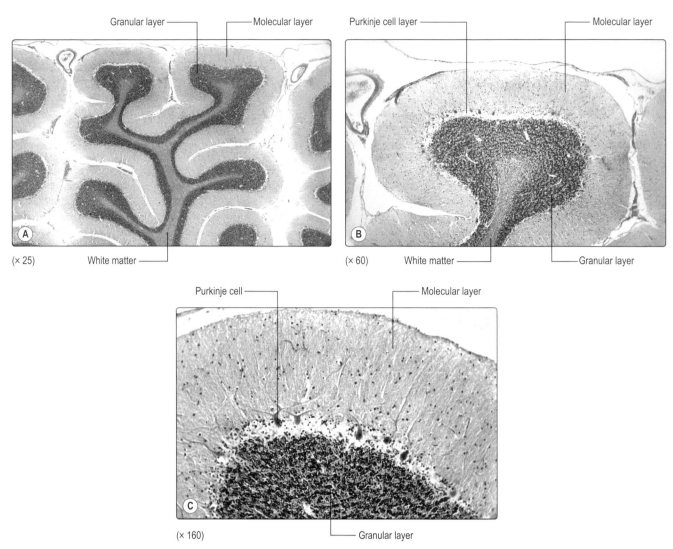

Granular layer — Molecular layer

Purkinje cell layer — Molecular layer

(× 25) White matter —

(× 60) White matter — Granular layer

Purkinje cell — Molecular layer

(× 160) Granular layer

Fig. 11.9 (A–C) Transverse sections of cerebellar folia showing the layers of the cerebellar cortex.

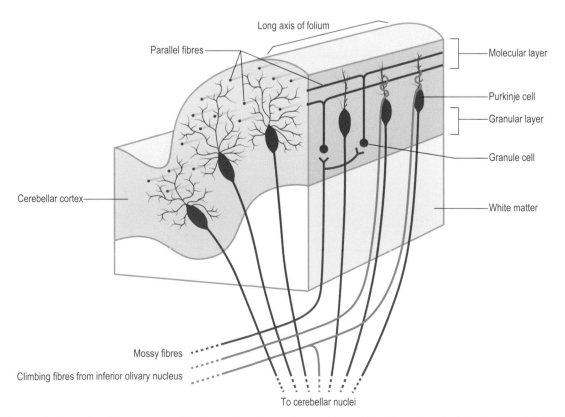

Long axis of folium

Parallel fibres

Molecular layer

Purkinje cell

Granular layer

Granule cell

Cerebellar cortex

White matter

Mossy fibres

Climbing fibres from inferior olivary nucleus

To cerebellar nuclei

Fig. 11.10 The cerebellar cortex. Diagram shows afferent and efferent connections and their relationships to the principal cells of the cerebellar cortex.

The Purkinje cell layer consists of a unicellular layer of the somata (cell bodies) of Purkinje neurones. The profuse dendritic arborisations of these cells (see Fig. 2.1B) extend towards the surface of the cortex, into the molecular layer (Fig. 11.10). The arborisations are flattened and oriented at right angles to the long axis of the folium. They are, therefore, traversed by numerous parallel fibres, from which they receive excitatory synaptic input. Inhibitory modulation of intracortical circuitry is provided by numerous other neurones known as Golgi, basket and stellate cells. The axons of Purkinje cells are the only axons to leave the cerebellar cortex. Most of these fibres do not leave the cerebellum entirely but end in the deep cerebellar nuclei. The other type of afferent fibre entering the cerebellar cortex, the climbing fibre, originates from the inferior olivary nucleus of the medulla. These fibres provide relatively discrete excitatory input to Purkinje cells. At the same time, axon collaterals of climbing fibres excite the neurones of the deep cerebellar nuclei. Purkinje cells utilise GABA as their neurotransmitter, which means that the output of the whole of the cerebellar cortex is mediated through the inhibition of cells in the cerebellar nuclei.

Cerebellar nuclei

Deep within the cerebellar white matter, above the roof of the fourth ventricle, lie four bilaterally paired nuclei. From medial to lateral, they are known as:

- Fastigial nucleus
- Globose nucleus
- Emboliform nucleus
- Dentate nucleus (Figs 11.6–11.8)

The dentate nucleus is by far the largest of the cerebellar nuclei and is the only one that can be discerned clearly with the naked eye (Fig. 11.6). It consists of a thin layer of nerve cells which, in three dimensions, is reminiscent of a crenated bag; as a result, it appears somewhat similar to the inferior olivary nucleus of the medulla, from which it receives afferent fibres. The cerebellar nuclei also receive extracerebellar afferents from the vestibular nuclei, reticular nuclei, pontine nuclei and spinocerebellar tracts, predominantly by means of collaterals of mossy fibres destined for the cerebellar cortex. From within the cerebellum, the nuclei receive dense innervation from the Purkinje cells of the cerebellar cortex itself. The cerebellar nuclei constitute the primary source of efferent fibres from the cerebellum to other parts of the brain. The

principal destinations of efferent fibres are the reticular and vestibular nuclei of the medulla and pons, the red nucleus of the midbrain and the ventral lateral nucleus of the thalamus.

Internal structure of the cerebellum

- Internally, the cerebellum consists of a surface layer of cortex, highly convoluted to form folia, beneath which lies white matter.

- Within the white matter lie cerebellar nuclei (fastigial, globose, emboliform and dentate).

- The nuclei are the origin of cerebellar efferent fibres.

Functional anatomy of the cerebellum

The cerebellum is often regarded as consisting of three functional subdivisions, based upon phylogenetic, anatomical and functional considerations (Fig. 11.5).

- The **archicerebellum**, or oldest portion in phylogenetic terms, is equated with the **flocculonodular lobe** and the associated **fastigial** nuclei.
- The **paleocerebellum** approximates to the midline **vermis** and surrounding **paravermis**, together with the **globose** and **emboliform** nuclei.
- The **neocerebellum** comprises the remainder (and vast majority) of the **cerebellar hemisphere** and the **dentate nuclei**.

Archicerebellum

The archicerebellum is primarily concerned with the maintenance of balance (equilibrium). It has extensive connections with the vestibular and reticular nuclei of the brainstem, through the inferior cerebellar peduncles (Fig. 11.11). Vestibular information is carried from the vestibular nuclei to the cortex of the ipsilateral flocculonodular lobe. Cortical efferent (Purkinje cell) fibres project to the fastigial nucleus which, in turn, projects back to the vestibular nuclei and to the reticular formation. A significant proportion of fastigial efferents cross to the contralateral side of the brainstem. The influence of the archicerebellum upon the lower motor system is, therefore, bilateral and principally mediated by means of descending vestibulospinal and reticulospinal projections.

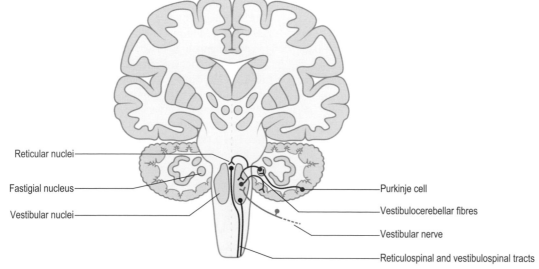

Fig. 11.11 Connections of the archicerebellum. Contralateral projections of the fastigial nucleus are not shown.

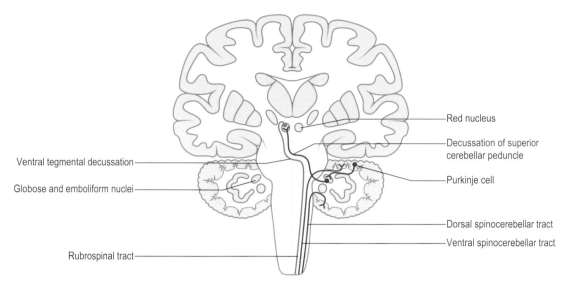

Fig. 11.12 Connections of the paleocerebellum.

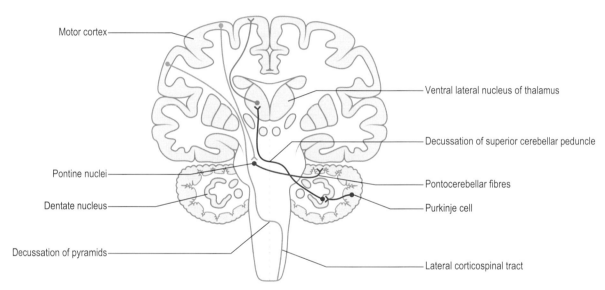

Fig. 11.13 Connections of the neocerebellum.

Paleocerebellum

The paleocerebellum influences muscle tone and posture. Afferents consist principally of dorsal and ventral spinocerebellar tract neurones that carry information from muscle, joint and cutaneous receptors and enter the cerebellum through the inferior and superior cerebellar peduncles, respectively (Fig. 11.12). Fibres terminate largely in the cortex of the ipsilateral vermis and adjacent paravermis. Cerebellar cortical efferents from these areas pass to the globose and emboliform nuclei and also to the fastigial nucleus. The globose and emboliform nuclei project via the superior cerebellar peduncle to the contralateral red nucleus of the midbrain, where they influence the activity of cells giving rise to the descending rubrospinal tract.

Neocerebellum

The neocerebellum is concerned with muscular coordination, including the trajectory, speed and force of movements. The principal afferent pathway to the neocerebellum consists of pontocerebellar fibres that originate in the pontine nuclei, located in the basal portion of the pons (Fig. 11.13). Pontocerebellar neurones are influenced by widespread regions of the cerebral cortex, involved in the planning and execution of movement, via corticopontine fibres that end in the pontine nuclei. Pontocerebellar fibres cross to the opposite side of the brainstem, entering the cerebellum through the middle cerebellar peduncle. Pontocerebellar fibres terminate predominantly in the lateral parts of the cerebellar hemisphere. Output from the neocerebellar cortex is directed to the dentate nucleus. The dentate is the largest of the cerebellar nuclei and it, in turn, projects to the contralateral red nucleus and ventral lateral nucleus of the thalamus. These efferent fibres form the major part of the superior cerebellar peduncle, or brachium conjunctivum (see Figs 9.11, 9.12). The ascending fibres decussate in the caudal midbrain just before reaching the red nucleus. Some fibres relay in the red nucleus with rubrothalamic cells, but most bypass the red nucleus and proceed directly to the ventral lateral thalamus. The ventral lateral nucleus of the thalamus projects to the cerebral cortex, principally to the motor cortex of the frontal lobe. The neocerebellum thus exerts its role in the coordination of movement primarily through an action on cerebral cortical areas that give rise to descending corticospinal and corticobulbar pathways.

Functional anatomy of the cerebellum

- The archicerebellum corresponds to the flocculonodular lobe and fastigial nucleus. Its principal connections are with the vestibular and reticular nuclei of the brainstem and it is concerned with the maintenance of equilibrium.

- The paleocerebellum corresponds to the vermis and paravermal area, together with the globose and emboliform nuclei. It receives fibres from the spinocerebellar tracts and projects to the red nucleus of the midbrain.

- The neocerebellum corresponds to most of the cerebellar hemisphere and the dentate nucleus. It receives afferents from the pons and projects to the ventral lateral nucleus of the thalamus.

Lesions of the cerebellum

A midline lesion of the cerebellum (such as a tumour) leads to loss of postural control; as a result, it is impossible to stand or sit without toppling over, despite preserved coordination of the limbs themselves.

Because of the pattern of ipsilateral and decussated pathways that enter and leave the cerebellum, unilateral lesions of the cerebellar hemisphere cause symptoms on the same side of the body. This is in contrast to cerebral lesions (e.g. in the cerebral cortex, internal capsule or basal ganglia), which give rise to contralateral symptoms.

A unilateral cerebellar hemispheric lesion causes ipsilateral incoordination of the arm (**intention tremor**) and of the leg, causing an unsteady gait, in the absence of weakness or sensory loss.

Bilateral dysfunction of the cerebellum, caused by alcoholic intoxication, hypothyroidism, inherited cerebellar degeneration/ataxia, multiple sclerosis or paraneoplastic disease, causes slowness and scanning of speech (**dysarthria**), incoordination of both arms and a staggering, wide-based, unsteady gait (**cerebellar ataxia**).

Cerebellar lesions also impair coordination of eye movements. The eyes exhibit a characteristic, involuntary and rhythmic to-and-fro motion (**nystagmus**), greatest in amplitude when gaze is directed to the same side as the lesion. Nystagmus is a very common feature of multiple sclerosis. The combination of nystagmus with scanning dysarthria and intention tremor constitutes '**Charcot's triad**', which is highly diagnostic of the disease.

12 | Thalamus

Rostral to the midbrain lies the forebrain (prosencephalon, cerebrum; see Fig. 1.13). The forebrain consists of the bilaterally paired diencephalon and cerebral hemisphere on each side and is by far the largest derivative of the three basic embryological divisions of the brain. The diencephalon is continuous with the rostral part of the midbrain and lies between the brainstem and the cerebral hemisphere. From dorsal to ventral, the diencephalon is comprised of the epithalamus, thalamus, subthalamus and hypothalamus, of which the thalamus is the largest. The **thalamus** consists of numerous nuclei, most of which have extensive reciprocal connections with the cerebral cortex. Of particular note are:

- Nuclei that transmit general and special sensory information to corresponding regions of the sensory cortices
- Nuclei that receive impulses from the cerebellum and basal ganglia and interface with motor regions of the frontal lobe
- Nuclei that have connections with associative and limbic areas of the cerebral cortex

The diencephalon is almost entirely surrounded by the cerebral hemisphere; consequently, little of its structure can be seen externally, apart from the ventral portion of the **hypothalamus**, which can be seen on the base of the brain (Fig. 12.1). Immediately caudal to the optic chiasm is a small midline elevation, the **tuber cinereum**. From its apex extends the **infundibulum** or pituitary stalk, which attaches to the pituitary gland. Caudal to the tuber cinereum, a pair of rounded

eminences, the mammillary bodies, are located on either side of the midline. These contain the mammillary nuclei of the hypothalamus. The hypothalamus lies below the thalamus, extending medial and ventral to the subthalamus. It has important connections with the limbic system, a controlling influence upon the activity of the autonomic nervous system and a central role in neuroendocrine function, partly through its relationship with the pituitary gland. The hypothalamus is discussed further in Chapter 16.

The other parts of the diencephalon can be seen in sagittal and coronal sections of the brain (Figs 12.2, 12.3). The diencephalon forms the lateral wall of the third ventricle. The dorsal part of the ventricular wall is formed by the thalamus and the ventral part by the hypothalamus. The **epithalamus** is a relatively small part of the diencephalon located, in its most caudal and dorsal region, immediately rostral to the superior colliculus of the midbrain. It consists principally of the **pineal gland** and the **habenula** (**habenular nuclei**). The pineal gland (Fig. 12.2 and see Fig. 13.12) is an endocrine organ. It synthesises the hormone melatonin. The pineal gland has been implicated in control of the sleep/waking cycle (circadian rhythm) and in regulation of the onset of puberty. The habenula (habenular nuclei; Fig. 12.2 and see Fig. 13.11) has connections with the limbic system (Chapter 16).

The **subthalamus** lies beneath the thalamus and dorsolateral to the hypothalamus, with its ventrolateral aspect against the internal capsule. It contains two notable cell groups, the **subthalamic nucleus** and the **zona incerta**. The subthalamic nucleus is located

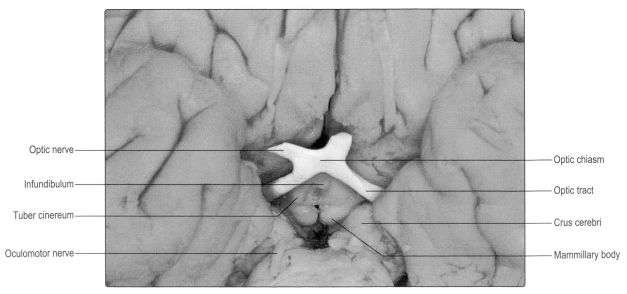

Optic nerve
Infundibulum
Tuber cinereum
Oculomotor nerve

Optic chiasm
Optic tract
Crus cerebri
Mammillary body

Fig. 12.1 Ventral aspect of the diencephalon.

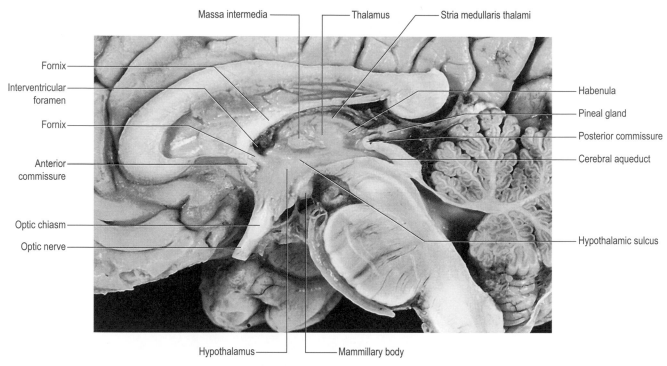

Fig. 12.2 **Median sagittal section of the brain showing the relationships of the diencephalon.**

in the ventrolateral part of the subthalamus, immediately medial to the internal capsule (see Figs 13.9, 14.8). It has the shape of a biconvex lens in coronal section. The subthalamic nucleus has prominent connections with the globus pallidus and the substantia nigra and is important in the control of movement. It is discussed in more detail in Chapter 14. The zona incerta is a rostral extension of the brainstem reticular formation. Several important fibre systems traverse the subthalamus en route to the thalamus. These include ascending sensory projections (medial lemniscus, spinothalamic tracts, trigeminothalamic tracts), cerebellothalamic fibres from the dentate nucleus and pallidothalamic fibres from the internal segment of the globus pallidus. The latter group of fibres envelop the zona incerta as the lenticular fasciculus and thalamic fasciculus (see Fig. 14.8).

Topographical anatomy of the thalamus

External features

The thalamus has been likened in size and shape to a small hen's egg. Together with the hypothalamus, it forms the lateral wall of the third ventricle, the transition between the two being marked by a faint groove, the hypothalamic sulcus. In most individuals, the two thalami are joined across the thin slit of the ventricle by the **interthalamic adhesion** or **massa intermedia**. A fascicle of nerve fibres, the **stria medullaris (thalami)**, which has limbic connections, courses along the dorsomedial margin of the thalamus (Fig. 12.2). Along this line, the ependymal lining of the third ventricle spans the narrow lumen to form the ventricular roof.

The anterior pole of the thalamus extends as far as the interventricular foramen, through which the third and lateral ventricles are in continuity. Lateral to the thalamus lies the posterior limb of the internal capsule and anterolateral lies the head of the caudate nucleus (Fig. 12.4). The dorsal aspect of the thalamus thus forms part of the floor of the body of the lateral ventricle. Another fascicle of nerve fibres with limbic connections, the **stria terminalis**, marks the boundary between thalamus and

caudate (Figs 12.3B, 12.4). Ventral to the thalamus lie the subthalamus and hypothalamus; caudal to it lies the midbrain.

Internal organisation

Within the thalamus is located a thin layer of nerve fibres composed of some of the afferent and efferent connections of thalamic nuclei. This is called the **internal medullary lamina** (Figs 12.3, 12.5, 12.6). The lamina is roughly Y-shaped when viewed from above and provides the basis for dividing the main part of the thalamus into three nuclear masses: **anterior**, **medial** and **lateral**. Each of these cellular complexes is further subdivided into a number of individually named nuclei. The lateral nuclear group, in particular, has important connections with sensory and motor regions of the cerebral cortex. Embedded within the internal medullary lamina are several cell groups, known collectively as the **intralaminar nuclei** (Fig. 12.5). Lateral to the main mass of thalamic nuclei lies another sheet of nerve fibres, the **lateral medullary lamina** (Fig. 12.3B), which consists of thalamocortical and corticothalamic fibres. Between this and the internal capsule is located a thin stratum of neurones that constitute the **reticular nucleus** of the thalamus (Fig. 12.3B).

Anatomy of the thalamus

- The thalamus is the largest component of the diencephalon, which is situated between the brainstem and the cerebral hemisphere.

- Almost all thalamic nuclei have rich reciprocal connections with the cerebral cortex.

- The thalamus is divided into three principal nuclear masses (anterior, medial and lateral) by

  the internal medullary lamina. The lateral nuclear group have connections with sensory and motor cortices.

- Embedded within the internal medullary lamina lie intralaminar nuclei.

- On the lateral aspect of the thalamus lies the thin reticular nucleus.

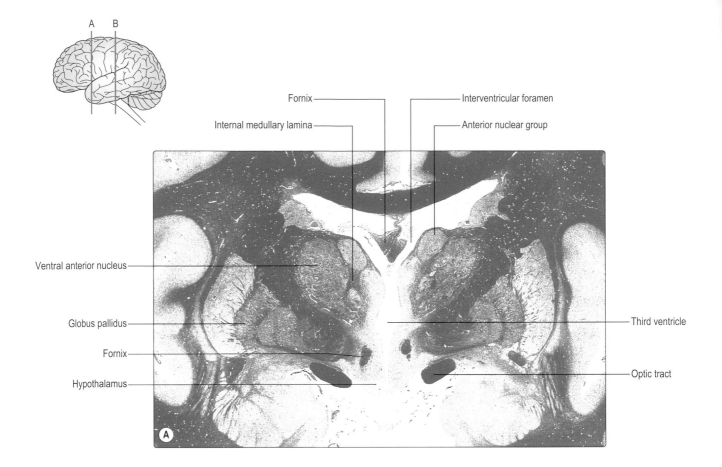

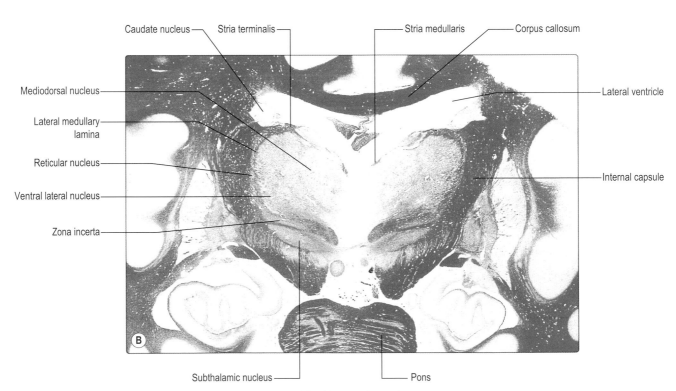

Fig. 12.3 (A,B) Coronal sections through the diencephalon. Luxol fast blue stain for myelin.

thalamic nuclei include the nuclei of the dorsal tier of the lateral nuclear complex as well as the whole of the anterior and medial complexes.

Lateral nuclear group

The lateral nuclear group contains all of the so-called 'specific' thalamic nuclei. These are located in the ventral part of the complex and include the ventral anterior, ventral lateral, ventral posterior, lateral geniculate and medial geniculate nuclei (Figs 12.5, 12.6).

Ventral posterior nucleus

The ventral posterior (VP) nucleus lies between the ventrolateral nucleus and the pulvinar. Within the ventral posterior nucleus there is termination of all the ascending pathways from the spinal cord and brainstem that carry general sensory information from the contralateral half of the body to a conscious level. These pathways include the spinothalamic tracts, medial lemniscus and trigeminothalamic tracts. The termination of these fibres in the ventral posterior nucleus is highly organised somatotopically.

An extensive, lateral portion of the nucleus receives information from the trunk and limbs via the spinothalamic tracts and medial lemniscus. This is referred to as the ventral posterolateral (VPL) division (Fig. 12.6). A smaller, medial portion of the ventral posterior nucleus receives information from the head, via the trigeminothalamic tract, and is termed the ventral posteromedial nucleus (VPM). This area also receives taste information from the nucleus solitarius of the medulla and vestibular information from the vestibular nuclei. The ventral posterior nucleus projects to the primary somatosensory cortex in the postcentral gyrus of the parietal lobe.

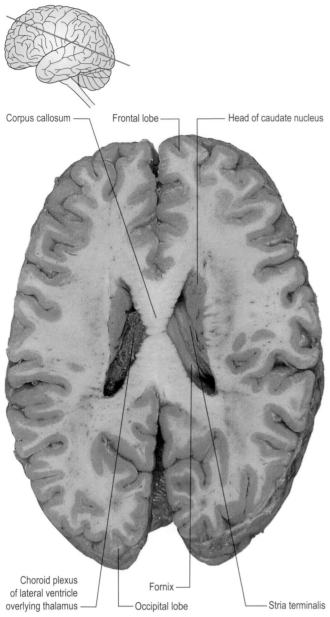

Corpus callosum — Frontal lobe — Head of caudate nucleus

Choroid plexus of lateral ventricle overlying thalamus — Fornix — Occipital lobe — Stria terminalis

Fig. 12.4 Dorsal aspect of the diencephalon. The choroid plexus has been removed on the right side.

Thalamic lesions

Strokes and tumours destroying the thalamus lead to loss of sensation in the contralateral face and limbs, accompanied by a distressing discomfort in the paradoxically anaesthetic areas (**thalamic pain**).

Thalamic lesions may mimic focal cortical defects because of the richness of thalamocortical connections.

Functional organisation of thalamic nuclei

All the nuclei of the thalamus, with the exception of the reticular nucleus, project to the ipsilateral cerebral cortex and the whole of the cortex receives input from the thalamus. Similarly, all thalamic nuclei receive corticofugal fibres that are ordered in a basically reciprocal fashion. In some cases, precise, point-to-point projections exist between individual thalamic nuclei and restricted cortical zones with well-defined sensory or motor functions. This organisation typifies the relationship between the thalamic nuclei and cortical regions that subserve the general and special senses and the motor regions that receive cerebellar and basal ganglia input (Fig. 12.6). Such thalamic nuclei are often referred to as the 'specific' nuclei.

The specific nuclei all lie within the ventral part (tier) of the lateral nuclear group. Other thalamic nuclei receive less functionally distinct afferent input that does not include overtly sensory or motor pathways; in turn, these connect with wider areas of cortex, including associative and limbic domains. These are often referred to as the 'non-specific' nuclei. Non-specific

Lateral geniculate nucleus

The geniculate nuclei are located near the posterior pole of the thalamus, ventral to the pulvinar. Here, they form small eminences on the surface, known as the geniculate bodies. The lateral geniculate nucleus is a part of the visual system and receives further discussion in Chapter 15. It is the site of termination of the optic tract, which carries the axons of retinal ganglion cells. As a result of hemidecussation of optic nerve fibres in the optic chiasm, each lateral geniculate nucleus receives axons that have originated from the ipsilateral temporal hemiretina and the contralateral nasal hemiretina. Each nucleus thus receives visual information relating to the contralateral half of the visual field (see Fig. 15.5). The lateral geniculate nucleus sends fibres, via the retrolenticular part of the internal capsule (see Fig. 13.25) and the optic radiation, to the primary visual cortex of the occipital lobe.

Medial geniculate nucleus

The medial geniculate nucleus is part of the auditory system, which is described in Chapter 10. It receives ascending fibres from the inferior colliculus of the midbrain, via the inferior brachium, or brachium of the inferior colliculus (see Fig. 9.13). The medial geniculate nucleus projects, via the retrolenticular part of the internal capsule and the auditory radiation, to the primary auditory cortex of the temporal lobe.

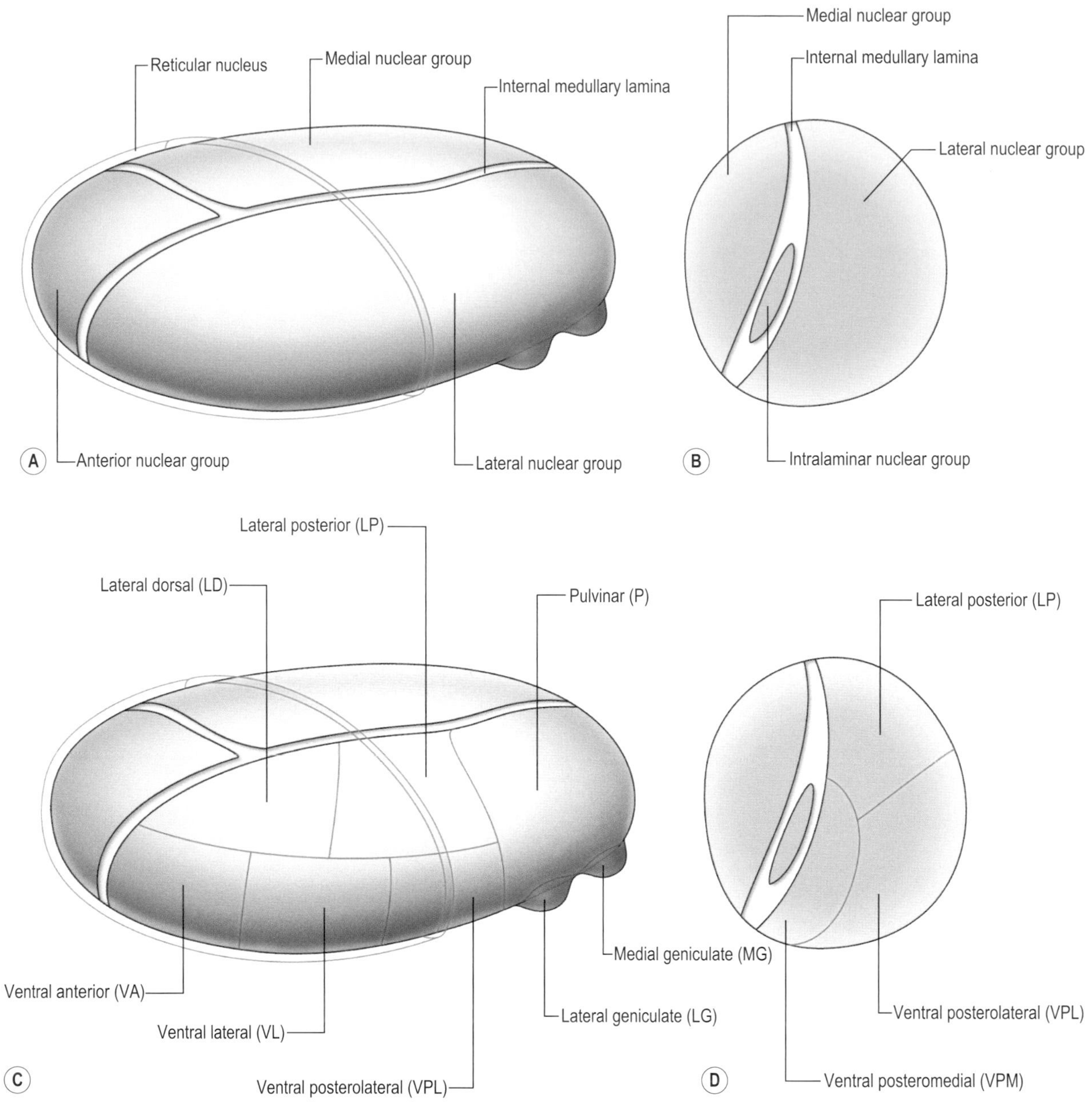

Fig. 12.5 The left thalamus viewed from the anterolateral aspect (A,C) and in coronal section (B,D), showing the principal nuclear groups (A,B) and the divisions of the lateral nuclear group (C,D).

Ventral anterior nucleus

The ventral anterior (VA) nucleus occupies the rostral part of the lateral nuclear mass. It consists of two subdivisions: the larger, principal part (VApc) and the smaller, magnocellular part (VAmc). The principal subcortical afferents to this region are output fibres of the ipsilateral basal ganglia system, which originate from the internal segment of the globus pallidus (GPi) and its homologue, the pars reticulata of the substantia nigra (SNr). Fibres from the globus pallidus terminate in VApc, while those from the substantia nigra end in VAmc. The ventral anterior nucleus of the thalamus has reciprocal connections with motor regions of the frontal lobe, particularly the premotor and supplementary motor cortices.

Ventral lateral nucleus

The ventral lateral (VL) nucleus lies immediately caudal to the ventral anterior nucleus in the ventral tier of the lateral nuclear complex. It consists of three subdivisions: pars oralis (VLo), pars medialis (VLm) and pars caudalis (VLc). Subcortical afferents to the ventral lateral nucleus originate mainly from the ipsilateral globus pallidus and substantia nigra, and from the contralateral

dentate nucleus of the cerebellum. Pallidal and nigral afferents terminate in VLo and VLm, while those from the cerebellum terminate in VLc. The ventral lateral nucleus, like the ventral anterior nucleus, has reciprocal connections with motor areas of the frontal lobe and especially with the primary motor cortex of the precentral gyrus. The ventral anterior and ventral lateral nuclei are an important part of the mechanism by which the basal ganglia and cerebellum exert their influence on normal movement and through which abnormalities of movement are mediated in basal ganglia and cerebellar disorders.

Surgical treatment of disorders of the basal ganglia and cerebellum

Neurosurgically placed lesions in the region of the ventral anterior and ventral lateral nuclei have been used to alleviate some of the motor symptoms associated with disorders of the basal ganglia (rigidity, tremor at rest, dyskinesias) and cerebellum (intention tremor). Such **thalamotomy** has been largely superseded by drug therapy in basal ganglia disease but is still used to relieve cerebellar tremor, e.g. in multiple sclerosis.

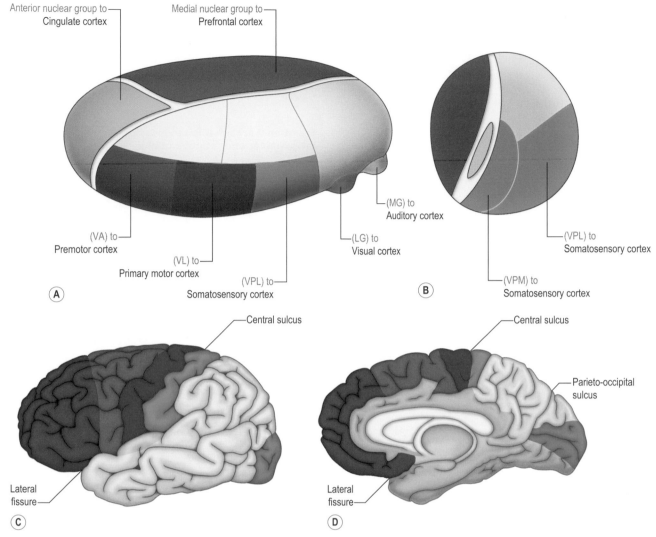

Fig. 12.6 Organisation of thalamic nuclei and their principal relationships with the cerebral cortex. The thalamus is viewed from its anterolateral aspect (A) and in coronal section (B). Colours indicate the relationships between thalamic nuclei and corresponding cerebral cortical regions on the lateral (C) and medial (D) aspects of the cerebral hemisphere.

> ### Functional organisation of the lateral nuclear group
>
> - 'Specific' thalamic nuclei have well-defined sensory or motor functions and highly organised connections with sensory and motor regions of the cerebral cortex. They all lie within the ventral tier of the lateral nuclear mass and include:
>
>   - Ventral posterior nucleus: receives general sensory afferents in the medial lemniscus, spinothalamic tract and trigeminothalamic tract; sends efferents to the primary somatosensory cortex of the parietal lobe.
>   - Lateral geniculate nucleus: receives visual afferents in the optic tract; projects to the primary visual cortex of the occipital lobe.
>   - Medial geniculate nucleus: receives auditory afferents from the inferior colliculus; sends efferents to the primary auditory cortex of the temporal lobe.
>   - Ventral anterior and ventral lateral nuclei: receive afferents from the cerebellum and basal ganglia; send efferents to motor cortical areas of the frontal lobe.
>
> - 'Non-specific' nuclei connect with wider areas of cortex, including associative and limbic regions.

Within the dorsal tier of the lateral nuclear complex lie a number of so-called 'non-specific' nuclei. Among these, the lateral dorsal nucleus is part of the limbic system. It receives afferents from the hippocampus and sends efferents to the cingulate gyrus. The lateral posterior nucleus has connections with the sensory association cortex of the parietal lobe. The **pulvinar** is a large region at the most posterior part of the thalamus. It has extensive connections with association cortices of the parietal, temporal and occipital lobes.

Anterior nuclear group

The most anterior portion of the thalamus, extending to its rostral pole, is the anterior nuclear complex. It consists of three subdivisions: the anteroventral, anteromedial and anterodorsal nuclei. The individual connections of these will not be discussed here since their specific functional significance is unclear. The anterior nuclear group is, however, part of the limbic system. It receives a large afferent projection from the mammillary body of the hypothalamus via the mammillothalamic tract. The anterior complex projects principally to the cingulate gyrus on the medial surface of the cerebral hemisphere (see Fig. 16.7). It is involved in the control of instinctive drives, in the emotional aspects of behaviour and in memory.

Medial nuclear group

The medial nuclear group forms a large region consisting primarily of the mediodorsal nucleus (dorsomedial nucleus) and some much smaller components, such as the nucleus reuniens. Subcortical afferents to the mediodorsal nucleus come from the hypothalamus, amygdala and from other thalamic nuclei, including the intralaminar nuclei and nuclei of the lateral complex. Extensive reciprocal connections exist between the mediodorsal nucleus and the prefrontal cortex. It is concerned mainly with the control of mood and the emotions.

Intralaminar nuclei

Several nuclei lie embedded within the internal medullary lamina of the thalamus. These include the centromedian and parafascicular nuclei, the centromedian being the largest intralaminar nucleus in humans. The intralaminar nuclei receive ascending afferents from the brainstem reticular formation and also from the spinothalamic and trigeminothalamic systems. In turn, they project to widespread regions of the cerebral cortex and to the caudate nucleus and putamen of the basal ganglia. The intralaminar nuclei are part of the mechanism for activation of the cerebral cortex. When they are stimulated, alpha rhythm activity, which is associated with repose and sleep, is disrupted and the electroencephalogram (EEG) becomes desynchronised. Lesions of the intralaminar nuclei reduce the perception of pain and the level of consciousness.

Reticular nucleus

The reticular nucleus is a thin layer of cells located on the lateral aspect of the thalamus between the external medullary lamina and the internal capsule. This nucleus receives collaterals of both thalamocortical and corticothalamic fibres, which pass between other thalamic nuclei and the cerebral cortex.

Functional organisation of anterior, medial, intralaminar and reticular nuclei

- The anterior nuclear group of the thalamus is part of the limbic system. This region receives fibres from the mammillary body of the hypothalamus and projects to the cingulate gyrus.

- Within the medial nuclear group, the mediodorsal nucleus has extensive reciprocal connections with the cortex of the frontal lobe.

- The intralaminar nuclei receive input from the reticular formation and ascending sensory systems. They project to the cerebral cortex and the striatum and are responsible for activation of the cerebral cortex.

- The reticular nucleus receives collaterals of thalamocortical and corticothalamic fibres.

Cerebral hemisphere and cerebral cortex

13

The cerebral hemisphere is derived from the embryological telencephalon (Chapter 1). It is the largest part of the forebrain and it reaches the greatest degree of development in the human brain. Superficially, the cerebral hemisphere consists of a layer of grey matter, the cerebral cortex, which is highly convoluted to form a complex pattern of ridges (**gyri**; singular, **gyrus**) and furrows (**sulci**; singular, **sulcus**). This serves to maximise the surface area of the cerebral cortex, about 70% of which is hidden within the depths of sulci (Figs 13.1, 13.2). Beneath the surface, axons running to and from the cells of the cortex form an extensive mass of white matter. Deep within the hemisphere lie additional masses of grey matter, most notably the thalamus and the basal ganglia (consisting of the caudate nucleus, putamen and globus pallidus). Figs 13.3–13.12 show a rostro-caudal series of coronal sections through the brain in which the major internal structures can be identified.

The vast majority of those nerve fibres that pass between the cerebral cortex and subcortical structures are condensed, deep within the hemisphere, into a broad sheet called the **internal capsule** (Figs 13.4–13.11, 13.13–13.15; see also Figs 1.25–1.28, 1.30, 13.24). Between the internal capsule and the cortical surface, fibres radiate in and out to produce a fan-like arrangement, the **corona radiata**. The principal subcortical grey matter is located in close proximity to the internal capsule, the thalamus and caudate nucleus lying medially and the putamen and globus pallidus lying laterally (Figs 13.1–13.14). Within the cerebral hemisphere lies the large C-shaped cavity of the lateral ventricle, which is considered with the rest of the ventricular system in Chapter 6.

The two cerebral hemispheres are separated by a deep cleft, the **great longitudinal fissure**, which accommodates the meningeal falx cerebri. In the depths of the fissure, the hemispheres are united by the **corpus callosum**, an enormous sheet of commissural nerve fibres which run between corresponding areas of the two cortices (Figs 13.2–13.15; see also Figs 13.21–13.23, 13.25).

Gyri, sulci and lobes of the cerebral hemisphere

Certain gyri and sulci on the surface of the hemisphere are relatively consistently located in different individuals and are the basis for dividing the hemisphere into four lobes, namely the **frontal**, **parietal**, **temporal** and **occipital lobes**. Their principal topographical features and functional significance are described below. The most conspicuous and deepest cleft on the lateral surface of the hemisphere is the **lateral fissure** (Fig. 13.1). This separates the temporal lobe below from the frontal and parietal lobes above. Within the depths of the lateral fissure lies a cortical area known as the **insula** (Figs 13.6–13.12, 13.14, 13.17). The parts of the frontal, parietal and temporal lobes that overlie the insula are called the **opercula**. Also on the lateral surface of the hemisphere, a single, often uninterrupted sulcus can usually be identified, running between the great longitudinal fissure and the lateral fissure. This is the **central sulcus**, which marks the boundary between the frontal and parietal lobes (Figs 13.1, 13.16). The central sulcus extends for a short distance onto the medial surface of the hemisphere, within the great longitudinal fissure (Figs 13.2, 13.16).

The frontal lobe constitutes the entire region in front of the central sulcus. Immediately in front of the sulcus, and running

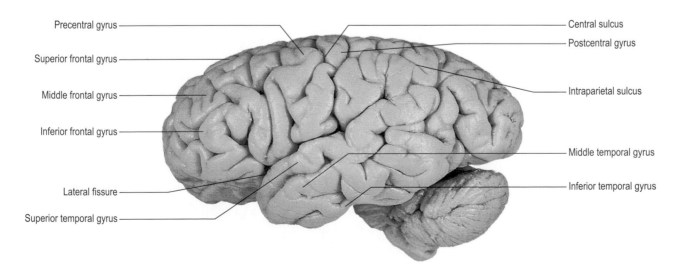

Fig. 13.1 Lateral aspect of the cerebral hemisphere showing major gyri and sulci.

parallel to it, lies the **precentral gyrus**, which is the **primary motor region** of the cerebral cortex. In front of the precentral gyrus, the rest of the frontal lobe consists of a more variable pattern of convolutions, of which the **superior**, **middle** and **inferior frontal gyri** can usually be identified (Fig. 13.1).

Behind the central sulcus, and above the lateral fissure, lies the parietal lobe. Its most anterior part is the **postcentral gyrus**, which is the site of the **primary somatosensory cortex**. Behind the postcentral gyrus, on the lateral surface of the hemisphere, the intraparietal sulcus divides the rest of the parietal lobe into superior and inferior parietal lobules (Figs 13.1, 13.16).

The boundary between the parietal lobe and the posteriorly located occipital lobe is not coincident with a single sulcus on the lateral surface of the hemisphere; however, it is clearly marked by the deep **parieto-occipital sulcus** on the medial surface (Figs 13.2, 13.16). The occipital lobe does not bear any important landmarks on its lateral surface but, on the medial surface, the prominent **calcarine sulcus** indicates the location of the **primary visual cortex** (Figs 13.2, 13.16).

The temporal lobe lies beneath the lateral fissure, merging posteriorly with the parietal and occipital lobes. On its lateral surface, the temporal lobe is divided into three principal gyri that run roughly parallel to the lateral fissure: the **superior**, **middle** and **inferior temporal gyri** (Fig. 13.1). The superior temporal gyrus includes the **primary auditory cortex**. Most of this functional region is situated on the superior bank of the gyrus, within the lateral fissure, where the **transverse temporal gyri**, or **Heschl's convolutions**, provide a more precise localisation (Fig. 13.17).

On the medial surface of the hemisphere, certain portions of the frontal, parietal and temporal lobes also constitute components of the limbic system. Curving around the corpus callosum, and running parallel to it, lies the **cingulate gyrus** (Figs 13.2, 13.16), separated from the rest of the hemisphere by the **cingulate sulcus**. The cingulate gyrus passes posteriorly and inferiorly round the posterior portion, or splenium, of the corpus callosum to become continuous with the **parahippocampal gyrus** of the temporal lobe. Deep to the parahippocampal gyrus, within the temporal lobe, lies the **hippocampus** (Figs 13.8–13.12). This structure is formed by an in-curling of the inferomedial part of the temporal lobe. The cingulate gyrus, parahippocampal gyrus and hippocampus are sometimes referred to as the **limbic lobe** of the cerebral hemisphere.

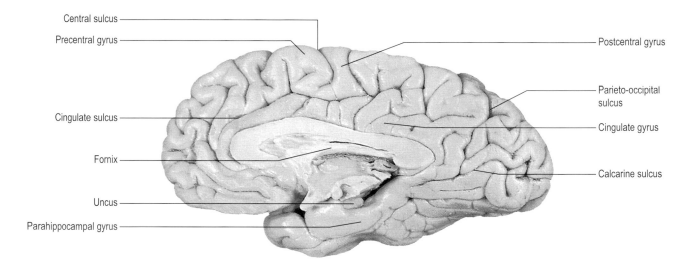

Fig. 13.2 Median sagittal section of the cerebral hemisphere showing major gyri and sulci. The brainstem and cerebellum have been removed to show the inferomedial aspect of the temporal lobe.

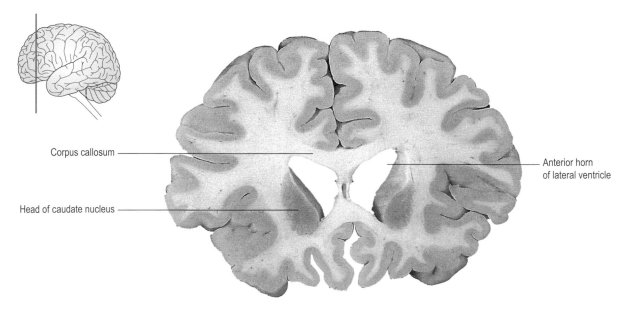

Fig. 13.3 Coronal section of the cerebral hemisphere.

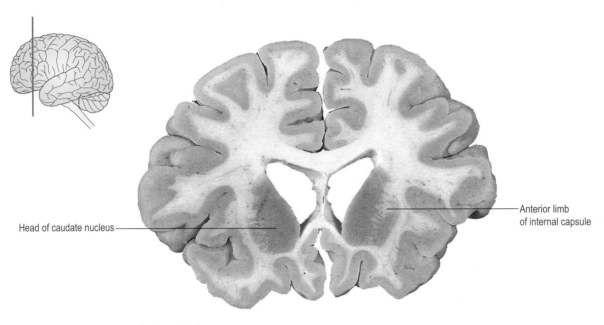

Fig. 13.4 Coronal section of the cerebral hemisphere.

Head of caudate nucleus

Anterior limb of internal capsule

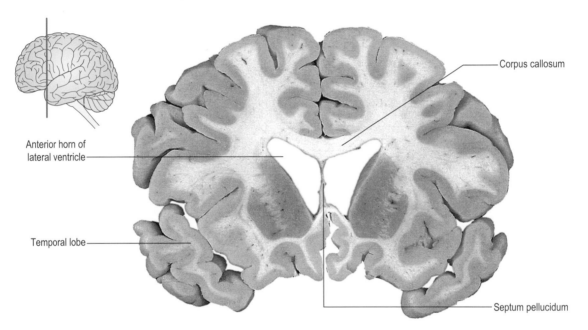

Corpus callosum

Anterior horn of lateral ventricle

Temporal lobe

Septum pellucidum

Fig. 13.5 Coronal section of the cerebral hemisphere.

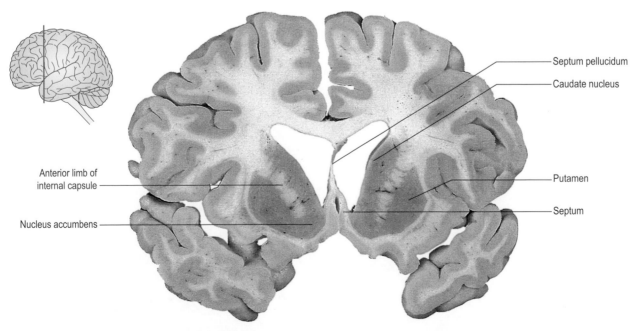

Septum pellucidum

Caudate nucleus

Anterior limb of internal capsule

Nucleus accumbens

Putamen

Septum

Fig. 13.6 Coronal section of the cerebral hemisphere.

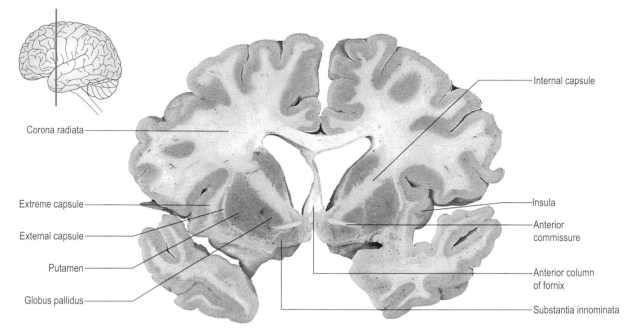

Corona radiata

Internal capsule

Extreme capsule

External capsule

Putamen

Globus pallidus

Insula

Anterior commissure

Anterior column of fornix

Substantia innominata

Fig. 13.7 Coronal section of the cerebral hemisphere.

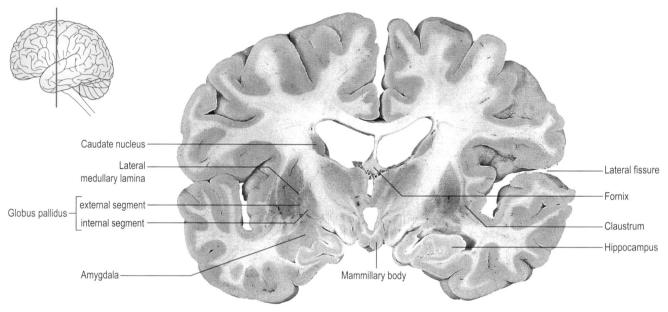

Caudate nucleus

Lateral medullary lamina

Globus pallidus — external segment — internal segment

Amygdala

Lateral fissure

Fornix

Claustrum

Hippocampus

Mammillary body

Fig. 13.8 Coronal section of the cerebral hemisphere.

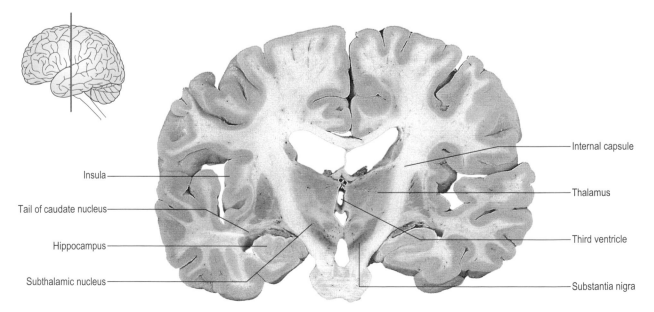

Insula

Tail of caudate nucleus

Hippocampus

Subthalamic nucleus

Internal capsule

Thalamus

Third ventricle

Substantia nigra

Fig. 13.9 Coronal section of the cerebral hemisphere.

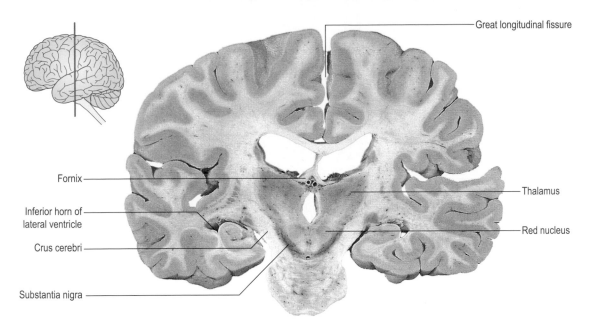

Fig. 13.10 Coronal section of the cerebral hemisphere.

Labels: Great longitudinal fissure; Fornix; Inferior horn of lateral ventricle; Crus cerebri; Substantia nigra; Thalamus; Red nucleus

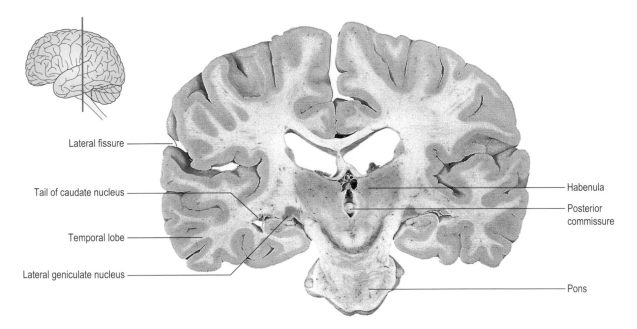

Fig. 13.11 Coronal section of the cerebral hemisphere.

Labels: Lateral fissure; Tail of caudate nucleus; Temporal lobe; Lateral geniculate nucleus; Habenula; Posterior commissure; Pons

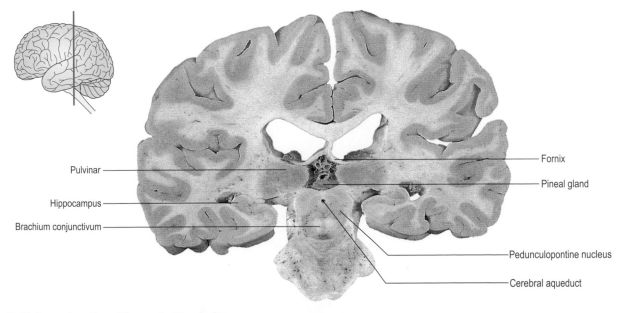

Fig. 13.12 Coronal section of the cerebral hemisphere.

Labels: Pulvinar; Hippocampus; Brachium conjunctivum; Fornix; Pineal gland; Pedunculopontine nucleus; Cerebral aqueduct

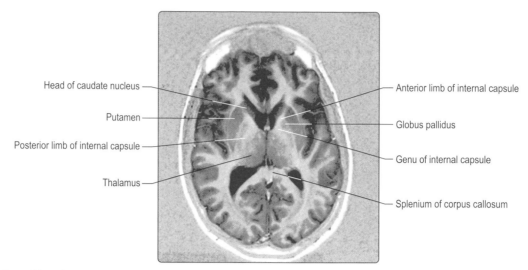

Head of caudate nucleus

Putamen

Posterior limb of internal capsule

Thalamus

Anterior limb of internal capsule

Globus pallidus

Genu of internal capsule

Splenium of corpus callosum

Fig. 13.13 Horizontal (axial) magnetic resonance image of the living brain. *(Courtesy of Professor A Jackson, Wolfson Molecular Imaging Centre, University of Manchester, Manchester, UK.)*

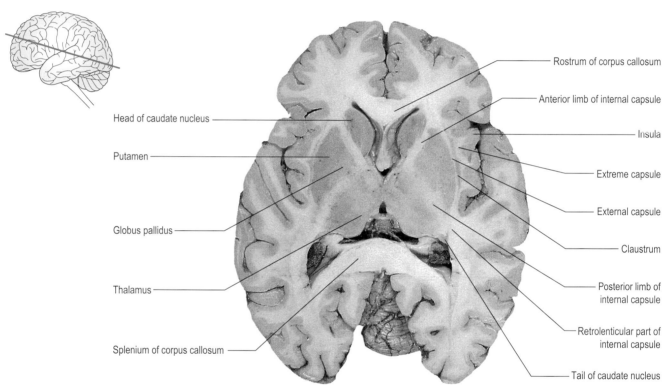

Head of caudate nucleus

Putamen

Globus pallidus

Thalamus

Splenium of corpus callosum

Rostrum of corpus callosum

Anterior limb of internal capsule

Insula

Extreme capsule

External capsule

Claustrum

Posterior limb of internal capsule

Retrolenticular part of internal capsule

Tail of caudate nucleus

Fig. 13.14 Horizontal section of the brain.

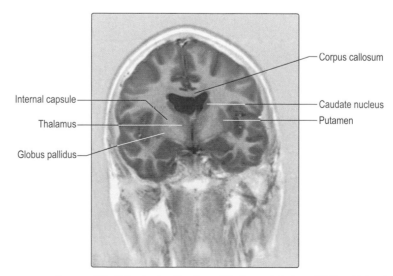

Internal capsule

Thalamus

Globus pallidus

Corpus callosum

Caudate nucleus

Putamen

Fig. 13.15 Coronal magnetic resonance image of the living brain. *(Courtesy of Professor A Jackson, Wolfson Molecular Imaging Centre, University of Manchester, Manchester, UK.)*

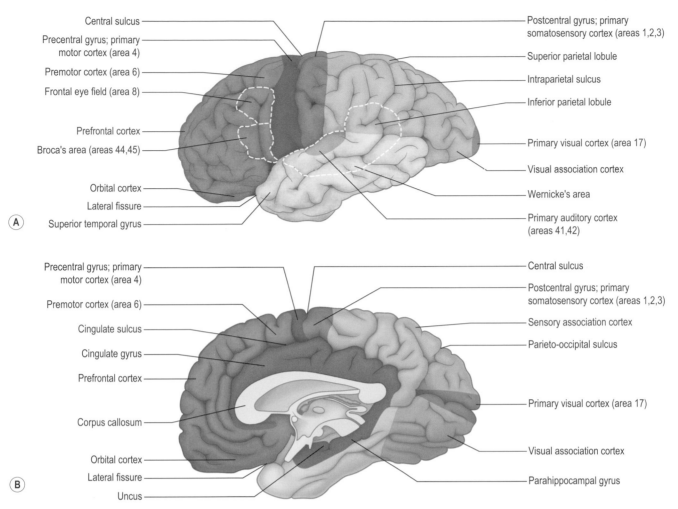

Fig. 13.16 Major functional areas of the cerebral cortex. (A) Lateral aspect of left cerebral hemisphere; (B) medial aspect of right cerebral hemisphere in sagittal section.

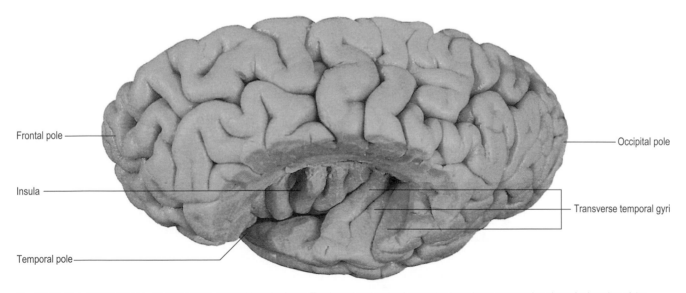

Fig. 13.17 Superolateral aspect of the left cerebral hemisphere. The frontal and parietal operculae have been removed to show the location of the transverse temporal gyri (Heschl's convolutions) and the insula.

Gyri, sulci and lobes of the cerebral hemisphere

- The cerebral hemisphere consists of:
  - Superficial cerebral cortex, convoluted to form gyri and sulci

- Underlying white matter, consisting of cortical afferent and efferent fibres
- Deep nuclear masses: the thalamus and basal ganglia

- The two cerebral hemispheres are separated by the great longitudinal fissure and joined by the corpus callosum.

- The hemisphere is divided into four lobes (frontal, parietal,

temporal and occipital) on the basis of surface topography.

- Principal landmarks that indicate the divisions between lobes are the lateral fissure, central sulcus and parieto-occipital sulcus.

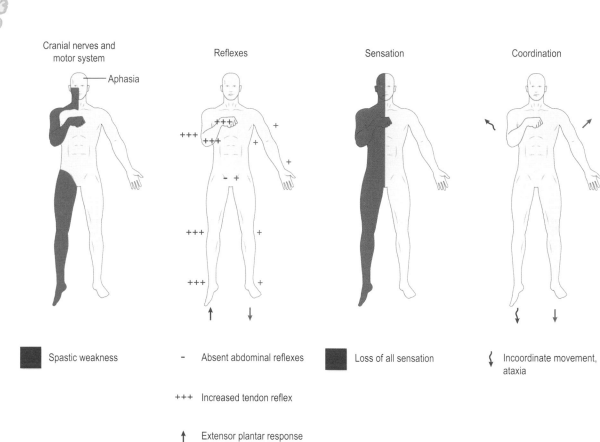

Cranial nerves and motor system

Aphasia

Reflexes

Sensation

Coordination

■ Spastic weakness

− Absent abdominal reflexes

■ Loss of all sensation

⟨ Incoordinate movement, ataxia

+++ Increased tendon reflex

↑ Extensor plantar response

Fig. 13.18 Unilateral cerebral hemisphere lesion. Refer also to Fig. 1.48.

🛈 Focal cerebral lesions

Focal cerebral lesions, e.g. a stroke or tumour, produce three kinds of symptoms:

1. **Focal epileptic seizures.** The repetitive discharges of groups of neurones in the cerebral cortex produce paroxysmal attacks lasting for brief periods and reflecting the functional properties of the neurones concerned. The patient experiences sudden attacks of abnormal movements or sensations (**simple focal seizures**) or brief alterations in perception, mood and behaviour (**complex partial seizures**). Focal seizures may trigger **generalised** (**tonic–clonic**) seizures.
2. **Sensory/motor deficits.** There is a loss of sensation or movement, detectable on clinical neurological examination.
3. **Psychological deficits.** There are breakdowns in psychological processes such as language, perception and memory, demonstrable on psychological evaluation.

If the focal lesion is space-occupying, the syndrome of **raised intracranial pressure** results (see Fig. 5.2).

A **unilateral cerebral hemisphere lesion** causes mental impairment (e.g. aphasia), a contralateral spastic hemiparesis, hyperreflexia and an extensor plantar response (upper motor neurone lesion) and contralateral hemisensory loss (Fig. 13.18). A vascular insult to the internal capsule, such as an infarction or haemorrhage, leads to the rapid development of this syndrome, known as **stroke**.

The regional localisation of neuropsychological functions in the cerebral cortex is summarised in Fig. 1.49.

Cerebral cortex

Histological structure

The cerebral cortex forms the outer surface of the cerebral hemisphere. It consists of a layer, several millimetres in thickness, of nerve cell bodies, dendritic arborisations and synaptic interconnections. In the early part of the twentieth century, the Swedish anatomist Brodmann produced a numbered, cytoarchitectural map of the cerebral cortex based upon its regional histological characteristics. Although largely superseded by the elucidation of function, in some instances, there is good correspondence between **Brodmann's areas** and functionally defined regions of the cortex. In such cases, Brodmann's numbers are retained in common use for descriptive purposes.

Long ago in evolutionary history, the cerebral cortex originally arose in relation to olfactory function. Phylogenetically old parts of the cortex (referred to as **archicortex** and **paleocortex**), such as the hippocampus and other parts of the temporal lobe, retain throughout evolution an association with the olfactory system and have a primitive, three-layered cytoarchitecture. These regions have important functions in the emotional aspects of behaviour and in memory. Together with other parts of the cortex and certain subcortical nuclei they constitute the limbic system (Chapter 16). However, most of the cerebral cortex is a more recent acquisition in phylogenetic terms and is referred to as the **neocortex**. Although its detailed cytological structure varies from region to region, it is generally recognised as consisting of six layers (Fig. 13.19):

- **Layer I**, the most superficial layer, contains few nerve cell bodies but many dendritic and axonal processes in synaptic interaction.
- **Layer II** contains many small neurones, which establish intracortical connections.
- **Layer III** contains medium-sized neurones giving rise to association and commissural fibres.
- **Layer IV** is the site of termination of afferent fibres from the specific thalamic nuclei.

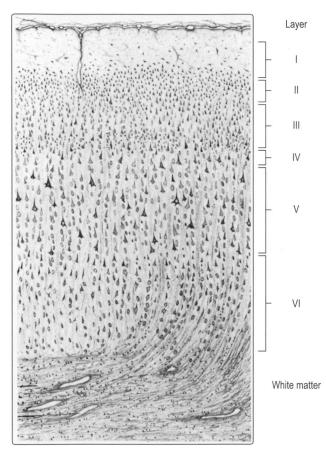

Layer

I

II

III

IV

V

VI

White matter

Fig. 13.19 Histological structure of the cerebral cortex. *(From Mitchell, GAG and Patterson, EL. Basic Anatomy. London: Livingstone; 1954. Courtesy of Churchill Livingstone.)*

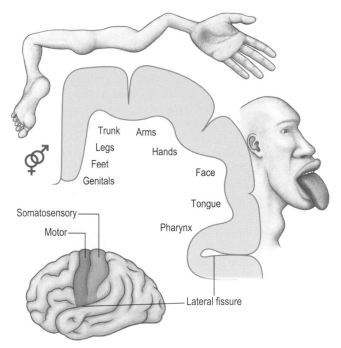

Trunk Arms
Legs Hands
Feet
Genitals Face
Tongue
Somatosensory
Motor Pharynx

Lateral fissure

Fig. 13.20 Schematic coronal section through the cerebral hemisphere illustrating the approximate somatotopic representation of the contralateral body half in the motor and sensory cortices.

- **Layer V** is the origin of projection fibres to extracortical targets, such as the basal ganglia, thalamus, brainstem and spinal cord. In the primary motor cortex of the frontal lobe, this layer contains the giant Betz cells, which project fibres into the pyramidal tract.
- **Layer VI** also contains association and projection neurones.

Functional organisation

The cerebral cortex is necessary for conscious awareness and thought, memory and intellect. It is the region to which all sensory modalities ultimately ascend (mostly via the thalamus) and where they are consciously perceived and interpreted in the light of previous experience. The cerebral cortex is also the highest level at which the motor system is represented. It is here that actions are conceived and initiated.

- The posterior part of the cerebrum receives sensory information from the outside world in the primary sensory areas of the parietal lobe (somatosensory), occipital lobe (vision) and temporal lobe (hearing).
- In adjacent cortical zones, the information is elaborated and interpreted, thus permitting identification of objects by touch, sight and hearing in a modality-specific process of perception. Areas of cortex at the junction of the three cerebral lobes, known as association cortex, are critical for the multimodal and spatial recognition of the environment.
- The medial portions of the cerebral hemisphere (limbic system) enable the storage and retrieval of information processed in the posterior hemispheric regions.
- The anterior part of the cerebrum (frontal lobe) is concerned with the organisation of movement (primary motor area; premotor and supplementary motor areas) and the strategic

guidance of complex motor behaviour over time (prefrontal area).
- In the majority of individuals, areas of association cortex in frontal, parietal and temporal lobes of the left hemisphere are responsible for the comprehension and expression of language. The left hemisphere is, therefore, said to be **dominant** for language.

The regional localisation of neuropsychological functions in the cerebral cortex is summarised in Fig. 1.49.

Frontal lobe

The frontal lobe lies anterior to the central sulcus. Immediately anterior to the central sulcus, and running parallel to it, is the precentral gyrus. Functionally, this is known as the **primary motor cortex** (Figs 13.1, 13.2, 13.16). It corresponds to Brodmann's area 4. Within the cortex of the precentral gyrus, the contralateral half of the body is represented in a precise somatotopic fashion (Fig. 13.20). The representation of the body is inverted, with the head area located in the most inferior part of the precentral gyrus, just above the lateral fissure. Progressing superiorly, successive areas of cortex represent the digits, hand, arm, shoulder and trunk. The lower limb is represented on the medial surface of the hemisphere, above the corpus callosum. The area of cortex devoted to a particular body part is proportional, not to its size, but to the degree of precision with which movements can be executed. Therefore the larynx, tongue, face and digits of the hand are represented by disproportionately large regions.

Stimulation of the primary motor cortex elicits contraction of discrete muscle groups on the opposite side of the body. The function of this region is the control of voluntary, skilled movements, sometimes referred to as fractionated movements; 30% of corticospinal (pyramidal tract) and corticobulbar fibres arise from neurones of the primary motor cortex, about 3% originating from giant pyramidal (Betz) cells. The principal subcortical afferents to the primary motor cortex originate from the ventral lateral nucleus of the thalamus (see Fig. 12.6), which in turn receives input mainly from the dentate nucleus of the cerebellum and from the globus pallidus of the basal ganglia.

The region immediately anterior to the primary motor cortex is known as the **premotor cortex** (Brodmann's area 6; Fig. 13.16). On the lateral surface of the hemisphere, this includes the posterior portions of the superior, middle and inferior frontal gyri. On the medial surface of the hemisphere, the premotor cortex includes a region referred to as the **supplementary motor cortex**. Here, like the primary motor cortex, there is somatotopic representation of the body although, unlike the primary motor cortex, representation appears to be bilateral in both hemispheres.

Stimulation of premotor cortical areas induces movement that is less focused than that elicited from the primary motor cortex and involves groups of functionally related muscles. Movement evoked from the supplementary motor cortex tends to be postural in nature, involving axial and proximal musculature. Premotor cortical areas are thought to function in the programming of, and preparation for, movement and in the control of posture. The premotor cortex exerts its actions partly via the primary motor cortex, with which it is connected by short association fibres, and partly via corticospinal and corticobulbar fibres. About 30% of the latter originate in the premotor cortex although, unlike the primary motor cortex, giant Betz cells are absent from premotor areas. The principal subcortical input to premotor cortical regions, including the supplementary motor cortex, is the ventral anterior nucleus of the thalamus. This, in turn, receives fibres from the globus pallidus and substantia nigra.

Immediately in front of the premotor cortex, on the lateral surface of the hemisphere, are located two other important regions. In the middle frontal gyrus lies the **frontal eye field** (Brodmann's area 8). This region controls voluntary conjugate deviation of the eyes, as occur when scanning the visual field. Unilateral damage to this area causes conjugate deviation of the eyes towards the side of the lesion. In the inferior frontal gyrus of the dominant hemisphere (usually the left) lies the motor speech area, also known as **Broca's area** (Brodmann's areas 44 and 45). Broca's area has important interconnections with parts of the ipsilateral temporal, parietal and occipital lobes that are involved in language function.

The extensive regions of the cortex of the frontal lobe that lie anterior to premotor areas are referred to as the **prefrontal cortex**. The prefrontal cortex has rich connections with parietal, temporal and occipital cortex through long association fibres running in the subcortical white matter (Fig. 13.22). Subcortical afferents to the prefrontal cortex arise mainly in the mediodorsal and anterior nuclei of the thalamus. The prefrontal cortex has cognitive functions of a high order. These include intellectual, judgemental and predictive faculties and the planning of behaviour.

Parietal lobe

The parietal lobe lies behind the frontal lobe and is bounded posteriorly and inferiorly by the occipital and temporal lobes, respectively. The most anterior part of the parietal lobe is the postcentral gyrus, running parallel to the central sulcus (Figs 13.1, 13.2, 13.16). Functionally, this region is the **primary somatosensory cortex** (Brodmann's areas 1, 2 and 3). This is the region of termination of thalamocortical neurones that constitute the third and final relay in the chain of neurones carrying general sensation to a conscious level. The thalamic origin of these neurones is the ventral posterior nucleus, which in turn receives fibres of the medial lemniscus (fine touch and proprioception), spinal lemniscus (coarse touch and pressure), spinothalamic tracts (pain and temperature) and trigeminothalamic tracts (general sensation from the head).

Within the somatosensory cortex, the contralateral half of the body is represented in an inverted, somatotopic pattern which resembles that in the primary motor cortex of the frontal lobe

Frontal lobe lesions

Left frontal lobe lesions cause:

- Focal seizures. Paroxysmal jerking movements of the contralateral limbs are termed 'simple motor' or '**Jacksonian**' seizures.
- Sensory/motor deficit. There is weakness of the face and upper motor neurone signs in the limbs on the opposite side to the lesion (**contralateral hemiplegia**).
- Psychological deficit. Speech is produced with great effort and poor articulation, in brief utterances with word errors (**paraphasia**). Repetition of words is impaired but powers of comprehension are relatively preserved. This is known as **Broca's aphasia**. There is also impairment of reading and writing (**alexia** and **agraphia**). Degenerative disease of the left frontal lobe results in a **progressive non-fluent aphasia**, akin to Broca's aphasia.

Premotor areas of the frontal lobes are responsible for the organisation of skilled movements. Unilateral and bilateral lesions of the premotor cortex lead to the inability to carry out skilled movements in the absence of paralysis, sensory loss or cerebellar incoordination (**apraxia**).

Bilateral prefrontal lesions cause:

- Profound disturbance of behaviour and personality
- Impaired problem-solving and judgement

Progressive atrophy of the frontal lobes occurs in the degenerative disorder of **frontotemporal dementia**.

(Fig. 13.20). Similarly, the amount of cortex devoted to a particular body part is disproportionate to the size of the latter; in the case of the sensory cortex, it reflects rather the richness of sensory innervation. Therefore the pharynx, tongue, face, lips and the palmar surface of the hands and digits are particularly well represented. Adjacent to the mouth area is a region where taste is perceived.

The surface of the parietal lobe posterior to the primary somatosensory cortex constitutes the parietal **association cortex**. The superior parietal lobule is responsible for the interpretation of general sensory information and for conscious awareness of the contralateral half of the body. Lesions here impair the interpretation and understanding of sensory input and may cause neglect of the opposite side of the body. The inferior parietal lobule interfaces between somatosensory cortex and the visual and auditory association cortices of the occipital and temporal lobes, respectively, and in the dominant hemisphere it contributes to language functions.

Parietal lobe lesions

Left parietal lobe lesions cause:

- Focal seizures – paroxysmal attacks of abnormal sensations, spreading down the contralateral side of the body (sensory seizures).
- Sensory/motor deficit – a contralateral hemisensory loss and inferior visual field loss.
- Psychological deficit – an inability to name objects (**anomia**) and a loss of literacy, with inability to read (**alexia**), to write (**agraphia**) and to calculate (**acalculia**).

Right parietal lobe lesions cause:

- Focal seizures – paroxysmal attacks of sensory disturbance affecting the contralateral side of the body (simple sensory seizures).
- Sensory/motor deficit – contralateral hemisensory loss and an inferior visual field loss.
- Psychological deficit – an inability to copy and construct designs because of spatial disorientation (**constructional apraxia**).

Bilateral parietal lobe lesions lead to disorientation in space and inability to perceive, copy and match objects (**apperceptive agnosia**). This occurs in the degenerative disorder of Alzheimer's disease.

Temporal lobe

The lateral surface of the temporal lobe is divided into superior, middle and inferior temporal gyri, which run parallel to the lateral fissure. Within the superior temporal gyrus is located the **primary auditory cortex** (Brodmann's areas 41 and 42). More exactly, most of this functional zone lies in the superior bank of the gyrus, normally hidden within the lateral fissure. Its precise location is marked by the small transverse temporal gyri, or Heschl's convolutions (Fig. 13.17).

The primary auditory cortex is responsible for the conscious perception of sound and, within it, there is so-called 'tonotopical' representation of the cochlear duct. The primary auditory cortex receives input from the medial geniculate nucleus of the thalamus. The ascending acoustic projection undergoes partial decussation in the brainstem on its way to the medial geniculate nucleus (see Fig. 10.22). At the cortical level, therefore, the organs of hearing are bilaterally represented so that unilateral lesions of the primary auditory cortex cause partial deafness in both ears. Auditory information is further processed and interpreted in the **auditory association cortex**, which lies surrounding and immediately posterior to the primary auditory cortex. In the dominant hemisphere, this region is also known as **Wernicke's area**. This region is crucial for understanding the spoken word and has important connections with other language areas of the brain.

The location of the cortical representation of the vestibular system is uncertain. There is evidence that it lies in the superior temporal gyrus anterior to the primary auditory cortex or in the inferior parietal lobule.

The inferomedial part of the temporal lobe is curled inwards to form the **hippocampus**. This structure lies in the floor of the inferior horn of the lateral ventricle, deep to the parahippocampal gyrus (Figs 13.8–13.12, 13.16). As part of the limbic system, the principal functions of the hippocampus are in relation to memory and the emotional aspects of behaviour. Close to the anterior end of the hippocampus and the temporal pole lies a mass of subcortical grey matter, the **amygdala**, which is also part of the limbic system. The amygdala and adjacent parts of the inferomedial temporal cortex receive fibres from the olfactory tract and are responsible for the conscious appreciation of the sense of smell. These connections receive further consideration in Chapter 16.

 Temporal lobe lesions

Left temporal lobe lesions cause:

- Focal seizures – paroxysmal attacks of unresponsiveness (**absences**), purposeless behaviour (**automatism**), olfactory and complex visual and auditory hallucinations and disturbances of mood and memory (**déjà vu**). These attacks are referred to as complex partial seizures.
- Sensory/motor deficit – a contralateral superior visual field loss.
- Psychological deficit – speech that is fluent and rapid but contains word errors (**paraphasia**) and is incomprehensible. There is profound word-finding difficulty, impaired repetition of words and profound loss of comprehension. This is known as **Wernicke's aphasia**.

Bilateral lesions of the medial temporal gyri (including the hippocampi) cause **amnesia** (loss of memory for past autobiographical/episodic events and impaired new learning). This occurs in alcoholic Wernicke's (metabolic) encephalopathy, when it is referred to as Korsakoff's amnesia. The hippocampi are particularly atrophied in the degenerative disorder of **Alzheimer's disease**.

Bilateral lesions of temporal neocortex lead to loss of meaning of words (verbal semantics) and understanding of visual percepts, despite preserved copying and visual matching of objects (**associative agnosia**). In addition, faces cannot be recognised (**prosopagnosia**). This occurs in the degenerative disorder of **semantic dementia**.

Occipital lobe

The occipital lobe lies behind the parietal and temporal lobes. On the medial surface of the hemisphere, the boundary with the parietal lobe is marked by the deep parieto-occipital sulcus. Also on the medial surface, the calcarine sulcus marks the location of the **primary visual cortex** (Brodmann's area 17; Fig. 13.16), which is responsible for visual perception. It occupies the gyri immediately above and below the calcarine sulcus, much of it being hidden in the depths of the sulcus. This region receives fibres from the lateral geniculate nucleus of the thalamus by way of the optic radiation of the internal capsule. Each lateral half of the visual field is represented in the primary visual cortex of the contralateral hemisphere. The upper half of the visual field is represented below the calcarine sulcus, and the lower half is represented above the sulcus. The rest of the occipital lobe constitutes the **visual association cortex**. This region is concerned with the interpretation of visual images. Lesions of the primary visual cortex cause blindness in the corresponding part of the visual field, while damage to the visual association cortex causes deficits in visual interpretation and recognition. The visual system is considered in more detail in Chapter 15.

 Occipital lobe lesions

Occipital lobe lesions cause:

- Focal seizures – paroxysmal visual hallucinations of a simple, unformed nature, such as lights and colours (simple partial seizures)
- Sensory/motor deficit – a contralateral visual field loss (**contralateral homonymous hemianopia**)

Bilateral occipital lobe lesions lead to **cortical blindness**, of which the patient is unaware (**Anton's syndrome**). This occurs following cerebral hypoxia.

Language areas of the cerebral hemisphere

Certain higher cognitive functions are dealt with primarily, or even exclusively, by one of the cerebral hemispheres, which is then referred to as being 'dominant' for that function. In the great majority of people the left hemisphere is dominant for language and mathematical ability. The right hemisphere excels at spatial perception and musical proficiency. Cerebral dominance becomes established during the first few years after birth. During this formative period, both hemispheres exhibit linguistic ability and if one hemisphere sustains damage it may be compensated for by the plasticity of the developing brain and the child learns to speak normally. Later in life, this flexibility becomes greatly diminished and damage to the dominant hemisphere often causes loss of speech, in addition to the other deficits produced by hemispheric lesions.

The language areas of the brain are organised around the lateral fissure of the cerebral hemisphere. In the frontal lobe, Broca's area occupies the posterior part of the inferior frontal gyrus, adjacent to the motor cortical area for the head and neck. This region is concerned with expressive aspects of language (articulation). In the temporal lobe, the auditory association cortex, or Wernicke's area, is responsible for comprehension of the spoken word.

Nearby regions of the temporal lobe and parietal lobe, most notably the angular gyrus and supramarginal gyrus of the inferior parietal lobule, provide a functional interface between auditory and visual association areas important in naming, reading, writing and calculation.

The cerebral cortex

- The frontal lobe lies immediately in front of the central sulcus. The precentral gyrus is the primary motor region. Anterior to this lie the premotor and supplementary motor cortices and, in the left hemisphere, Broca's (motor speech) area. The prefrontal cortex is concerned with complex cognitive functions.

- The parietal lobe lies posterior to the central sulcus. The postcentral gyrus is the primary somatosensory region. It receives afferents from the ventral posterior nucleus of the thalamus, which is the site of termination of the spinothalamic tracts, trigeminothalamic tract and medial lemniscus. Behind this region lies the sensory association cortex, which is responsible for the interpretation of general sensory information.

- The temporal lobe lies beneath the lateral fissure. On the superior surface of the superior temporal gyrus, the transverse temporal gyri (Heschl's convolutions) mark the location of the primary auditory cortex, which receives input from the medial geniculate nucleus of the thalamus. Adjacent lies the auditory association cortex, which is responsible for the interpretation of auditory information and which, in the left hemisphere, constitutes Wernicke's area.

- The occipital lobe makes up the posterior part of the hemisphere. On the medial surface, the calcarine sulcus indicates the location of the primary visual cortex, which receives afferents from the lateral geniculate nucleus of the thalamus. The rest of the occipital lobe is the visual association cortex, which is responsible for the interpretation of visual information.

White matter of the cerebral hemisphere

Beneath the cortical surface lies an extensive mass of nerve fibres, all of which have their origin or termination, and sometimes both, within the cortex. The fibres are classified into three types, depending upon their origin and destination:

1. **Association fibres**, which interconnect cortical sites lying within one cerebral hemisphere.
2. **Commissural fibres**, which run from one cerebral hemisphere to the other, connecting functionally related structures.
3. **Projection fibres**, which pass between the cerebral cortex and subcortical structures such as the thalamus, striatum, brainstem and spinal cord.

Association fibres

Some association fibres (Figs 13.21, 13.22) are short and link nearby areas of cortex by arching beneath adjacent cerebral sulci ('U' fibres). Other association fibres are longer and travel through the white matter to link distant areas of cerebral cortex. The primary sensory areas in the parietal, temporal and occipital lobes are linked by long association fibres to the association areas of the cerebral cortex. These, in turn, are connected to each other.

The large **superior longitudinal fasciculus** interconnects the frontal and occipital lobes. A subsidiary of this bundle, known as

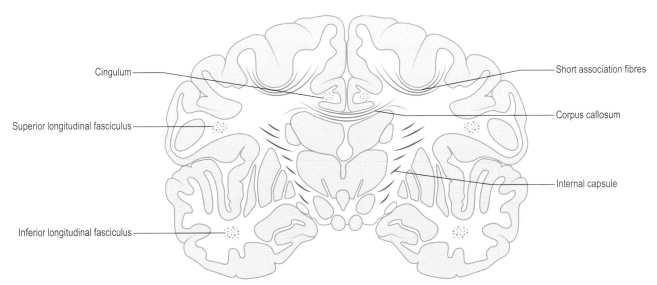

Fig. 13.21 Coronal section of the cerebral hemisphere. The diagram shows the location of the principal association, commissural and projection fibres.

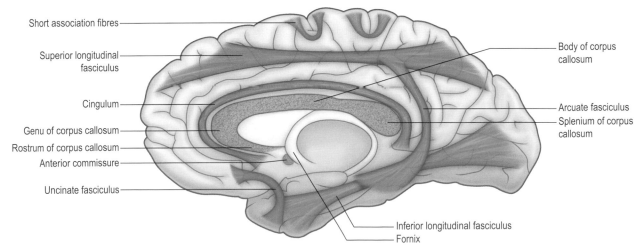

Fig. 13.22 Principal association and commissural fibres of the cerebral hemisphere projected onto a median sagittal section.

the **arcuate fasciculus**, links gyri in the frontal and temporal lobes, which are important for language function.

The **inferior longitudinal fasciculus** runs between the occipital and temporal poles and contributes to the function of visual recognition.

The **uncinate fasciculus** connects the anterior and inferior parts of the frontal lobe with the temporal gyri, which are important structures in the regulation of behaviour. The **cingulum** lies within the cingulate gyrus and courses parallel with the corpus callosum, connecting the frontal and parietal lobes with the parahippocampal and adjacent temporal gyri.

Commissural fibres

The major interhemispheric commissure is the corpus callosum (see Figs 1.14, 1.18, 13.3–13.12, 13.21). Much smaller ones are the anterior commissure (Fig. 13.7 and see Fig. 12.2), the posterior commissure (Fig. 13.11 and see Fig. 12.2) and the hippocampal commissure (commissure of the fornix) (see Fig. 16.5).

The **corpus callosum** spans between the two cerebral hemispheres and connects corresponding regions of neocortex, with the exception of the temporal cortices. The parts of the corpus callosum, from rostral to caudal, are named the rostrum, genu, body and splenium (Figs 13.14, 13.22, 13.25). The corpus callosum is shorter anteroposteriorly than is the hemisphere; as a result, callosal fibres linking the two frontal or two occipital poles curve forwards or backwards as the anterior forceps (forceps minor) or posterior forceps (forceps major), respectively (Fig. 13.23). The **splenium** interconnects the occipital cortices and, therefore, contributes to visual functions.

Damage to the corpus callosum

Some patients with chronic epilepsy have undergone surgical section of the corpus callosum to relieve their seizures. Subsequently, such individuals betray few difficulties under normal circumstances. However, when these 'split-brain' patients undergo psychological testing, the two halves of the brain appear to behave relatively autonomously. For example, visual information directed to the right, non-dominant, hemisphere alone does not evoke a verbal response; as a result, individuals cannot name objects or read words presented solely to the left visual field.

Destruction of the splenium of the corpus callosum by stroke or tumour leads to the posterior disconnection syndrome of **alexia without agraphia**. Such individuals speak and write without difficulty but cannot understand written material (alexia). Disconnection of visual processing in the right hemisphere from the verbal processing of the dominant left hemisphere is thought to explain the syndrome.

The **anterior commissure** runs transversely in front of the (anterior) column of the fornix, near the interventricular foramen (Fig. 13.7 and see Fig. 12.2). It interconnects the inferior and middle temporal gyri and the olfactory regions of the two sides. The **posterior commissure** lies dorsal to the periaqueductal grey at the transition between the midbrain and diencephalon (Fig. 13.11 and see Fig. 12.2). It is thought to carry some of the decussating fibres that mediate the consensual light reflex and it is an important neuroradiological landmark. The **hippocampal commissure** (commissure of the fornix) consists of fibres passing between the posterior columns (crura) of the fornix of each side (Fig. 16.5).

Projection fibres

Projection fibres (Fig. 13.24) consist of afferent fibres conveying impulses to the cortex and efferent fibres conducting impulses away from it. The fibres projecting to and from the cerebral cortex have an expansive radial distribution within the hemisphere known as the **corona radiata** (see Fig. 1.30). Deeper within the hemisphere the fibres are concentrated into a dense sheet, called the **internal capsule**. Medial to the internal capsule lie the

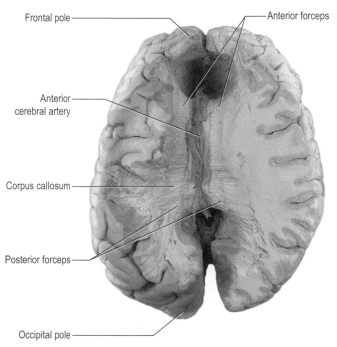

Fig. 13.23 Dissection of the brain from the superior aspect revealing the corpus callosum.

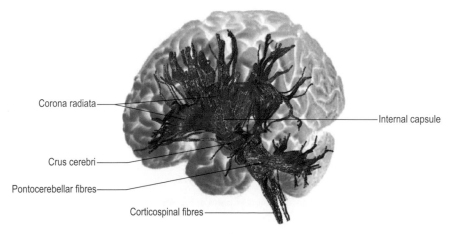

Fig. 13.24 Diffusion MRI tractography reconstruction of the projection fibres passing through the internal capsule. Tractography measures the diffusion of water along axonal fibres and allows reconstruction of their trajectories in the living human brain. *(Courtesy of Professor Marco Catani, Institute of Psychiatry, London, UK.)*

thalamus and caudate nucleus; lateral to it are the globus pallidus and putamen (see, for example Figs 13.8, 13.9, 13.13, 13.15). The internal capsule is concave laterally such that in horizontal section it has an angulated, "v", shape. This provides the basis for nominally dividing it into an anterior limb, genu, posterior limb and retrolenticular part (Figs 13.13, 13.14, 13.25).

The **anterior limb** contains connections between the mediodorsal nucleus of the thalamus and the prefrontal cortex, and also frontopontine fibres that project to the pontine nuclei in the basal portion of the pons.

The **genu** and **posterior limb** contain corticobulbar and corticospinal motor fibres. Also within the posterior limb are thalamocortical projections passing from the ventral posterior nucleus to the primary somatosensory cortex, and from the ventral anterior and ventral lateral nuclei to motor regions of the frontal lobe.

The **retrolenticular** part of the internal capsule lies posterior to the posterior limb and posterior to the globus pallidus/putamen (Fig. 13.14). It consists of fibres arising from the medial and lateral geniculate nuclei of the thalamus that pass to the auditory and visual cortices as the auditory and visual radiations, respectively. Visual thalamocortical fibres (also known as geniculocalcarine fibres) pass laterally round the lateral ventricle and, in doing so, follow one of two courses to the visual cortex

(see Fig. 15.6). Fibres that represent the lower half of the visual field project to the upper part of the visual cortex (above the calcarine sulcus of the occipital lobe). They may be interrupted in their course by lesions of the parietal lobe. Fibres that represent the upper half of the visual field loop forwards over the inferior horn of the lateral ventricle (Meyer's loop) and thence pass to the lower part of the visual cortex (below the calcarine sulcus). They may be damaged along their course by lesions of the temporal lobe.

White matter of the cerebral hemisphere

- Nerve fibres within the subcortical white matter are classified on the basis of their origin and termination.

- Association fibres link cortical regions within a single hemisphere. Important systems are: the superior longitudinal fasciculus, arcuate fasciculus, inferior longitudinal fasciculus and uncinate fasciculus.

- Commissural fibres pass between corresponding regions

of the two hemispheres. The principal commissural system is the corpus callosum.

- Projection fibres run between the cerebral cortex and various subcortical structures. They pass through the corona radiata and the internal capsule. Particularly important fibres in this category are corticospinal, corticobulbar and thalamocortical projections.

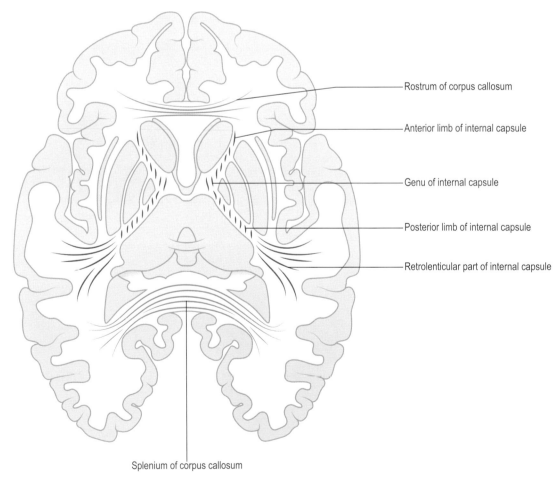

Rostrum of corpus callosum

Anterior limb of internal capsule

Genu of internal capsule

Posterior limb of internal capsule

Retrolenticular part of internal capsule

Splenium of corpus callosum

Fig. 13.25 Horizontal section of the cerebral hemisphere showing the parts of the internal capsule.

Progressive chronic encephalopathy (dementia)

Dementia syndromes are distinct from one another because degenerative brain diseases have specific topographical distributions in the brain and neuropsychological functions are regionally organized (Fig. 13.26 and see Fig. 1.49).

Cortical encephalopathies

The most common cortical dementia is **Alzheimer's disease**, a usually sporadic degenerative disease of the elderly. It affects medial temporal (hippocampal) structures causing amnesia and the posterior cerebral cortex causing aphasia, apperceptive visual agnosia, spatial disorientation and apraxia. In the late stages of illness, akinesia, rigidity and myoclonus supervene. In younger patients, a strongly familial disorder is **frontotemporal dementia (FTD)**, associated with atrophy of the anterior frontotemporal neocortex. The prominent clinical characteristic is behavioural change, which includes apathy, disinhibition, blunting of emotions, repetitive routines and dietary change. This is accompanied by 'executive' cognitive impairments in attention, planning and problem solving. Asymmetric involvement of the left frontal language area results in the degenerative disorder of **progressive non-fluent aphasia (PNFA)**. Utterances may be effortful and lacking in grammar. Bilateral degeneration of the temporal neocortex leads to the disorder of **semantic dementia (SD)** in which patients lose understanding of the meaning of words (semantic aphasia), faces and objects (associative agnosia) and other sensory stimuli, despite preserved elementary perception. FTD, PNFA and SD are associated with frontotemporal lobar degeneration pathology, which is distinct from that of Alzheimer's disease.

Subcortical encephalopathies

Subcortical encephalopathies affect structures such as the thalami, basal ganglia and cerebellum and the interconnecting white matter, causing physical and mental slowing and difficulty in motor and cognitive planning. Subcortical chronic vascular ischaemia (**multi-infarct dementia**) damages the white matter. **Huntington's disease**, **Parkinson's disease** and **progressive supranuclear palsy (PSP)** are degenerative disorders of the basal ganglia. PSP is a rare parkinsonian syndrome in which there is paralysis of voluntary eye movements.

Cortico-subcortical encephalopathies

Cortico-subcortical encephalopathies affect both cortical and subcortical structures. **Corticobasal degeneration** damages the superior parietal cortex and supplementary motor cortex asymmetrically, causing contralateral apraxia, rigidity, akinesia and myoclonus of the arm, which may behave autonomously ('alien limb'). **Cortical Lewy body disease** selectively damages not only the substantia nigra but also the posterior neocortex, leading to parkinsonism and myoclonus, together with cortical symptoms similar to those of Alzheimer's disease, but with chronic fluctuating confusion and visual hallucinations.

Multifocal encephalopathy

A **multifocal encephalopathy** occurs in **Creutzfeldt-Jakob disease** (CJD), a rare degenerative disorder that is rapidly fatal within months. Multiple neuropsychological deficits occur, such as occipital cortical blindness and aphasia, with cerebellar ataxia, pyramidal limb weakness, myoclonus and seizures.

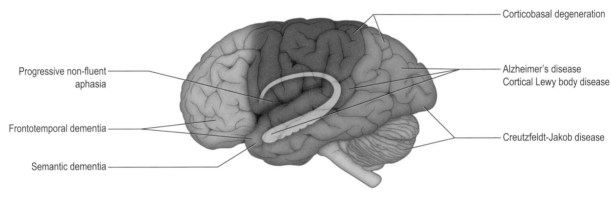

(A)

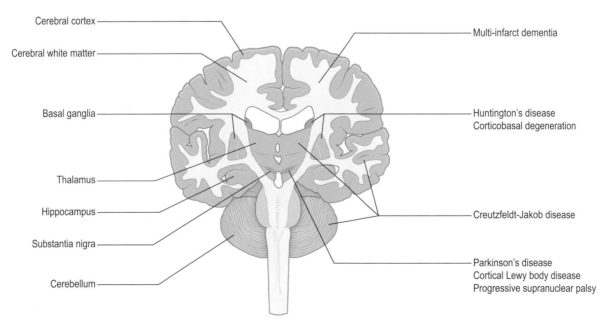

(B)

Fig. 13.26 Regional localisation of diseases causing dementia. (A) Cortical areas. Refer also to Fig. 1.49. (B) Subcortical areas.

14 | Basal ganglia

Within the cerebral hemisphere lie a number of nuclear masses. Apart from the thalamus (Chapter 12), the most prominent of these are the **caudate nucleus**, **putamen** and **globus pallidus**, which lie in close proximity to the internal capsule and are collectively referred to as the **basal ganglia**, **basal nuclei** or **corpus striatum** (Figs 14.1, 14.2; see also Figs 13.3–13.9, 13.14).

The basal ganglia are primarily concerned with the control of movement. Disorders of the basal ganglia are manifest by abnormalities of motor control, posture and muscle tone. The basal ganglia have important connections with other regions of the brain, particularly the cerebral cortex, the thalamus and subthalamic nucleus of the diencephalon, and the substantia nigra of the midbrain.

Terminology and topographical anatomy of the basal ganglia

The term 'basal ganglia' (nuclei) reflects the location of these structures deep within the hemisphere. The term 'corpus striatum' derives from the radially oriented striations, composed of fascicles of nerve fibres, which are readily seen in stained sections, particularly within the globus pallidus.

The globus pallidus is, in phylogenetic terms, the oldest part of the corpus striatum and is sometimes referred to as the **paleostriatum**. The abbreviation '**pallidum**' is more commonly used, particularly in composite terms for afferent and efferent connections, such as 'subthalamopallidal' or 'pallidothalamic'. The globus pallidus and the putamen together are sometimes collectively called the **lentiform** (or **lenticular**) **complex** (or nucleus), because they lie close together, forming an apparently single structure on gross anatomical examination. The name means 'lentil-shaped', but a closer analogy is a Brazil nut or the segment of an orange. The lentiform complex is three-sided, having a convex lateral surface and two other surfaces that converge to a medial apex, which lies against the genu of the internal capsule (Fig. 14.1). The terms 'lentiform' and 'lenticular' are rather archaic and of limited use, although they are still retained in certain anatomical names (such as the retrolenticular

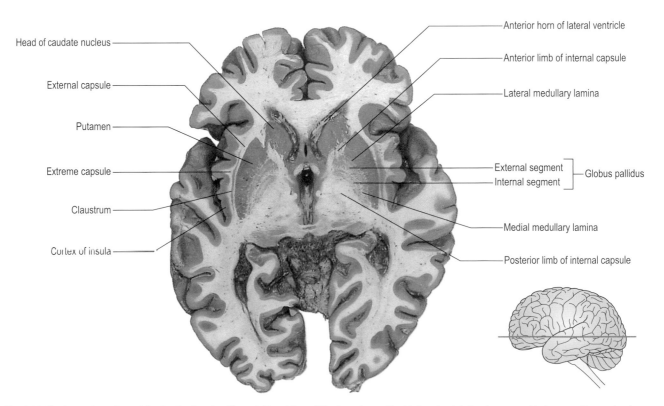

Fig. 14.1 Horizontal section of the brain showing the relationships of the basal ganglia. Mulligan's stain has been used to increase the contrast between cell-rich areas (green/blue) and white matter.

Labels (left side): Head of caudate nucleus · External capsule · Putamen · Extreme capsule · Claustrum · Cortex of insula

Labels (right side): Anterior horn of lateral ventricle · Anterior limb of internal capsule · Lateral medullary lamina · External segment / Internal segment — Globus pallidus · Medial medullary lamina · Posterior limb of internal capsule

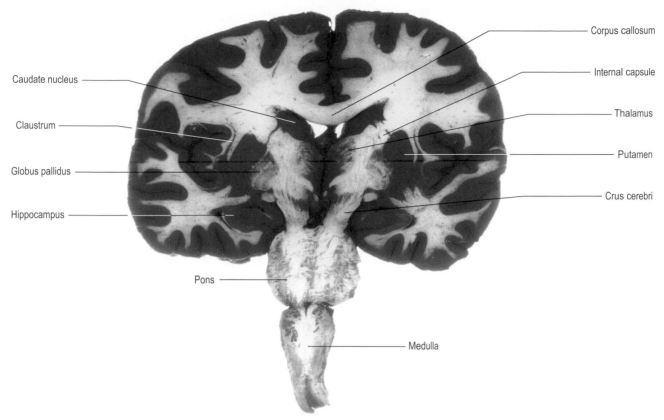

Fig. 14.2 Coronal section of the brain showing the relationships of the basal ganglia. Mulligan's stain has been used to increase the contrast between cell-rich areas (blue) and white matter.

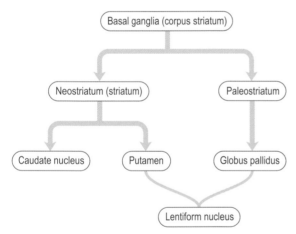

Fig. 14.3 Nomenclature of the basal ganglia.

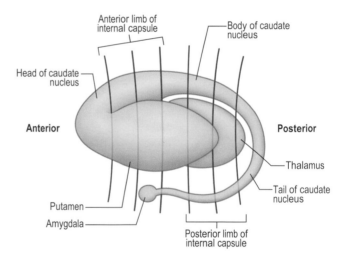

Fig. 14.4 Lateral aspect of the left caudate nucleus, putamen, amygdala and thalamus. The globus pallidus is obscured by the putamen. The course of the internal capsule is shown in red. The putamen and the head of the caudate nucleus are separated by the anterior limb of the internal capsule, except at their most rostral extent where the two are in continuity. The posterior limb of the internal capsule separates the globus pallidus and putamen from the thalamus.

part of the internal capsule). On phylogenetic, connectional and functional grounds, however, the putamen is more closely allied to the caudate nucleus than to the globus pallidus.

The caudate nucleus and putamen constitute the phylogenetically most recent parts of the basal ganglia and are best regarded as a single entity. Together, they are commonly referred to as the **neostriatum**, or simply as the **striatum**. The two components are almost (but not entirely) separated by the anterior limb of the internal capsule but their gross anatomical separation is not as significant as their neuronal and functional similarities. These rather confusing names of, and relationships between, the components of the basal ganglia are summarised in Fig. 14.3.

Some authorities include the substantia nigra and subthalamic nucleus in the definition of basal ganglia. This is justified for the pars reticulata of the substantia nigra since it shares much in common with the globus pallidus and both of these have close,

functionally important interconnections with the subthalamic nucleus.

Striatum

The **striatum** (neostriatum) consists of the caudate nucleus and the putamen. Their combined three-dimensional shape is reminiscent of a tadpole when viewed laterally (Fig. 14.4).

Caudate nucleus

The caudate nucleus is described as consisting of a large head, a body and a tapering, curved tail. The head of the caudate is almost completely separated from the putamen by the internal capsule but, at their rostral extremities, they are continuous through and beneath the anterior limb (Fig. 14.4; see also Figs 13.4–13.6). At this anterior level, the most ventral and medial part of the striatum constitutes the **nucleus accumbens** (see Fig. 13.6).

The nucleus accumbens has connections similar to the rest of the striatum and also has connections with the amygdala. The amygdala, which is located within the temporal lobe, near to the temporal pole and deep to the lentiform complex (see Fig. 13.8) also has a similar embryological derivation to the corpus striatum but is functionally different, being part of the limbic system (Chapter 16). The nucleus accumbens and amygdala provide an important interface between the basal ganglia and the limbic system and they fulfill a role in the physical expression of behaviour driven by affective and motivational states. The nucleus accumbens is associated with reward and gratification and is believed to be a part of the mechanism underlying addictive aspects of behaviour, including being an important site of action of addictive substances.

The head of the caudate nucleus forms a prominent bulge in the lateral wall of the anterior horn of the lateral ventricle (Fig. 14.1; see also Figs 13.3–13.7). The tail of the caudate passes posteriorly, progressively tapering as it does so and, following the curvature of the ventricle, descends into the temporal lobe where it lies in the roof of the inferior horn (Fig. 14.4; see also Figs 13.9–13.12, 13.14).

Putamen

The putamen lies lateral to the internal capsule and globus pallidus (Figs 14.1, 14.2; see also Figs 13.7, 13.8, 13.14). It is separated from the globus pallidus by a thin lamina of nerve fibres, the **lateral medullary lamina**. Lateral to the putamen lies more white matter, sandwiched within which lies a thin sheet of grey matter, known as the **claustrum**. This separates the white matter into two layers, the **external capsule** and the **extreme capsule** (Fig. 14.1). Lateral to the extreme capsule lies the cortex of the insula, deep within the lateral fissure of the hemisphere.

Globus pallidus

The globus pallidus lies medial to the putamen, separated from it by the lateral medullary lamina. Its medial apex nestles into the lateral concavity of the internal capsule (Fig. 14.1). The globus pallidus consists of two divisions, referred to as the **external** (or lateral) and the **internal** (or medial) **segments** (abbreviated as GPe and GPi, respectively). The segments are separated by a thin sheet of fibres, the **medial medullary lamina** (Fig. 14.1). The smaller internal segment shares many similarities, in terms of cytology and connections, with the pars reticulata of the substantia nigra in the midbrain (Chapter 9, p. 96). Although the two are separated anatomically by the internal capsule/crus cerebri, they are best regarded as a single entity, in the functional sense, as described below.

The basal part of the rostral forebrain, deep to the corpus striatum, also includes a region known as the substantia innominata (Fig. 14.7 and see Fig. 13.7). This complex region contains several groups of neurones, one of them being the **nucleus basalis** (of Meynert), the cells of which project widely to the cerebral cortex and utilise acetylcholine as their neurotransmitter. These neurones undergo degeneration in Alzheimer's disease.

Functional anatomy of the basal ganglia

Connections of the striatum

The caudate nucleus and putamen, together commonly referred to as the striatum, are best considered as a single entity since they share common neuronal organisation, neurotransmitter systems

---

Topographical anatomy of the basal ganglia

- The basal ganglia consist of the caudate nucleus, putamen and globus pallidus.
- These structures are primarily concerned with the control of posture and movement.
- The caudate nucleus lies in the wall of the lateral ventricle.
- The head of the caudate lies medial to the internal capsule and forms a prominent bulge in the lateral wall of the anterior horn of the ventricle.
- The curved, tapering tail of the caudate follows the curvature of the lateral ventricle into the temporal lobe.

- The putamen and globus pallidus lie lateral to the internal capsule, deep to the cortex of the insula.
- Topographically, the putamen and globus pallidus constitute the lentiform complex.
- Functionally, however, the caudate nucleus and putamen form a single entity, the neostriatum (striatum), while the globus pallidus forms the paleostriatum.
- The globus pallidus consists of external and internal segments.

---

and connections (Fig. 14.5). They are often regarded as the 'input' portions of the basal ganglia, since the majority of afferents from other parts of the brain end here, rather than in the globus pallidus.

Striatal afferents

Afferents to the striatum come from three principal sources: the cerebral cortex, the thalamus and the substantia nigra.

Corticostriatal fibres originate from widespread regions of the cerebral cortex, predominantly, but not exclusively, of the ipsilateral side. Fibres from the frontal and parietal lobes predominate. Motor regions of the frontal lobe project mainly to the putamen, where the body is represented in an inverted, approximately somatotopic fashion. More anterior regions of the frontal lobe, and other association cortices, project mainly to the caudate nucleus. For these reasons, the putamen is considered to be the most overtly motor part of the striatum, the caudate nucleus having more associative functions. Corticostriatal fibres are excitatory to striatal neurones and use glutamic acid as their transmitter.

The **thalamostriatal projection** comes from the intralaminar nuclei (centromedian and parafascicular nuclei) of the ipsilateral thalamus (Chapter 12).

The **nigrostriatal projection** originates from the **pars compacta** of the ipsilateral **substantia nigra** of the midbrain tegmentum (Chapter 9, p. 96). The transmitter used by this pathway is the monoamine dopamine, which has both excitatory and inhibitory effects upon striatal neurones. The neurones of the pars compacta contain the dark pigment neuromelanin (Fig. 14.6), which is produced as a byproduct of dopamine synthesis. The most rostral and ventral portion of the striatum, the nucleus accumbens, receives its dopaminergic input from the ventral tegmental area, which lies medial to the substantia nigra (see Fig. 9.13). This projection is part of the so-called **mesolimbic pathway** which also provides dopaminergic innervation of the amygdala. Other afferents to the striatum include a projection from neurones of the brainstem **raphé nuclei**, which utilise serotonin as their transmitter.

Striatal efferents

The principal neuronal type within the striatum is known as the medium spiny neurone. The axons of medium spiny neurones constitute the efferent projections of the striatum and they are directed principally to the two segments of the globus pallidus and to the pars reticulata of the substantia nigra (**striatopallidal** and **striatonigral fibres**, respectively). Although there is some

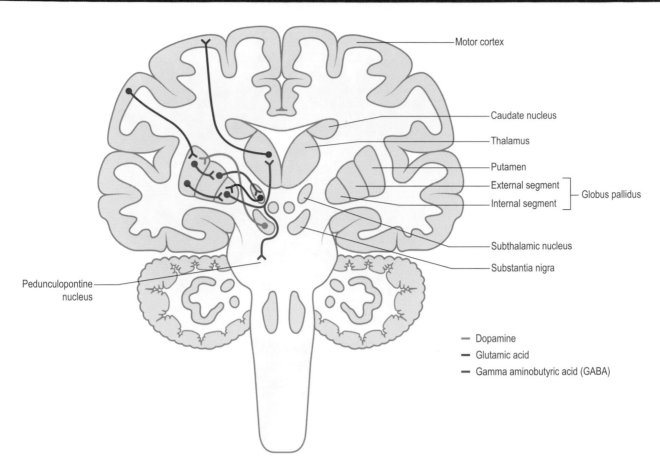

Fig. 14.5 Schematic diagram illustrating the principal connections of the basal ganglia and related nuclei. For the sake of clarity, the connections of the (neo)striatum are shown for the putamen only. The connections of the caudate nucleus are similar. Afferents to the striatum from the intralaminar thalamic nuclei and brainstem raphé nuclei have been omitted. All efferents from the basal ganglia system are shown to originate from the internal segment of the globus pallidus, those from the pars reticulata of the substantia nigra being omitted. Colours indicate the neurotransmitters used.

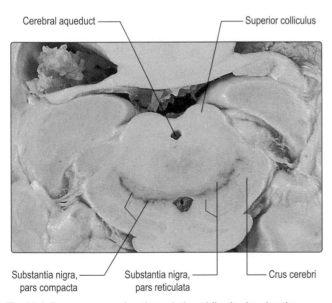

Fig. 14.6 Transverse section through the midbrain showing the substantia nigra.

collateralisation of axons, separate populations of striatal neurones generally project to each of the three output targets. These projections are all inhibitory upon pallidal and nigral neurones and utilise GABA as their primary transmitter. In addition, a number of neuropeptides are co-localised in these efferent neurones. The cells that project to the internal segment of the globus pallidus (GPi) and the substantia nigra contain both **substance P** and **dynorphin**. The projection to the external segment of the globus pallidus (GPe) contains **met-enkephalin**.

Connections of the striatum

- The caudate nucleus and putamen are the 'input' regions of the basal ganglia.

- They receive afferents from the cerebral cortex, intralaminar thalamic nuclei and the pars compacta of the substantia nigra.

- Efferent fibres arise from medium spiny neurones. Separate cell groups project to either of the two segments of the globus pallidus (GPe or GPi) or to the pars reticulata of the substantia nigra. The efferents are inhibitory and GABAergic.

Connections of the globus pallidus

The two segments of the globus pallidus have similar afferent connections to one another, but substantially different efferent projections. The internal segment of the globus pallidus is very similar in structure and function to the pars reticulata of the substantia nigra, from which it is separated by the internal capsule/crus cerebri. Together, the internal pallidum and pars reticulata of the substantia nigra are regarded as the 'output' portion of the basal ganglia, since they are the origin of the majority of basal ganglia efferent fibres that project to other levels of the neuraxis.

Pallidal afferents

Pallidal afferents arise principally from the striatum and from the subthalamic nucleus. Striatopallidal fibres are of two types, as previously noted, originating from different populations of striatal medium spiny neurones. Both utilise GABA as their primary transmitter. In addition, each contains characteristic peptide co-transmitters; fibres projecting to the external pallidal segment contain enkephalin, while those projecting to the internal pallidum contain substance P and dynorphin.

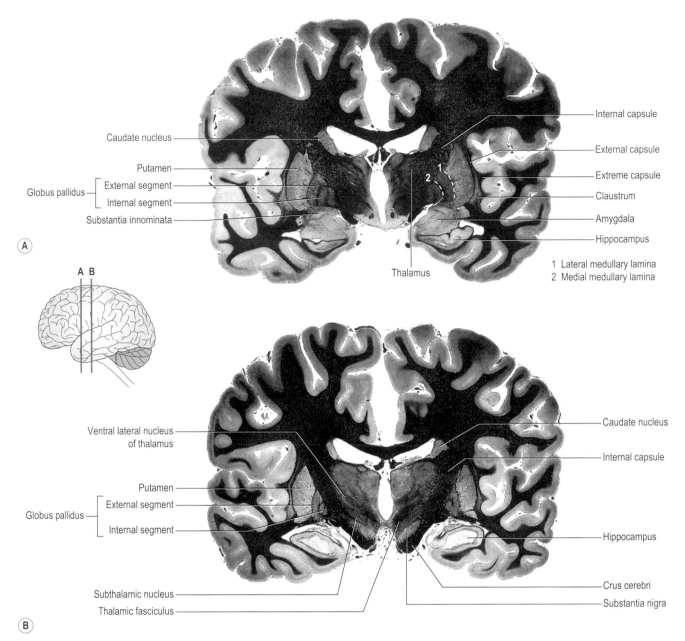

Fig. 14.7 (A,B) Coronal sections through the corpus striatum and diencephalon. Loyez method for myelin. *(Sections courtesy of the National Museum of Health and Medicine, Armed Forces Institute of Pathology, Washington, DC, USA.)*

The **subthalamopallidal projection** originates in the subthalamic nucleus of the caudal diencephalon (Figs 14.7, 14.8 and see Figs 12.3B, 13.9). This small structure is located beneath the thalamus, lying against the medial border of the internal capsule. In coronal sections, it has the appearance of a biconvex lens. Subthalamopallidal fibres pass laterally through the internal capsule, contributing to a fibre system known as the **subthalamic fasciculus** (Fig. 14.8), and terminate in both segments of the globus pallidus, although termination is more dense in the internal segment.

The subthalamopallidal pathway is excitatory to pallidal neurones, using glutamic acid as its transmitter. The subthalamic nucleus also sends similar fibres to the pars reticulata of the substantia nigra, the other 'output' part of the basal ganglia system. The subthalamopallidal and subthalamonigral pathways have a pivotal role in the normal function of the basal ganglia and in the pathophysiology of basal ganglia disorders (see below).

Pallidal efferents

The two pallidal segments have very different efferent projections. The external segment projects principally to the subthalamic nucleus. Such pallidosubthalamic fibres pass medially through the

internal capsule in the **subthalamic fasciculus**. This projection is inhibitory and uses GABA as its transmitter. The internal segment of the globus pallidus, together with the pars reticulata of the substantia nigra, projects primarily to the thalamus (ventral lateral, ventral anterior and centromedian nuclei), with a smaller projection to the brainstem tegmentum. These output neurones are all inhibitory and utilise GABA as their transmitter.

Pallidothalamic fibres take one of two routes from the GPi to reach their target (Fig. 14.8). Some fibres loop round the anterior margin of the internal capsule as the **ansa lenticularis**. Others pass through the internal capsule as the **lenticular fasciculus**. Medial to the internal capsule, as the latter fibres pass over the subthalamic nucleus, they are known as Forel's field H_2. Having passed either round or through the internal capsule, pallidothalamic fibres continue to course medially and then loop dorsally and laterally as the **thalamic fasciculus** (also known as Forel's field H_1) to enter the thalamus from its ventral aspect. In following this trajectory, pallidothalamic fibres circumnavigate a cellular region of the subthalamus known as the **zona incerta**, which lies between the thalamus and the subthalamic nucleus.

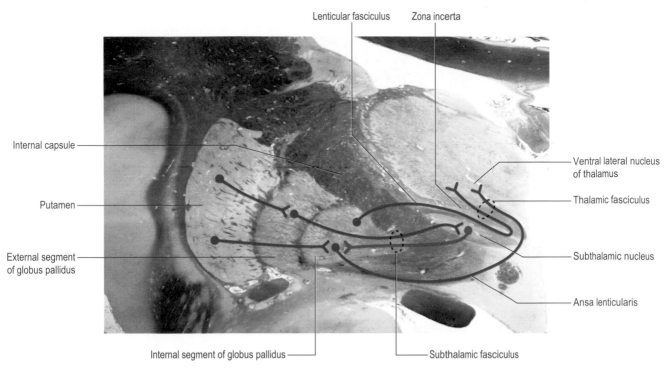

Fig. 14.8 **Coronal section through the corpus striatum and diencephalon illustrating the efferent projections of the globus pallidus.**

Pallidothalamic fibres constitute the main outflow from the basal ganglia. Their thalamic target nuclei (ventral anterior and ventral lateral nuclei) in turn project excitatory, glutamatergic fibres to the motor regions of the frontal lobe, principally the primary motor and supplementary motor cortices. A smaller contingent of medial pallidal efferent fibres passes caudally to terminate in the brainstem tegmentum in the **nucleus tegmenti pedunculopontinus (pedunculopontine nucleus)**, which lies at the boundary between midbrain and pons, near the lateral margin of the superior cerebellar peduncle (Fig. 14.5; see also Fig. 13.12). This region has been termed the **mesencephalic locomotor region** in lower mammals, since it is involved in the regulation of quadrupedal progression.

The pars reticulata of the substantia nigra is regarded as a homologue of the internal segment of the globus pallidus and, thus, has a similar status as the origin of basal ganglia output neurones. Like the internal pallidum, the pars reticulata receives fibres from the striatum and the subthalamic nucleus. The projection from the striatum is somatotopically organised, both in the pallidum and nigra, such that pallidal neurones are associated primarily with limb movements, whereas nigral cells control the axial musculature, including the extraocular muscles. As already noted, efferents from the internal pallidum project to the ventral anterior, ventral lateral and centromedian thalamic nuclei and to the pedunculopontine nucleus. Efferents of the pars reticulata of the substantia nigra also pass to a subregion of the ventral lateral thalamus, to the superior colliculus and to the brainstem reticular formation (including the pedunculopontine nucleus).

Normal functions of the basal ganglia

The basal ganglia are sometimes referred to as components of the so-called 'extrapyramidal motor system'. This term was coined to distinguish the symptoms seen clinically in diseases of the basal ganglia and related structures, such as the substantia nigra and subthalamic nucleus, from the symptoms observed following stroke in the internal capsule. Since the latter were thought to be caused by destruction of the pyramidal tract, the term 'extrapyramidal' seemed an appropriate descriptor for disorders of the basal ganglia. As understanding of the functional anatomy of motor control has increased, it has become apparent: (1) that the

Connections of the globus pallidus

- The globus pallidus consists of two segments: external and internal.

- Both pallidal segments receive GABAergic afferent fibres from the striatum and glutamatergic afferents from the subthalamic nucleus.

- The external pallidal segment projects GABAergic fibres to the subthalamic nucleus.

- The internal pallidal segment is homologous to the pars reticulata of the substantia nigra; the two structures are the 'output' regions of the basal ganglia.

- The internal pallidal segment projects GABAergic fibres to the thalamus (ventral anterior, ventral lateral and centromedian nuclei) and to the brainstem (pedunculopontine nucleus).

pyramidal and extrapyramidal 'systems' are intimately related rather than separate and (2) that so-called pyramidal signs are not all attributable to dysfunction of the pyramidal tract itself (see p. 28). The term 'extrapyramidal' is, therefore, somewhat outdated but is still in widespread use.

Current concepts of the role of the basal ganglia consider that their function is to facilitate behaviour and movements that are required and appropriate in any particular context and to inhibit unwanted or inappropriate movements. How this might be achieved can be explained with reference to the internal connections of the basal ganglia (Fig. 14.5).

When a movement is initiated from the cerebral cortex, impulses discharge not only through corticospinal and corticobulbar pathways but also through the corticostriatal projection to the neostriatum. These glutamatergic fibres cause excitation of striatal medium spiny neurones. The striatum has two routes by which it is able to control the activity of basal ganglia output neurones in the internal segment of the globus pallidus and the pars reticulata of the substantia nigra. One of these is the so-called 'direct pathway', consisting of striatopallidal and striatonigral neurones, which directly inhibit internal pallidal or pars reticulata neurones. This mechanism has been shown to operate in experimental electrophysiological studies in primates, where basal ganglia output neurones associated with a particular body part or muscle group show a pause in their action potential discharge during movement

Parkinson's disease   Chorea

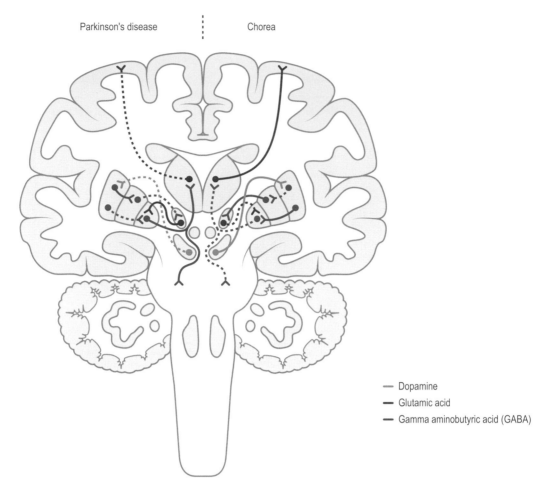

— Dopamine
— Glutamic acid
— Gamma aminobutyric acid (GABA)

Fig. 14.9 Schematic diagram illustrating how activities in basal ganglia and related nuclei become disordered in Parkinson's disease and chorea. Overactive pathways are shown by solid lines; underactive pathways are shown by interrupted lines. For identification of structures, see Fig. 14.5.

of that region. This has been shown to occur in the internal pallidum for limb movements and in the substantia nigra, pars reticulata, for eye movements. Since internal pallidal and pars reticulata output neurones are themselves inhibitory, this leads to disinhibition of target neurones, including those of the motor thalamus. The resulting increase in the activity of thalamic neurones causes excitation of the cells of the cerebral cortex. The effect of activation of the direct pathway is, therefore, to support or facilitate ongoing movements, through this positive feedback to the cortex.

The other route by which striatal neurones can influence the output of the basal ganglia is the so-called 'indirect pathway', via the subthalamic nucleus. A proportion of efferents from the striatum terminate in the external pallidal segment and their activation induces inhibition of external pallidal neurones. The principal efferent projection of the external pallidum is to the subthalamic nucleus which, therefore, becomes disinhibited. The resultant increase in discharge of subthalamic neurones causes activation of internal pallidal and nigral neurones and, in turn, inhibition of thalamic and cortical cells. This has the effect of inhibiting unwanted movements.

Pathophysiology of basal ganglia disorders

Basal ganglia dysfunction leads to abnormal motor control, alterations in posture and muscular tone and the emergence of abnormal, involuntary movements or dyskinesias. The combination of symptoms depends upon the nature and site of the lesion. The most common disorder of the basal ganglia is **Parkinson's disease**, which is characterised by poverty and slowness of movement (akinesia/bradykinesia), tremor and rigidity. It is caused by degeneration of the dopaminergic neurones of the substantia nigra, pars compacta, that project to the

striatum. Studies on the post mortem brains of patients with Parkinson's disease and experimental animal studies have provided insight into the pathophysiological mechanisms that underlie the appearance of parkinsonian symptoms, in particular akinesia (Fig. 14.9). Normally, dopamine appears to exert an excitatory influence upon striatal neurones of the 'direct' projection to the internal pallidal segment, and an inhibitory effect upon neurones of the 'indirect' pathway that projects to the external pallidal segment. Loss of striatal dopamine, therefore, causes abnormal underactivity of the direct pathway, leading to disinhibition of internal pallidal neurones. At the same time, loss of striatal dopamine causes overactivity of the indirect projection leading to inhibition of external pallidal neurones, disinhibition of the subthalamic nucleus and, thus, excessive excitatory drive of internal pallidal cells. Changes in both the direct and indirect pathways, thus, compound to exacerbate the abnormal overactivity of internal pallidal output cells, inhibiting the motor thalamic nuclei and motor cortical areas, inducing akinesia.

The archetypal basal ganglia disease in which excessive, unwanted, abnormal movements (dyskinesias) occur is **Huntington's disease** (Huntington's chorea), which is an inherited, progressive neurodegenerative disorder. Within the striatum, there is particular attrition of the cells that project to the external segment of the globus pallidus (the 'indirect' projection), at least early on in the condition. This leads to disinhibition of external pallidal neurones and inhibition of the subthalamic nucleus. Internal pallidal neurones, therefore, become abnormally underactive, and unwanted, involuntary movements (chorea) ensue. Similar abnormal movements occur as a complication of the long-term treatment of Parkinson's disease with L-DOPA. The underlying neural mechanism is similar but, in the latter case, there is both relative underactivity of the indirect pathway and overactivity of the direct pathway (Fig. 14.9). A very rare, but instructive, condition which dramatically demonstrates the central importance of the subthalamic nucleus in basal ganglia function is **ballism** (hemiballism, hemiballismus). This is caused by damage to the subthalamic nucleus, most often by stroke. It is characterised by gross choreic, flailing movements of the contralateral limbs due to removal of the excitatory drive upon basal ganglia output neurones.

Because of the anatomical arrangement of basal ganglia connections, unilateral basal ganglia lesions produce their effects on the contralateral side of the body, as is the case with cerebral hemisphere lesions, but distinct from cerebellar disorders.

Basal ganglia function and dysfunction

- The basal ganglia historically were referred to as parts of the extrapyramidal motor system to distinguish basal ganglia disorders from those of the pyramidal tract. However, the systems are intimately related.
- The basal ganglia facilitate purposeful behaviour and movement via the 'direct' pathway and inhibit unwanted movements via the 'indirect' pathway.
- Lesions of the basal ganglia produce effects on the contralateral side of the body.
- Diseases of the basal ganglia are typified by Parkinson's disease, in which there is poverty of movement, and Huntington's disease, which is associated with dyskinesias.

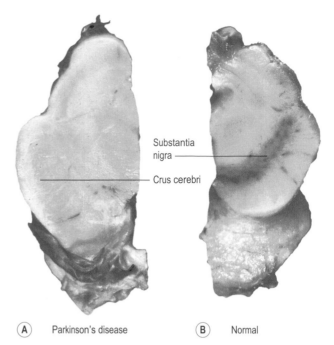

Fig. 14.10 (A, B) Approximately transverse sections through the lateral half of the midbrain, showing degeneration and depigmentation of the substantia nigra, pars compacta in Parkinson's disease. *(Courtesy of Professor D Mann, Clinical Neurosciences, Hope Hospital, University of Manchester, Manchester, UK.)*

Basal ganglia movement disorders

A **resting tremor** of the upper limb characterises the onset of the movement disorder of **Parkinson's disease**, in which the pars compacta of the substantia nigra degenerates (Fig. 14.10), leading to depletion of striatal dopamine (Fig. 14.11). The elderly patients develop progressive akinesia, motor rigidity, a flexed posture and difficulty in initiating movements. Treatment is with levodopa (L-DOPA) or dopamine receptor agonists. If drug therapy fails, stimulation of the subthalamic nucleus or GPi through implanted electrodes (deep brain stimulation) can help the patient.

A **postural tremor** of the upper limbs is seen in **benign essential tremor**; it is exacerbated by anxiety and relieved by alcohol. There is no progressive disability, in contrast to Parkinson's disease.

A violent ('bat's wing') postural tremor characterises **hepatolenticular degeneration** (**Wilson's disease**), an autosomal recessive disorder of copper metabolism, which also leads to progressive dementia, dystonia, cerebellar dysarthria and ataxia.

Chorea is the hallmark of **Huntington's disease,** an autosomal dominantly inherited degeneration of the neostriatum in which dystonia, akinesia and dementia progressively supervene.

Sydenham's chorea is now rare and is a manifestation of rheumatic fever, an immune disorder triggered by streptococcal infection. Affected children develop abnormal behaviour and generalised chorea (St Vitus' dance).

Dystonia characterises **hereditary dystonias**, which are neurodegenerative diseases of childhood in which involuntary movements are generalised. In adults, dystonia is sporadic and focal, affecting the upper limb (**writer's cramp**), lower limb, neck (**torticollis**), face and mouth (**orofacial dystonia**) and larynx (**spasmodic dysphonia**).

Both dystonia and chorea develop in the late stages of Parkinson's disease treated with levodopa (**levodopa-induced dyskinesia**) and in psychotic patients treated with neuroleptic drugs (**tardive dyskinesia**).

Myoclonus (sudden, involuntary muscle contractions chiefly affecting the head, neck and upper limbs) is the sole manifestation of **familial essential myoclonus**. Myoclonus is also seen in the neurodegenerative disorders of **Alzheimer's disease, Lewy body disease** and **Creutzfeldt-Jakob disease**.

Tics, which are simple and focal muscle twitches, most often involving the head and neck, are usually of no pathological significance in adolescence. However, in the familial **Tourette's syndrome** children and adolescents develop complex involuntary motor repertoires, which change their nature and site, and also suffer obsessive–compulsive disorders.

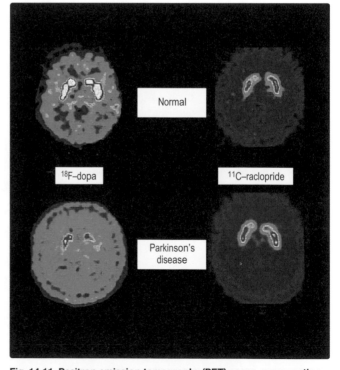

Fig. 14.11 Positron emission tomography (PET) scans, representing horizontal sections through the brain at the level of the striatum. Anterior is towards the top in each case. The top scans are from a normal individual and the bottom ones from a patient with Parkinson's disease. The scans on the left were made using the tracer [18F]-dopa. This is taken up by intact dopaminergic nerve terminals and, therefore, acts as an index of the integrity of the nigrostriatal pathway. There is reduced labelling in the striatum of the parkinsonian patient. The scans on the right were made using the tracer [11C]-raclopride. This binds to dopamine receptors located on striatal neurones that receive input from the nigrostriatal pathway. These receptors remain intact in parkinsonian patients. *(Courtesy of Professor D J Brooks, Hartnett Professor of Neurology, Imperial College, London, UK.)*

15 | Visual system

Vision is the most highly developed and versatile of all the sensory modalities and, arguably, the one on which humans are most dependent. The optic nerve and retina develop from the prosencephalic primary brain vesicle (p. 7) and, therefore, are regarded as an outgrowth of the brain itself. Vision commences with the formation of an image of the external world on the photoreceptive **retina**. The retina encodes visual information in the discharge of neurones that project to the brain through the **optic nerve**. Fibres of the optic nerve undergo hemidecussation in the **optic chiasm** and project to the lateral geniculate nucleus of the thalamus. Thalamocortical neurones in turn project to the primary visual cortex in the occipital lobe of the cerebral hemisphere, where visual perception occurs.

The eye

In the eye, the eyeball, or globe, is approximately spherical in shape (Fig. 15.1). Near its posterior pole emerges the optic nerve. The eyeball may be considered to consist of three concentric layers of tissue, the outermost of which is tough, fibrous and protective. Over most of the globe it forms an opaque white coat, the **sclera**, to which are attached the extraocular muscles that move the eyeball (see Fig. 10.5). Over the anterior pole of the globe it forms the transparent **cornea**, through which light enters the eye.

Near to the anterior margin of the sclera, two rings of smooth muscle extend into the lumen of the eyeball (Fig. 15.2). The most anterior of these is the **iris**, which has a central aperture, the **pupil**, through which light is admitted to the posterior part of the eye. Some of the muscle fibres of the iris are arranged in a circular fashion, while others are oriented radially. They are under the control of the autonomic nervous system. Circular fibres are innervated by postganglionic parasympathetic neurones, which act to constrict the pupil and reduce the amount of light falling upon the retina (see p. 102). Radial fibres are innervated by postganglionic sympathetic neurones which dilate the pupil.

Behind the iris lies the **ciliary body** containing **ciliary muscle**, which receives innervation from the parasympathetic nervous system. The central aperture within the annulus of the ciliary body is occupied by the transparent, biconvex **lens**, which focuses light upon the retina. The lens is held in place by a **suspensory ligament** that is attached to the peripheral margin of the lens and to the ciliary body. Contraction of the ciliary muscle alters the shape and, therefore, the focusing power (focal length) of the lens, a process known as accommodation (p. 102). The lens and suspensory ligament divide the lumen of the eyeball into an anterior and a posterior part. The anterior part, in front of the lens, contains a thin, watery fluid, **aqueous humour**, which is continuously secreted from the ciliary body. It is also reabsorbed into the ciliary body where it is drained by a small duct, the **canal of Schlemm**, through which it is returned to the venous system. The posterior part of the globe contains a gelatinous material known as **vitreous humour**. Behind the ciliary body, the inner surface of the sclera is lined by the **choroid**, the cells of which contain dark pigment that absorbs light and thus reduces reflection within the eye. Lining the inner surface of the choroid is the photoreceptive retina.

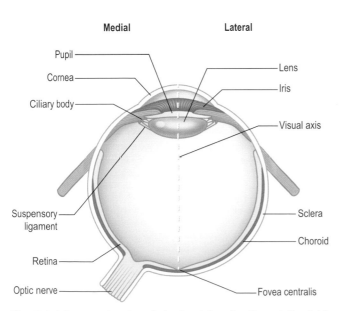

Fig. 15.1 Schematic drawing of a horizontal section through the right eyeball.

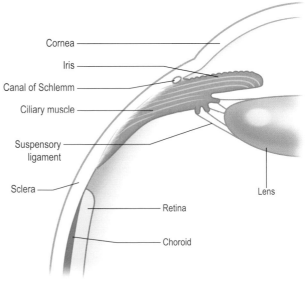

Fig. 15.2 Schematic drawing of the sclerocorneal junction of the eyeball.

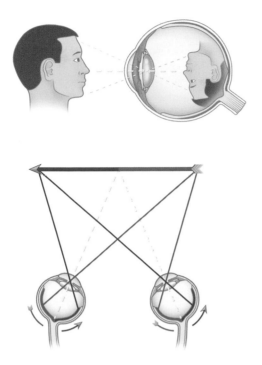

Fig. 15.3 The representation of the visual field upon the retinae.

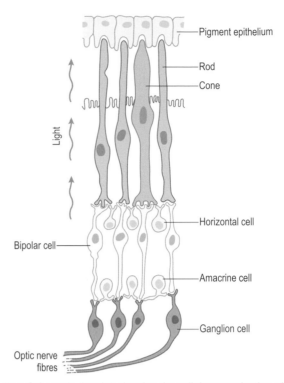

Fig. 15.4 Schematic drawing showing the cellular organisation of the retina.

Light passes from objects in the field of vision (**visual field**), through the narrow aperture of the pupil to subtend an image upon the retina. An object in the visual field, upon which attention is focused, subtends an image that is centred near the posterior pole of the eye along the line of the **visual axis** (Fig. 15.1). At this point, which is known as the **fovea centralis**, and the surrounding 1 cm, which is known as the **macula lutea**, the retina is specially modified for maximal visual acuity (resolving power). The basic optical properties of the eye, which may be likened to those of a pinhole camera, dictate that the image so formed is inverted in both lateral and vertical dimensions (Fig. 15.3). Furthermore, objects that lie in the left half of the visual field form an image upon the nasal (right) half of the left retina and the temporal (right) half of the right retina, and *vice versa*. Medial to the macula is a region where retinal axons accumulate to leave the eye in the optic nerve. This is known as the **optic disc**. Photoreceptors are absent from this region, which is also, therefore, referred to as the **blind spot**.

Retina

The retina consists of a non-neural and a neural portion. The non-neural part is represented by the **pigment epithelium**, a single layer of light-absorbing, pigmented cells lying adjacent to the choroid (Fig. 15.4). The neural part of the retina contains photoreceptors and neurones as well as neuroglia and a rich capillary network. The photoreceptive cells lie deepest within the retina and interdigitate with the pigment epithelium. Light entering the eye, therefore, passes through, and is refracted and partially absorbed by, these additional elements before reaching the photoreceptors. By means of a series of photochemical reactions and physicochemical changes, retinal photoreceptors transduce light energy into electrical energy (changes in membrane potential). Retinal photoreceptors are of two types, **rods** and **cones**, of which the rods are about 20 times more numerous. These cells share many structural similarities but have important functional distinctions. Rods are exquisitely sensitive to light. They are particularly important for vision in dim lighting conditions. Cones are responsible for colour vision and, because of their arrangement and neuronal connections, they confer high visual acuity.

Rods and cones are heterogeneously distributed across the retina. Rods greatly predominate in the peripheral parts of the

retina but their relative numbers decrease towards the macula, where cones are more abundant. At the fovea, only cones are present. Furthermore, at the fovea the neurones and capillaries, through which light has to pass to reach the photoreceptors, are displaced, so that the cones are directly exposed to light. This combination provides for maximal visual acuity.

In addition to photoreceptive cells, the retina contains the cell bodies of both the first- and second-order neurones of the central visual pathway (Fig. 15.4). The first-order neurones, or **bipolar cells**, lie entirely within the retina, while the axons of the second-order neurones, or **ganglion cells**, form the optic nerve. Information is transferred from photoreceptors to bipolar cells and then to ganglion cells, with greater convergence for rods than for cones. The retina also contains interneurones known as horizontal cells and amacrine cells. These modulate transmission between photoreceptors and bipolar cells, and between bipolar cells and ganglion cells, respectively.

The eye

- Objects in one lateral half of the visual field form images on the nasal half of the ipsilateral retina and the temporal half of the contralateral retina.

- The retina contains photoreceptors (rods and cones), first-order sensory neurones (bipolar cells) and second-order neurones (ganglion cells).

- The axons of retinal ganglion cells accumulate at the optic disc (blind spot) and pass into the optic nerve.

The central visual pathway

The axons of retinal ganglion cells assemble at the optic disc and pass into the optic nerve, which enters the cranial cavity through the optic canal. The two optic nerves converge to form the **optic chiasm** on the base of the brain (Fig. 15.5). The chiasm lies immediately rostral to the tuber cinereum of the hypothalamus and between the terminating internal carotid arteries (see Figs 7.2, 7.3). In the chiasm, axons derived from the nasal halves of the two retinae decussate and pass into the contralateral **optic tract**, while those from the temporal hemiretinae remain ipsilateral. The optic tracts diverge away from the chiasm and pass round the cerebral peduncle to terminate mainly in the **lateral geniculate nucleus** (within the lateral geniculate body) of the thalamus. A relatively small number of fibres leave the optic nerve, before reaching the lateral geniculate nucleus, to terminate in the **pretectal area** and the superior colliculus. These fibres are involved in mediation of the pupillary light reflex (Chapter 10). From the lateral geniculate nucleus, third-order thalamocortical neurones project through the retrolenticular part of the internal capsule and form the **optic radiation**, which terminates in the **primary visual cortex** of the occipital lobe. The primary visual cortex is located predominantly on the medial surface of the hemisphere in the region above and below the calcarine sulcus. Surrounding this area, the rest of the occipital lobe constitutes the visual association cortex. It is concerned with interpretation of visual images, recognition, depth perception and colour vision.

There is a precise point-to-point relationship between the retina and the visual cortex. Because of the importance of the macula in vision, it is represented by disproportionately large volumes (relative to its size) of the lateral geniculate nucleus and the visual cortex. Within the visual cortex the macula is represented most posteriorly, in the region of the occipital pole.

As previously noted, objects in either half (left or right) of the visual field produce images upon the nasal hemiretina of the ipsilateral eye and the temporal hemiretina of the contralateral eye (Fig. 15.3). Each optic nerve, therefore, carries information concerning both halves of the visual field (Fig. 15.5). Because of the decussation of fibres from the nasal hemiretinae at the optic chiasm, however, each optic tract, lateral geniculate nucleus and visual cortex receives information relating only to the contralateral half of the visual field. This combination of the images from both eyes is necessary for stereoscopic vision (depth perception). The upper half of the visual field forms images upon the lower halves of the retinae and the lower half of the visual field forms images upon the upper hemiretinae. As thalamocortical fibres leave the lateral geniculate nucleus they pass around the lateral ventricle, those representing the lower part of the visual field coursing superiorly to terminate in the visual cortex above the calcarine sulcus. Those which represent the upper part of the visual field sweep into the temporal lobe (**Meyer's loop**, Fig. 15.6) before terminating below the calcarine sulcus.

The visual field can be considered as being comprised of four quadrants (left/right, upper/lower; Fig. 15.7), each projecting to its own corresponding quadrant of the primary visual cortex (either left or right hemisphere and either above or below the calcarine sulcus). There is both lateral and vertical inversion in the projection of the visual field upon the visual cortex such that, for example, the upper left quadrant of the visual field is represented in the lower right quadrant of the visual cortex.

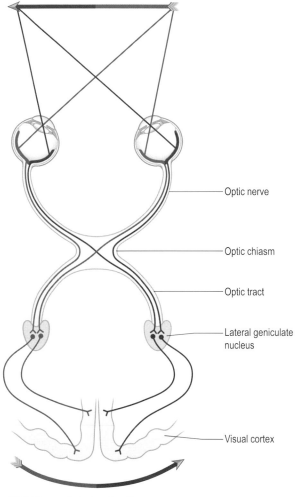

Optic nerve

Optic chiasm

Optic tract

Lateral geniculate nucleus

Visual cortex

Fig. 15.5 The central visual pathway.

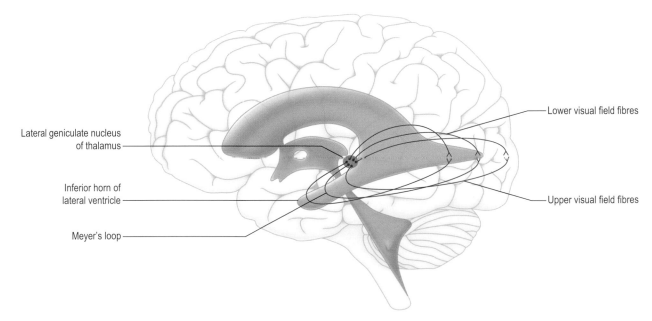

Lateral geniculate nucleus of thalamus

Inferior horn of lateral ventricle

Meyer's loop

Lower visual field fibres

Upper visual field fibres

Fig. 15.6 The course taken by thalamocortical fibres projecting from the lateral geniculate nucleus to the primary visual cortex.

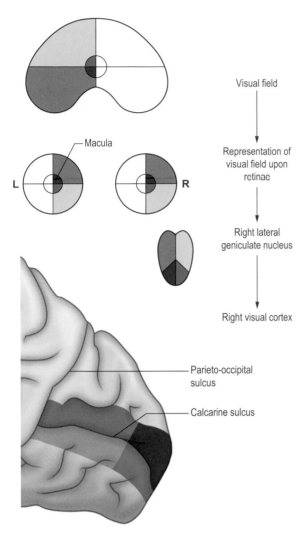

Visual field

↓

Representation of
visual field upon
retinae

↓

Right lateral
geniculate nucleus

↓

Right visual cortex

Macula

L

R

Parieto-occipital
sulcus

Calcarine sulcus

Fig. 15.7 Representation of the left half of the visual field at various levels in the visual pathway.

The central visual pathway

- At the optic chiasm, axons from the nasal halves of the two retinae decussate and pass into the contralateral optic tract.
- The optic tract contains axons that carry information relating to the contralateral half of the field of vision.
- Optic tract fibres end in the lateral geniculate nucleus of the thalamus.
- Third-order visual fibres from the lateral geniculate nucleus

pass through the retrolenticular part of the internal capsule and the optic radiation to terminate in the primary visual cortex.

- The primary visual cortex is located above and below the calcarine sulcus of the occipital lobe.
- The rest of the occipital lobe constitutes the visual association area.

Visual field deficits

Disease of the eyeball (cataract, intraocular haemorrhage, retinal detachment) and disease of the optic nerve (multiple sclerosis and optic nerve tumours) lead to loss of vision in the affected eye (**monocular blindness**). Compression of the optic chiasm by an adjacent pituitary tumour leads to **bitemporal hemianopia**. Vascular and neoplastic lesions of the optic tract, optic radiation or occipital cortex produce a contralateral **homonymous hemianopia** (Fig. 15.8). Because of the configuration of the optic radiation (Fig. 15.6), lesions in the parietal lobe can lead to unilateral lower visual field loss while lesions in the temporal lobe can lead to unilateral upper visual field loss (quadrantanopia).

Retinitis pigmentosa is an inherited metabolic disorder of the photoreceptor and retinal pigment epithelial cells. There is progressive night blindness, peripheral visual field constriction and pigmentation of the retina visible on ophthalmoscopy.

Senile **macular degeneration** is a degenerative disorder of the elderly leading to loss of central and colour vision.

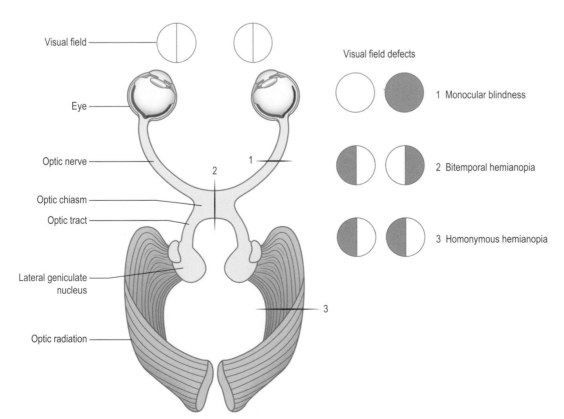

Fig. 15.8 Visual field deficits produced by lesions of the visual pathway.

16 | Hypothalamus, limbic system and olfactory system

In order to survive, there must be continual biochemical and physiological adjustments to preserve the internal environment of the body in a balanced and stable state (homeostasis). Interoceptor signals from the internal organs and body fluids initiate homeostatic responses to achieve this end and the hypothalamus is the structure responsible for orchestrating the task.

Exteroceptive information concerning the outside world strongly influences behaviour. This is relatively simple and stereotyped in lower animals and is directed towards satisfying the drives of thirst, hunger, sex and defence, in instinctive repertoires. These also depend upon the hypothalamus. The limbic system, which is strongly connected to the hypothalamus, is essential for adaptive behaviour, meaning the ability to learn new responses based on previous experience (memory). The complex and non-stereotyped behaviour of humans manages not only to preserve the individual within the physical landscape but also within a changing social environment ('individual homeostasis'). The association areas of the neocortex are capable of analysing exteroceptive information from the environment and from other individuals, enabling adaptive personal and social responses. These phylogenetically more recent structures are also partly connected to the limbic system.

As a result, the hypothalamus, limbic system and association neocortices act as interfaces in a hierarchical fashion between the internal structure of the individual and the environment. A reminder of this evolutionary ascent in humans is the olfactory system: vital for sensing the environment in lower animals, overwhelmed by visuospatial dominance in humans and intimately related to the limbic system.

Hypothalamus

Topographical anatomy of the hypothalamus

The hypothalamus is the most ventral part of the diencephalon, lying beneath the thalamus and ventromedial to the subthalamus (Fig. 16.1; see also Figs 12.1–12.3). It forms the floor and the lower part of the wall of the third ventricle, below the hypothalamic sulcus (see Fig. 12.2). On the base of the brain, parts of the hypothalamus can be seen occupying the small area circumscribed by the crura cerebri, optic chiasm and optic tracts (see Fig. 12.1). Between the rostral limits of the two crura cerebri,

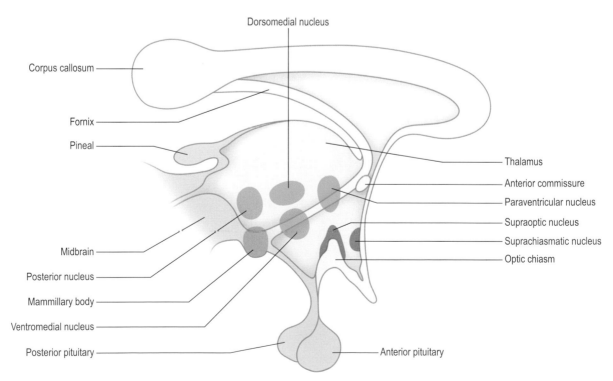

Fig. 16.1 Schematic drawing of a mid-sagittal section of the diencephalon. The diagram shows the medial aspect of the hypothalamus. The approximate locations of some of the principal hypothalamic nuclei are shown.

on either side of the midline, lie two distinct, rounded eminences, the **mammillary bodies**, which contain the hypothalamic **mammillary nuclei**. In the midline, immediately caudal to the optic chiasm, lies a small elevated area known as the **tuber cinereum**, from the apex of which extends the thin **infundibulum** (infundibular process), or **pituitary stalk**. This is attached to the **pituitary gland (hypophysis)**, a pea-sized structure which lies within the hypophyseal fossa (sella turcica) of the sphenoid bone (see Figs 5.1, 5.4). The pituitary gland consists of two major, cytologically distinct, parts: the posterior pituitary or **neurohypophysis** and the anterior pituitary or **adenohypophysis** (Figs 16.2, 16.3). The posterior pituitary is a neuronal structure,

being an expansion of the distal part of the infundibulum. The anterior pituitary is not neural in origin. The two parts are, however, closely linked by the **pituitary (hypophyseal) portal system** of vessels (Fig. 16.3), which are derived from the superior hypophyseal artery. Releasing factors, which are synthesised in the hypothalamus, pass to the adenohypophysis through these vessels to control the release of anterior pituitary hormones.

The hypothalamus is able to integrate interoceptive signals from internal organs and fluid-filled cavities and make appropriate adjustments to the internal environment by virtue of its input and output systems.

Input to the hypothalamus is both circulatory and neural in origin (Fig. 16.4). The circulating blood provides physical (temperature, osmolality), chemical (blood glucose, acid–base state) and hormonal signals of the state of the body, its growth and development and its readiness for action. (e.g. sex, suckling, defence, escape, etc.). Neural signals come from a number of sources. The largest input originates from limbic structures, the hippocampus and the amygdala. Fibres of hippocampal origin constitute the fornix, a large component of which terminates in the medial mammillary nucleus within the mammillary body (Figs 16.5–16.7). Fibres from the amygdala to the hypothalamus run in the stria terminalis (see Fig. 12.3). The nucleus solitarius of the medulla projects to the hypothalamus, conveying information collected by the autonomic nervous system concerning the

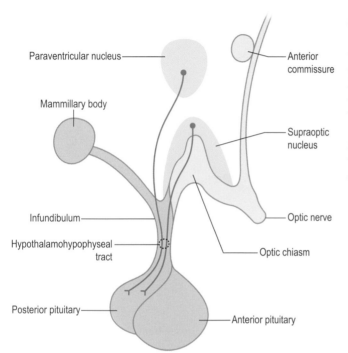

Fig. 16.2 Supraoptic and paraventricular nuclei projecting to the posterior pituitary via the hypothalamohypophyseal tract.

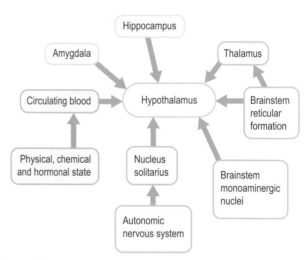

Fig. 16.4 Neural and non-neural inputs of the hypothalamus.

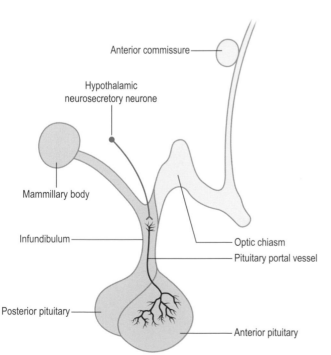

Fig. 16.3 Pituitary portal system linking anterior and posterior parts of the pituitary gland.

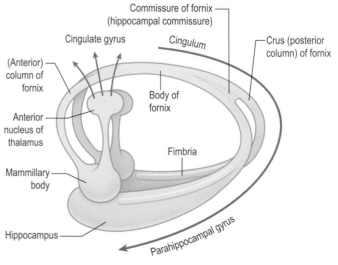

Fig. 16.5 The interconnection of limbic structures that constitute the Papez circuit.

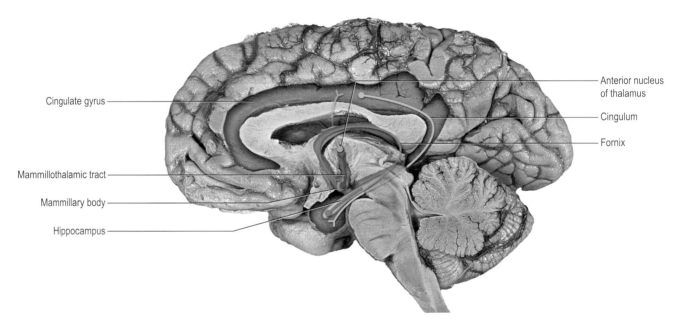

Fig. 16.6 Dissection of the medial aspect of the diencephalon to show the relationships of the fornix, mammillary body and mammillothalamic tract.

Cingulum

Corpus callosum

Anterior horn of lateral ventricle

(Anterior) column of fornix

Body of fornix

Anterior nucleus of thalamus

Mammillothalamic tract

Mammillary body

Cingulate gyrus

Mammillothalamic tract

Mammillary body

Hippocampus

Anterior nucleus of thalamus

Cingulum

Fornix

Fig. 16.7 The Papez circuit projected onto the medial aspect of the cerebral hemisphere.

pressure within the smooth-muscled walls of organs (baroreceptors) and the chemical constituents of the fluid-filled cavities (chemoreceptors). The state of arousal is communicated by connections that originate in the brainstem. Monoaminergic projections ascend in the medial forebrain bundle (see Fig. 9.14) and the reticular formation provides input both directly and indirectly via the thalamus.

The hypothalamus generates responses to these varied stimuli by, again, both circulatory and neural means (Fig. 16.8). An intimate relationship with the pituitary gland and privileged access to its circulation (portal system) confers the role of 'orchestrator of the endocrine system' on the hypothalamus, as it directs hormonal synthesis and release. The neural output of the hypothalamus is directed to widespread regions of the neuraxis. Descending fibres pass to the brainstem and some reach the spinal cord. In this way, connection is made with various brainstem nuclei, including the reticular formation, influencing wakefulness and sleep, and control is exerted over preganglionic sympathetic and parasympathetic neurones of the autonomic nervous system.

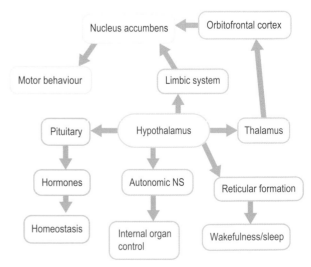

Fig. 16.8 Neural and non-neural outputs of the hypothalamus.

Ascending connections pass to the limbic system, both directly and, via the thalamus, to the orbital frontal cerebral cortex. The hypothalamus can initiate appropriate motor behavioural repertoires of an instinctive kind through its connections with the limbic system and limbic part of the corpus striatum (the nucleus accumbens). Furthermore, it can influence, or even override, more complex adaptive behaviour because of its close links with the limbic system and the orbital frontal association cortex.

Hypothalamic nuclei

The hypothalamus consists of many nuclear divisions, only some of which will be described here (Fig. 16.1). The region lying medial and ventral to the structures of the subthalamus is known as the **lateral hypothalamus**. It is traversed longitudinally by many fibres, including the medial forebrain bundle. The lateral hypothalamic area is important in the control of food and water intake and is, in part, equivalent to the physiologically defined 'feeding centre'. Lateral hypothalamic lesions cause aphagia and adipsia.

The medial region of the hypothalamus contains various nuclei, only some of which have well-defined functions. Anteriorly lie the supraoptic, paraventricular and suprachiasmatic nuclei. The supraoptic and paraventricular nuclei both produce systemically acting hormones, which are released from the posterior pituitary into the general circulation. The **supraoptic nucleus** produces vasopressin (antidiuretic hormone; ADH). The supraoptic nucleus contains osmosensitive neurones that are activated by changes in the osmolality of circulating blood. An increase in osmolality causes release of vasopressin. This acts upon the tubules of the kidney to increase water reabsorption, thus maintaining water homeostasis. The **paraventricular nucleus** synthesises oxytocin. In the female, activation of the paraventricular nucleus, and release of hormone, is induced by suckling. This stimulates milk production by the mammary gland and causes contraction of uterine muscle. The axons of cells in the supraoptic and paraventricular nuclei pass to the neurohypophysis in the hypothalamohypophyseal tract (Fig. 16.2). The neuroendocrine products are transported in this tract to the neurohypophysis, where they are released into the capillary bed and, thus, reach the general circulation. The **suprachiasmatic nucleus** is concerned with the control of diurnal rhythms and the sleep/waking cycle. It receives some afferent fibres directly from the retina.

More caudally, dorsomedial and ventromedial nuclei lie deep to the lateral wall of the third ventricle. The **dorsomedial nucleus** has connections with the suprachiasmatic nucleus and is involved in the control of circadian rhythms. The **ventromedial nucleus**, like the lateral hypothalamus, is concerned with the control of food and fluid intake. The ventromedial nucleus is equated with the physiologically defined 'satiety centre' and lesions of this region cause abnormally increased food intake. In the most caudal part of the hypothalamus lie the posterior nucleus and the **medial mammillary nucleus**, the latter being located within the mammillary body. The mammillary body is part of the limbic system, receiving afferents from the hippocampus via the fornix and projecting to the anterior nucleus of the thalamus and the brainstem.

The hypothalamus is the brain centre for regulation of the autonomic nervous system. Generally, activation of the posterior hypothalamic domain is associated with sympathetic responses, whereas activation of the anterior hypothalamus is associated with parasympathetic activity.

The hypothalamus also synthesises releasing factors and release-inhibiting factors, which control the release of hormones by the adenohypophysis. The adenohypophysis produces adrenocorticotropic hormone (ACTH), luteinising hormone (LH),

follicle-stimulating hormone (FSH), thyroid-stimulating hormone (TSH), growth hormone and prolactin, which are released into the general circulation. The factors that control them are released from the terminals of hypothalamic neurones into the capillary bed of the pituitary portal system (Fig. 16.3). These vessels, which are intrinsic to the hypophyseal stalk, convey the released agents to the adenohypophysis, where they act upon the hormone-secreting cells. Within this system, the neurotransmitter dopamine is synthesised by neurones of the hypothalamic **arcuate nucleus** and is released within the neurohypophysis by axons travelling in the hypothalamohypophyseal tract (see Fig. 9.14). Dopamine acts to inhibit the release of prolactin by the adenohypophysis. The synthesis of hypothalamic releasing factors is under feedback regulation by hormones produced by target organs.

Hypothalamus

- The hypothalamus is part of the diencephalon; it is connected to the pituitary gland via the infundibulum.

- The hypothalamus has autonomic, neuroendocrine and limbic functions and is involved in the coordination of homeostatic mechanisms.

- The hypothalamus produces hormones that are released from the posterior pituitary and also releasing factors that control the release of hormones from the anterior pituitary.

- The supraoptic and paraventricular nuclei of the hypothalamus produce vasopressin and oxytocin, respectively.

- Vasopressin and oxytocin are transported to the posterior pituitary in the hypothalamohypophyseal tract.

- The anterior pituitary produces: adrenocorticotropic hormone, luteinising hormone, follicle-stimulating hormone, thyroid-stimulating hormone, growth hormone and prolactin. Factors that control their secretion are released into the pituitary portal system of the pituitary stalk and carried to the anterior pituitary.

- The lateral hypothalamus and the ventromedial nucleus regulate eating and drinking.

- The suprachiasmatic nucleus controls circadian rhythms.

 Tumours of the hypothalamus and pituitary gland

Tumours and other diseases of the hypothalamus and associated pituitary gland lead to under- or over-production of circulating hormones. These, in turn, produce disorders of growth (**dwarfism, gigantism** and **acromegaly**), sexual function (**precocious puberty, hypogonadism**), body water control (**diabetes insipidus** and **pathological drinking**), eating (**obesity** and **bulimia**) and adrenal cortical control (**Cushing's disease** and **adrenal insufficiency**). Since the pituitary gland is closely adjacent to the optic chiasm, tumours of the gland (**pituitary adenomas**) may also lead to bitemporal visual field loss (see Fig. 15.8).

Limbic system

The limbic system consists of a number of phylogenetically ancient cortical and subcortical structures, with complex and widespread connections that provide the fundamental neural basis for instinctive and emotional aspects of behaviour and for memory. It has rich interconnections with the hypothalamus (Figs 16.4, 16.8), through which emotional states are influenced by, and mediate, changes in physiological and biochemical conditions. The limbic system earns its title from the location of some of its major cortical components on the medial rim of the cerebral hemisphere (*le grand lobe limbique*). It consists of a number of structures with complex interconnections and several major fibre pathways that project to the hypothalamus (Fig. 16.9).

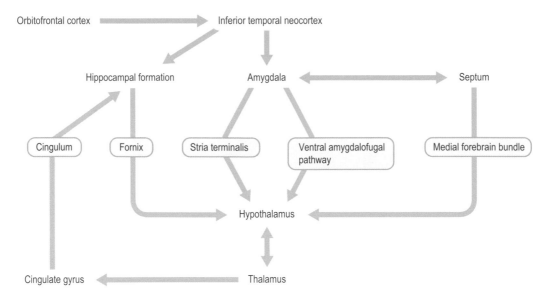

Fig. 16.9 The major components of the limbic system and their relationship with the hypothalamus. Nerve fibre pathways are indicated by shaded boxes.

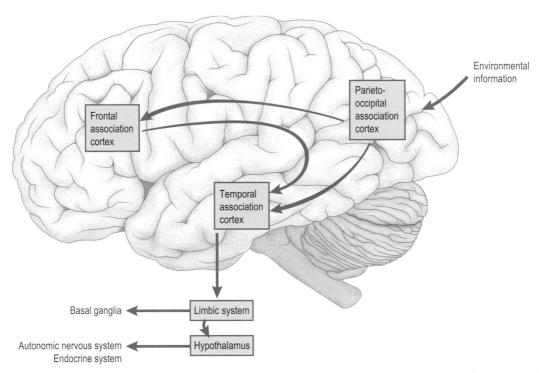

Fig. 16.10 The basic link between associative areas of neocortex, the limbic system, the hypothalamus and their major output pathways.

The powerful input to the limbic system from the neocortical association areas links complex 'goal-directed' behaviour to more primitive, instinctive behaviour and internal homeostasis in a cascade of neural connections (Figs 16.10, 16.11). In a simplified way, we may conceive of information from the outside world being collected in modality-specific ways (e.g. vision, hearing, touch) and refined in the parieto-occipital association areas (perceptuospatial function). This information is then conveyed to the frontal association areas involved in planned behaviour (regulation) and also to the inferior temporal association areas, where information can reach supramodal status and meaning (semantic processing). Entry of information into the limbic system is either directly to the amygdala or indirectly to the hippocampal formation, via the entorhinal cortex (see Fig. 16.14). The amygdala is vital to the motivational and emotional connotations of experience. The information flow into the hippocampal formation permits a link to previous experience, since the hippocampal formation is essential to remembering and learning (episodic memory).

The limbic system is able to influence motor responses appropriate to its informational analyses, through projections to the nucleus accumbens, which forms part of the basal ganglia, and autonomic responses through projections to the hypothalamus.

Limbic system: motivation and emotion

Goal-directed behaviour depends on the motivational states that initiate it and the emotional states associated with its outcome. It develops in relation to the rewards, punishment or avoidance of punishment of behaviours in the past. In lower animals behavioural repertoires are relatively simple, innate and respond rapidly to environmental stimuli. Even monkeys cannot delay a behavioural response to an environmental stimulus for more than a few minutes. In man, also, motivational/emotional states permit rapid responses to environmental stimuli such as dangers.

However, the development of the association areas of the neocortex permits adapted behaviour to be set and achieved over prolonged periods, e.g. years.

Motivational states can, in man and animals, be instinctual, for example fear, flight, feeding and sexual behaviour, and permit self-preservation within the environment. Primary emotions occur in humans (and possibly higher apes) in individual responses to the environment and evinced in the same facial expressions of joy and distress, surprise and disgust, fear and anger that occur in all human cultures.

In humans, 'social emotions' are experienced and expressed between individuals, for example love and hate, jealously and envy, pride and guilt, empathy and sympathy. Moods represent prolonged affective states, which may reflect appropriate responses to the environment or be pathological, for example depression, anxiety and elation.

The expression of emotional states is both motoric and autonomic. The movements of facial expression, pitch and tone of voice and limb gesture convey emotions and are involuntary and under the control of the basal ganglia (nucleus accumbens). Autonomic responses comprise blushing, hair standing on end, goose pimples, sweating, pallor and tears. They depend on the autonomic output of the hypothalamus.

Amygdala

The amygdala lies near the temporal pole, between the inferior horn of the lateral ventricle and the lentiform complex (Fig. 16.12; see also Fig. 13.8). It receives afferents from the inferior temporal association cortex, the thalamus, septum and the olfactory tract. In addition, it receives catecholamine- and serotonin-containing projections from the brainstem via the **medial forebrain bundle** (see Figs 9.14–9.16). The principal efferent projection from the amygdala is the **stria terminalis** (see Fig. 12.3), which runs in the wall of the lateral ventricle, following the curvature of the caudate nucleus, to terminate ultimately in the hypothalamus. The **ventral amygdalofugal pathway** also projects to the hypothalamus. An efferent projection to the nucleus accumbens, the 'limbic' part of the basal ganglia, permits motor behavioural responses.

Septum

The septum, or septal region, lies in the basal part of the forebrain (Fig. 16.12 and see Fig. 13.6). The septum is a cellular region, not to be confused with the septum pellucidum, which is a thin, non-neural lamina separating the anterior horns of the lateral ventricles (see Fig. 13.6). The septum interconnects with the amygdala and projects to the hypothalamus via the medial

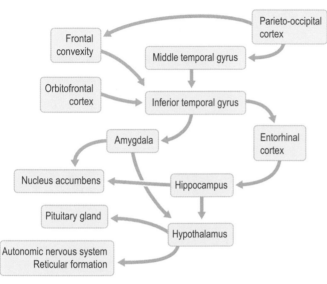

Fig. 16.11 The interconnections between associative neocortical regions and the component parts of the limbic system.

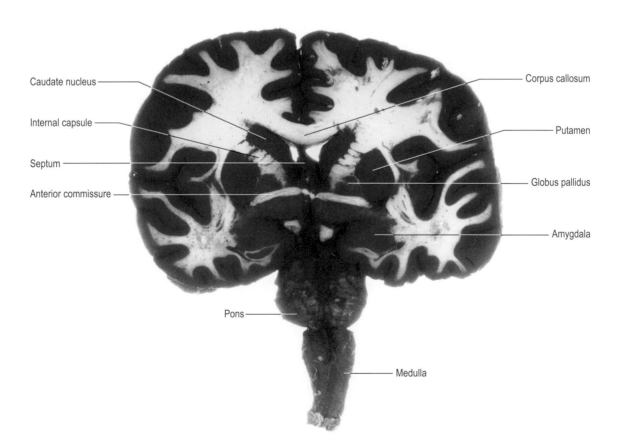

Fig. 16.12 Coronal section of the brain showing the location of the amygdala and anterior commissure and their relationships with the basal ganglia. Mulligan's stain (see Fig. 1.7).

forebrain bundle. The septum also influences the monoaminergic nuclei in the brainstem. It does so via fibres that run in the **stria medullaris thalami** (see Figs 12.2, 12.3) to end in the **habenular nuclei** of the diencephalon (see Fig. 12.2). The habenular nuclei in turn project, via the fasciculus retroflexus, to the interpeduncular nucleus, a small nucleus in the ventral midbrain, which has connections with other regions of the brainstem as well as the hypothalamus. In this way, two major pathways link the septum, the hypothalamus and the monoaminergic nuclei of the brainstem.

Orbital frontal cortex

The frontal neocortex comprises the frontal convexity and the orbital frontal cortex (i.e. that region lying above the orbit). The frontal convexity receives 'afferent' information about the world from the posterior association cortex. Projections from the posterior association cortex to the inferior temporal neocortex also permit entry of this information into the limbic system (amygdala and hippocampal formation). The orbital frontal cortex also receives input from the frontal convexity but is more powerfully connected to the limbic system. Not only are there projections from orbital frontal to inferior temporal neocortex via the uncinate fasciculus, but the orbital fontal cortex projects directly to the hypothalamus.

Thus, the frontal convexity is related to cognitive executive functions and the planning of behaviour in response to environmental information collected in the posterior neocortex. By contrast, the orbital frontal cortex is strongly related to the structures that mediate the instinctive, motivational and emotional drives influencing behaviour. In the healthy subject, the 'cognitive' and 'affective' aspects of behaviour act together in problem-solving in the environment. Both mechanisms are subject to the results of previous experience, which have engendered rewards and punishments: that is, they depend on the memory systems of the limbic system.

Disorders of motivation and emotion

In **frontotemporal dementia (FTD)**, a neurodegenerative disorder, there is atrophy of the prefrontal neocortex and amygdala. The patients have cognitive executive deficits causing poor planning and organisation and they undergo a personality change with personal, occupational and social breakdown because of damage to the prefrontal cortex. They also experience loss of primary and social emotions and they lose their sense of danger due to damage to the amygdala. These patients become profoundly apathetic when the disease spreads through the dorsolateral frontal regions. In some FTD patients, there is selective involvement of the orbital frontal neocortex. When this occurs, cognitive executive functions are relatively spared, but the patient's behaviour is disinhibited, overactive and uncontrolled.

Limbic system: memory

Memory processes are of three kinds. **Episodic** memory refers to the learning and recollection of autobiographical events in the individual's life and is dependent on the hippocampal formation and its connections. **Semantic memory** is the acquired knowledge of the meaning of verbal and perceptual concepts, i.e. knowledge of the world. Semantic memory is dependent on the functioning of the middle and inferior temporal gyri of the neocortex. **Procedural memory** refers to the learning of sensorimotor skills, for example learning to drive a car or play a musical instrument, and is dependent on cortico-subcortical motor systems and not on the hippocampal formation or the temporal neocortex.

Hippocampal formation

The hippocampal formation consists of the hippocampus itself, the dentate gyrus and parts of the parahippocampal gyrus. The **hippocampus** is formed by an infolding of the inferomedial part of the temporal lobe into the lateral ventricle, along the line of the choroid fissure (Figs 16.13, 16.14; see also Figs 13.8–13.12). The **dentate gyrus** lies between the parahippocampal gyrus and the hippocampus (Fig. 16.14).

The hippocampal formation receives afferents principally from the inferior temporal cortex via the entorhinal cortex (area) of the temporal lobe (Fig. 16.14). It also receives fibres from the contralateral entorhinal cortex and hippocampus via the fornix system and hippocampal commissure (commissure of the fornix). The principal efferent pathway from the hippocampus is the **fornix** (Figs 16.5–16.7; see also Figs 12.2, 13.2, 13.7–13.12). The fornix is a prominent C-shaped fascicle of fibres that links the hippocampus with the mammillary body of the hypothalamus and with the septum. Efferent fibres converge on the ventricular

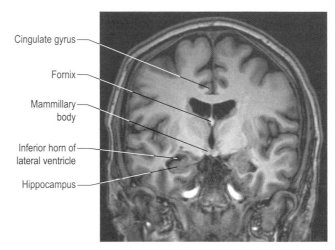

Fig. 16.13 Coronal MRI scan of the brain showing the hippocampus and other components of the limbic system. *(Courtesy of Professor A Jackson, Wolfson Molecular Imaging Centre, University of Manchester, Manchester, UK.)*

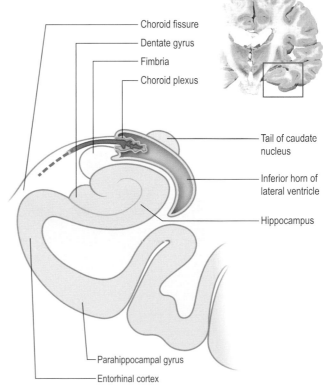

Fig. 16.14 Transverse section through the hippocampus and inferior horn of the lateral ventricle.

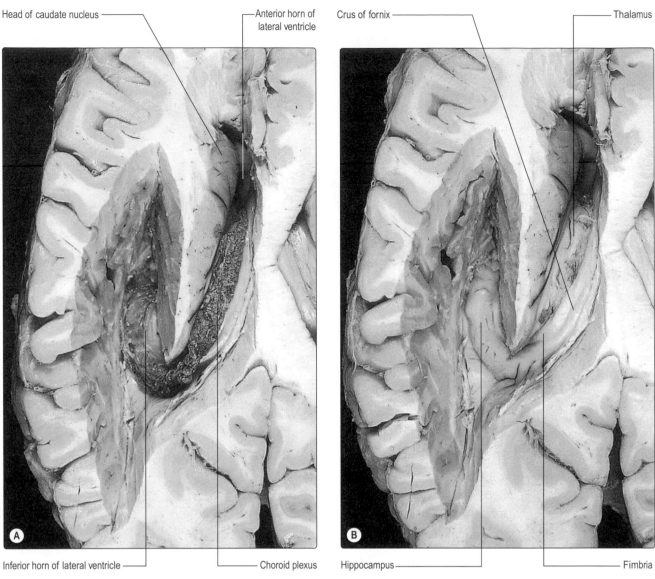

Head of caudate nucleus — Anterior horn of lateral ventricle

Crus of fornix — Thalamus

Inferior horn of lateral ventricle — Choroid plexus

Hippocampus — Fimbria

Fig. 16.15 The hippocampus–fimbria–fornix system. The brain is viewed from above. The cerebral cortex and white matter, including the corpus callosum, have been removed to reveal the lateral ventricle and its contents. (A) Choroid plexus of lateral ventricle intact; (B) choroid plexus removed.

surface of the hippocampus as the **fimbria**. This passes posteriorly and superiorly, to become continuous with the crus (posterior column) of the fornix, which then curves forward beneath the splenium of the corpus callosum (Fig. 16.15). The two crura unite in the midline, beneath the corpus callosum, to form the body of the fornix (Fig. 16.6). Some fibres cross to the opposite side through the small hippocampal commissure (commissure of the fornix). As it passes forwards beneath the corpus callosum, the body of the fornix divides into two columns. These curve downwards, forming the anterior border of the interventricular foramen, and enter the hypothalamus, where the majority of fibres terminate in the mammillary body. The mammillary body, in turn, projects to the anterior nuclear group of the thalamus via the mammillothalamic tract (Fig. 16.6) and to the brainstem via the mammillotegmental tract. The anterior nuclei of the thalamus have major connections with the cingulate gyrus. Hippocampal efferents also project to the nucleus accumbens, enabling motor responses.

Cingulate gyrus

The cingulate gyrus and the **parahippocampal gyrus** are in continuity with one another around the splenium of the corpus callosum (see Figs 13.2, 13.16). The cingulate gyrus projects to the parahippocampal gyrus via the fibres of the cingulum (Figs 13.22, 16.5, 16.6). The principal structures of the limbic system are thus

linked by a series of connections, which constitute the **Papez circuit** (Fig. 16.7).

Disorders of memory

In **Alzheimer's disease**, there is severe atrophy of the hippocampal formation (Fig. 16.16) leading to amnesia for relatively recent events and the inability to learn new information of an autobiographical kind, i.e. loss of episodic memory.

In **semantic dementia**, a neurodegenerative disorder, there is atrophy of the middle and inferior temporal neocortical gyri. The patients progressively lose the meaning of words and percepts, i.e. their knowledge of the world (semantic memory). For example, they do not know the name or meaning of objects and cannot recognise faces (associative agnosia). However, they have relative preservation of memory for their own autobiographical experiences, i.e. their episodic memory is preserved, because the hippocampal formation is not primarily affected in the disease.

Limbic system: emotion and memory

Memory of events and their past motivational and emotional connotations are the only guide to future complex social behaviour and are also the essential links that preserve the individual in permitting rapid response to potentially threatening situations. Input from both functional aspects of the limbic system is essential in problem-solving or executive functions, the

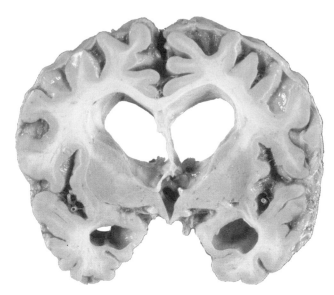

Fig. 16.16 Coronal section through the cerebral hemisphere of a patient dying with Alzheimer's disease. The section shows enlarged lateral ventricles and atrophic cortical gyri and hippocampus. *(Courtesy of Professor D Mann, Clinical Neurosciences, Hope Hospital, University of Manchester, Manchester, UK.)*

cognitive aspects of which are dependent on the functioning of the dorsolateral aspect of the frontal association neocortex.

The orbital aspect of the frontal neocortex is intimately linked to the limbic system and the processing of motivational and emotional states.

In rapid responses to environmental stimuli, the association areas of the neocortex involved in cognitive functioning can be bypassed and incoming sensory information can enter the limbic system via the thalamus so that relatively automatic behavioural responses such as fight or flight can be initiated via the basal ganglia (nucleus accumbens).

The cooperation between the two parts of the limbic system explains the fact that highly emotional experiences are readily learned and then remembered. It is important for survival of the individual to have recollection of precedents in experience that have previously led to reward or punishment, e.g. the avoidance of dangerous animals, plants and environments.

 Limbic lobe disorders

Alcohol abuse, in a setting of dietary deficiency of thiamine, leads to capillary haemorrhages in the upper brainstem and limbic structures. The patient falls into confusion and coma (**Wernicke's encephalopathy**). Partial recovery may occur, with failure to remember previous experience (retrograde amnesia) or to learn new facts (anterograde amnesia). This is known as **Korsakoff's psychosis**. A similar amnesic syndrome occurs when bilateral, surgical temporal lobectomy incorporates the hippocampal formations.

Temporal lobe, or **complex partial, seizures** arising close to the amygdala and hippocampi can lead to complex experiences of smell, mood and memory.

Olfactory system

Olfactory receptors are specialised, ciliated nerve cells that lie in the olfactory epithelium of the nasal cavity. Their axons assemble into numerous small fascicles (the true olfactory nerves) that enter the cranial cavity through the foramina of the **cribriform plate** of the ethmoid bone (see Fig. 5.1) and then attach to the olfactory bulb on the inferior surface of the frontal lobe (Fig. 16.17; see also Fig. 10.1). Preliminary processing of olfactory information occurs within the olfactory bulb, which contains interneurones and large **mitral cells**; axons from the latter leave the bulb in the **olfactory tract**.

The olfactory tract passes backwards on the basal surface of the frontal lobe and, just before reaching the level of the optic chiasm, most olfactory tract fibres are deflected laterally, in the **lateral olfactory stria** (Fig. 16.17). These fibres pass into the depths of the lateral fissure, which they cross to reach the temporal lobe. They terminate mainly in the **primary olfactory cortex** of the **uncus** (Fig. 16.17; see also Fig. 13.2), on the inferomedial aspect of the temporal lobe, and in the subjacent amygdala. Adjacent to the uncus, the anterior part of the parahippocampal gyrus, or **entorhinal area**, constitutes the olfactory association cortex. The primary and association cortices are also collectively referred to as the **pyriform cortex** and are responsible for the appreciation of olfactory stimuli. The olfactory projection is unique among the sensory systems in that it consists of a sequence of only two neurones between the sensory receptors and cerebral cortex and does not project via the thalamus.

Limbic system

- The amygdala is located near to the temporal pole. It receives projections from the olfactory system and the temporal cortex, and has reciprocal connections with the septum.

- The hippocampal formation is made up of the hippocampus, dentate gyrus and parahippocampal gyrus of the temporal lobe. It receives fibres from the entorhinal cortex and projects via the fornix to the mammillary body of the hypothalamus.

- The principal components of the limbic system are interconnected in the Papez circuit.

Olfactory system

- Olfactory nerve fibres terminate in the olfactory bulb.

- Second-order fibres run in the olfactory tract and terminate in the primary olfactory cortex of the uncus in the temporal lobe.

- Adjacent to this, the anterior part of the parahippocampal gyrus, or entorhinal cortex, constitutes the olfactory association cortex.

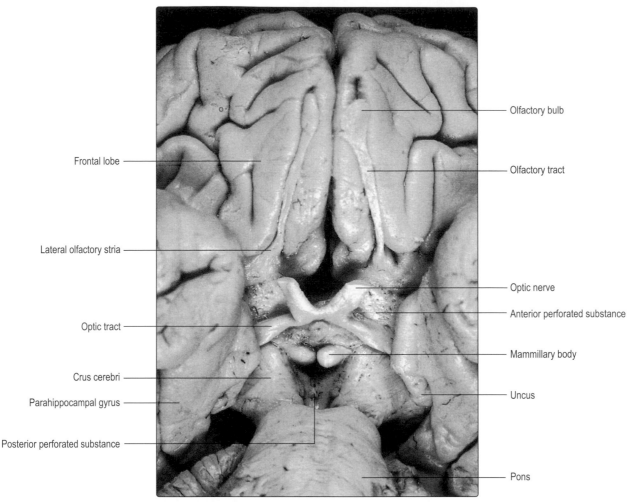

Frontal lobe

Lateral olfactory stria

Optic tract

Crus cerebri

Parahippocampal gyrus

Posterior perforated substance

Olfactory bulb

Olfactory tract

Optic nerve

Anterior perforated substance

Mammillary body

Uncus

Pons

Fig. 16.17 Ventral surface of the brain. The illustration shows the olfactory bulb and tract, the lateral olfactory stria and the primary olfactory area of the cerebral cortex (uncus).

 Anosmia

Anosmia follows damage to the olfactory nerves. There is loss not only of the sense of smell but also of the flavour of foods. However, elementary aspects of taste, e.g. sweet, salt, bitter and sour, are preserved. Anosmia frequently follows head trauma and can occur when tumours of the meninges (**meningiomas**) invade the olfactory nerves.

In **Alzheimer's disease**, there is atrophy of the uncus. Patients can detect the presence of odours but they cannot identify them, nor match the same odours, nor discriminate different odours (**apperceptive agnosia** for smell). In **semantic dementia**, there is atrophy of the amygdala and the inferior temporal neocortex. Patients can detect odours, match and discriminate between them, but are unable accurately to name, describe or identify them (**associative agnosia** for smell).

Glossary

Acalculia – Inability to calculate

Accommodation – Act of refocussing the visual image

Acromegaly – Overgrowth of the skeleton and organs caused by excessive release of growth hormone from a pituitary tumour

Action potential – Transient reversal of the resting potential that is propagated along the axon

Acuity – Resolving power

Adenoma – Benign tumour

Adhesion – Scarring of tissues, fixing them together

Adipsia – Inability, or loss of desire, to drink

Aetiology – Relating to the cause of disease

Afferent – Carrying towards (e.g. cerebellar afferent neurones carry impulses to the cerebellum)

Agnosia – Inability to recognise objects

Agraphia – Inability to write

Akinesia – Loss, or slowness, of movement

Alexia – Inability to read

Amnesia – Loss of memory

Anastomosis – Intercommunication between vessels (e.g. circulus arteriosus or circle of Willis)

Aneurysm – Abnormal dilatation of an artery

Angiography – Demonstration of the arterial system after injection of a radio-opaque medium

Angioma – Congenital swollen collection of blood vessels

Anomia – Inability to name objects

Antidiuretic – An agent that reduces the volume of urine produced by the kidney

Aphagia – Inability, or loss of desire, to eat

Aphasia – Loss of ability to use language

Apperceptive agnosia – Inability to perceive

Apraxia – Loss of skilled movements (praxis) despite preservation of power, sensation and coordination

Arachnoid mater – Middle of the three meningeal layers enveloping the central nervous system

Areflexia – Loss of reflexes

Arthritis – Inflammation of one or more joints

Associative agnosia – Inability to recognise the meaning of percepts

Astrocyte (astroglial cell) – A type of neuroglial cell (q.v.) that may form the blood–brain barrier

Ataxia – Loss of ability to coordinate voluntary movements

Atrophy – Wasting or degeneration

Axon – The nerve fibre carrying impulses away from the cell body

Baroreceptor – Neuronal sensory ending that detects changes in arterial blood pressure

Biopsy – Tissue sample taken from a patient for the diagnosis of disease

Blood–brain barrier – A selectively permeable barrier between the circulating blood and the brain believed to be formed by astrocytes

Bradykinesia – Slowness of movement

Brainstem – The stalk-like portion of the brain connecting the cerebral hemispheres with the spinal cord

Bulbar palsy – Weakness of tongue, pharynx and larynx resulting from disease of the lower cranial nerves

Bulimia – Overeating disorder

Cataract – Opacity of the lens of the eye, leading to deterioration of vision

Cell body – The part of the neurone that contains the nucleus and possesses dendritic and axonal processes

Central nervous system – The brain and spinal cord

Cephalic – Relating to the head

Cerebrospinal fluid (CSF) – The clear watery fluid that surrounds the brain and spinal cord

Cerebrum – The largest, most highly developed part of the brain comprised of two cerebral hemispheres

Chemoreceptor – Neuronal sensory ending that detects changes in the chemical composition of circulating blood

Chiasm (chiasma) – Decussation or crossing over of nerve fibres (e.g. optic chiasm)

Chorea – Involuntary, abnormal movements of the face and/or limbs

Collateral – A side-branch of a nerve or blood vessel

Coma – Prolonged and unnatural state of unconsciousness

Computed tomography (CT) – Imaging technique utilising X-rays to visualise the structure of the nervous system

Concussion – Loss of consciousness caused by head injury

Contralateral – Relating to the opposite side

Contusion – Bruising

Convulsion – Involuntary contraction or spasm of muscles

Cordotomy – Neurosurgical procedure to destroy specific pathways in the spinal cord

Craniopharyngioma – Congenital tumour of the base of the brain

Craniotomy – Neurosurgical procedure to open the cranial cavity

Cushing's disease – Overgrowth of the adrenal glands causing excessive release of corticosteroid hormones

Decussation – Crossing over of nerve fibres from one side of the CNS to the other (e.g. pyramidal decussation)

Déjà vu – False emotional conviction that current events have occurred before

Dementia – Loss of mental abilities

Demyelination – Loss of the myelin sheath surrounding neuronal axons

Dendrite – Branching process of a neurone that receives information from other neurones and conducts electrical changes to the cell body

Diabetes insipidus – Failure of the posterior pituitary gland causing reduced release of antidiuretic hormone

Diabetes mellitus – A disorder of carbohydrate metabolism caused by lack of insulin

Dorsal root ganglion – Location of cell bodies of primary afferent neurones entering the spinal cord through the dorsal roots of spinal nerves

Dura mater – Outermost of the three meningeal layers that envelop the central nervous system

Dysarthria – Inability to pronounce

Dysphagia – Inability to swallow

Dysphonia – Inability to produce the voice

Echocardiography – The use of ultrasound to display the action of the heart

Efferent – Carrying away from (e.g. striatal efferent fibres carry impulses away from the striatum)

Electroencephalography (EEG) – Technique to detect the surface electrical activity of the brain

Electromyography – Technique to determine the electrical activity of muscles

Emetic – Causing nausea and vomiting

Encephalopathy – Disorder of the brain

Entrapment neuropathy – Nerve injury caused by compression of a nerve within a tunnel or at a change in direction

Ependymal cells (ependyma) – Epithelial cells lining the ventricular system

Epilepsy – Paroxysmal attack of disturbed consciousness and sensorimotor function resulting from abnormal electrophysiological discharges of the brain

Fasciculation – Spontaneous contraction of denervated motor units, visible on inspection

Fasciculus – Bundle of nerve fibres (e.g. medial longitudinal fasciculus)

Febrile – Refers to raised body temperature (fever)

Fibrillation – Spontaneous contraction of denervated muscle fibres, detected on electromyography

Foramen – An opening (e.g. foramen magnum)

Ganglion – A collection of nerve cell bodies outside the CNS (e.g. dorsal root ganglion)

General paralysis of the insane (GPI) – Disease of the frontal lobes caused by late neurosyphilis

Glia – *See* Neuroglia

Glioma – Tumour derived from glial cells

Haematoma – Blood clot

Haemorrhage – Escape of blood from a ruptured blood vessel

Hallucination – Abnormal perceptual experience

Hemianopia – Loss of sight affecting one half of the visual field (e.g. bi-temporal hemianopia)

Hemiparesis – Weakness of one side of the body

Hemiplegia – *See* Hemiparesis

Hepatolenticular degeneration (Wilson's disease) – Inherited disease of copper metabolism affecting the liver and brain

Herpes zoster – Virus causing shingles (q.v.)

Huntington's disease – Inherited degenerative disease of the brain causing chorea (q.v.) and dementia (q.v.)

Hydrocephalus – Abnormally large amount of cerebrospinal fluid within the ventricles of the brain

Hyperacusis – Increased hearing sensitivity

Hyperreflexia – Abnormal increase in reflex activity

Hypertonia – Abnormal increase in muscle tone

Hypertrophy – Enlargement of tissues

Hypothyroidism – Underactivity of the thyroid gland causing reduced release of thyroid hormone

Hypotonia – Abnormal decrease in muscle tone

Idiopathic – Of unknown cause

Infarction – Death of tissue resulting from impairment of its circulation

Intervertebral – Between two vertebrae

Ipsilateral – Relating to the same side

Ischaemia – Restriction of blood supply to a tissue or organ causing inadequate supply of oxygen

Kinaesthesia – Perception of movement

Lamina – A thin layer (e.g. internal medullary lamina)

Lesion – Site of disease or damage

Levodopa –(**L-DOPA, L-dihydroxyphenylalanine**) The metabolic precursor of dopamine, used in the treatment of Parkinson's disease

Lobectomy – Surgical resection of lobe of the brain

Lumen – A space or cavity

Lymphoma – Tumour of the lymphoid system

Magnetic resonance imaging (MRI) – Technique for imaging structure that does not employ ionising radiation

Mastication – The act of chewing

Meninges – Connective tissue sheaths surrounding the CNS, namely dura mater, arachnoid mater and pia mater

Meningioma – A tumour arising from the fibrous coverings (meninges) of the brain

Meningitis – Inflammation of the meninges

Metastasis – Spread of tumour to distant sites

Microglia – A type of neuroglial cell (q.v.), having a mainly phagocytic function in the response to brain damage or injury

Migraine – Paroxysmal headache

Miosis – Pupillary constriction

Motor neurone disease – Degenerative disease of upper and lower motor neurones, causing paralysis

Multiple sclerosis – Immune disease of the CNS, causing relapsing disorder of nervous function

Muscular dystrophy – Inherited degeneration of muscles, causing progressive paralysis

Myasthenia gravis – Immune disorder of the neuromuscular junction, causing muscular fatigue

Myelin – A sheath of protein and phospholipid around the axons of certain neurones

Myoclonus – Sudden, involuntary muscle contractions

Myopathy – Disease of muscle

Narcolepsy – Paroxysmal sleep attacks

Necrosis – Death of tissue

Neoplasia – Tumorous overgrowth of tissue

Neurofibromatosis – Inherited disease causing tumours of meninges, CNS, peripheral nerves and skin

Neuroglia (neuroglial cell) – Non-neural supporting cells of the CNS comprised of oligodendrocytes, astrocytes, microglia and ependymal cells (q.v.)

Neuroleptic – Dopamine receptor antagonist drugs used to treat psychosis

Neuroma – Tumour derived from nerve cells

Neurone – The principal functional cell of the nervous system, specialised to integrate and transmit nerve impulses

Neuropathy – Disease of nerve cells

Neurosyphilis – Infection of the nervous system by a spirochaete

Neurotransmitter – Chemical substance stored within vesicles (q.v.) in presynaptic nerve endings and released on depolarisation to act upon postsynaptic receptors

Nociception – Sensitivity to noxious stimuli

Nucleus – Structure within a cell that contains chromosomal DNA; also a collection of nerve cell bodies within the CNS (e.g. dentate nucleus)

Nystagmus – To-and-fro movements of the eyes

Oedema – Swelling caused by accumulated fluid

Oligodendrocyte (oligodendroglia) – A type of neuroglial cell (q.v.) that produces the myelin sheath in the CNS

Oligodendroglioma – Tumour derived from oligodendroglia

Ophthalmoplegia – Weakness of the extraocular muscles controlling eye movements

Ophthalmoscopy – Clinical examination of the eye with an ophthalmoscope

Pallidum – Globus pallidus

Palsy – Weakness

Papilloedema – Swelling of the optic nerve(s)

Paraesthesia – Tingling sensations ('pins and needles')

Paralysis – Muscle weakness of varying severity

Paraphasia – Use of incorrect word

Paraplegia – Weakness or paralysis of the legs

Paresis – Muscular weakness

Parkinson's disease – Disease of the basal ganglia causing akinesia (q.v.), rigidity (q.v.) and tremor (q.v.)

Paroxysm – Sudden attack

Pathognomonic – Specifically characteristic of a particular disease, disorder or condition

Peripheral nervous system – All parts of the nervous system excluding the brain and spinal cord (CNS)

Photophobia – Intolerance to light

Pia mater – Innermost of the three meningeal layers that envelop the central nervous system

Plexus – Structure consisting of interwoven nerves (e.g. brachial plexus) or blood vessels (e.g. choroid plexus)

Poliomyelitis – Viral infection of motor neurones of the spinal cord and brainstem

Positron emission tomography (PET) – Technique for imaging the function of the brain

Praxis – The function of skilled (developed or learned) voluntary movement

Prolapse – Displacement from normal anatomical position

Proprioception – The detection of position and movement of body parts

Pseudobulbar palsy – Weakness of the tongue, pharynx and larynx caused by disease of the corticobulbar tracts

Psychosis – Abnormal mental state with altered precepts (hallucinations) and false ideas (delusions)

Ptosis – Abnormal drooping of the eyelid

Quadriplegia – Paralysis affecting all four limbs

Radiculopathy – Disease of the nerve roots

Receptor – Specialised element of the cell membrane that binds neurotransmitter substances (or exogenous drugs) bringing about a change in membrane permeability or an intracellular response

Resting potential – The electrical potential across the membrane of a nerve cell at rest

Rheumatic fever – Immune disease of the joints, heart and brain following bacterial infection

Rigidity – Increased resistance to passive movement of the limbs throughout their range

Schizophrenia – Disease of the brain causing psychosis (q.v.)

Seizure – Sudden disturbance of consciousness or sensorimotor function

Shingles – Infection of the ganglia of cranial and spinal nerves by herpes zoster virus (q.v.)

Single photon emission tomography (SPECT) – Technique for imaging the function of the brain

Somatic – Relating to body parts other than the viscera

Somatotopic – The orderly representation of body parts in the CNS

Spasticity – Increased resistance to passive movement of the limbs when muscles are initially stretched

Spondylosis – Degeneration of the spine

Stroke – Sudden neurological deficit caused by disease of the circulation to the brain

Sydenham's chorea – Manifestation of rheumatic fever (q.v.) affecting the basal ganglia and causing involuntary movements

Synapse – The gap between neurones across which nerve impulses pass by release of a neurotransmitter

Synaptic vesicle – Structure within the presynaptic ending that contains neurotransmitter substance which is released on depolarisation

Syncope – Fainting attack

Syndrome – Group of signs and symptoms which characterise a disease

Syringobulbia – Expanding cavity (syrinx) within the medulla

Syringomyelia – Expanding cavity within the spinal cord

Syrinx – An abnormal cavity in the spinal cord or medulla

Terminal bouton – Specialised presynaptic ending of an axon

Thalamotomy – Neurosurgical destruction of part of the thalamus

Thrombosis – Coagulation of blood in artery or vein

Tract – An aggregation of nerve cell processes having more or less the same origin and destination (e.g. corticospinal tract)

Tremor – Trembling of head or limbs

Tumour – A swelling or morbid enlargement; a mass of abnormal tissue resulting from uncontrolled cell growth (neoplasm)

Vesicle – *See* Synaptic vesicle

Index

Page numbers followed by "*f*" indicate figures, "*t*" indicate tables, and "*b*" indicate boxes.